SUBSTANCE MISUSE IN PSYCHOSIS

The Wiley Series in

CLINICAL PSYCHOLOGY

Hermine L. Graham, *Alex Copello,* *Max J. Birchwood* *and Kim T. Mueser (Editors)*	Substance Misuse in Psychosis: Approaches to Treatment and Service Delivery
Jenny A. Petrak *and Barbara Hedge (Editors)*	The Trauma of Sexual Assault: Treatment, Prevention and Practice
Gordon J.G. Asmundson, *Steven Taylor* *and Brian J. Cox (Editors)*	Health Anxiety: Clinical and Research Perspectives on Hypochondriasis and Related Conditions
Kees van Heeringen *(Editor)*	Understanding Suicidal Behaviour: The Suicidal Process Approach to Research, Treatment and Prevention
Craig A. White	Cognitive Behaviour Therapy for Chronic Medical Problems: A Guide to Assessment and Treatment in Practice
Steven Taylor	Understanding and Treating Panic Disorder: Cognitive-Behavioural Approaches
Alan Carr	Family Therapy: Concepts, Process and Practice
Max Birchwood, *David Fowler* *and Chris Jackson (Editors)*	Early Intervention in Psychosis: A Guide to Concepts, Evidence and Interventions
Dominic H. Lam, *Steven H. Jones,* *Peter Hayward,* *and Jenifer A. Bright*	Cognitive Therapy for Bipolar Disorder: A Therapist's Guide to Concepts, Methods and Practice

Titles published under the series editorship of:

J. Mark G. Williams *School of Psychology, University of Wales,*
Bangor, UK

Peter Salmon	Psychology of Medicine and Surgery: A Guide for Psychologists, Counsellors, Nurses and Doctors
William Yule *(Editor)*	Post-Traumatic Stress Disorders: Concepts and Therapy

A list of earlier titles in the series follows the index.

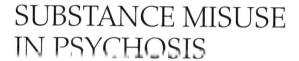

SUBSTANCE MISUSE IN PSYCHOSIS

Approaches to Treatment and Service Delivery

Edited by

Hermine L. Graham
The COMPASS Programme, Birmingham and University of Birmingham, UK

Alex Copello
Substance Misuse Services, Birmingham and University of Birmingham, UK

Max J. Birchwood
The Early Intervention Service, Birmingham, UK

Kim T. Mueser
New Hampshire—Dartmouth Psychiatric Research Center, New Hampshire, USA

JOHN WILEY & SONS, LTD

This publication is designed to provide accurate and authoritative information in regard to the
subject matter covered. It is sold on the understanding that the Publisher is not engaged in
rendering professional services. If professional advice or other expert assistance is required, the
services of a competent professional should be sought.

Other Wiley Editorial Offices

John Wiley & Sons Inc., 111 River Street,
Hoboken, NJ 07030, USA

Jossey-Bass, 989 Market Street, San Francisco,
CA 94103-1741, USA

Wiley-VCH Verlag GmbH, Boschstr. 12,
D-69469 Weinheim, Germany

John Wiley & Sons Australia Ltd, 33 Park Road,
Milton, Queensland 4064, Australia

John Wiley & Sons (Asia) Pte Ltd, 2 Clementi Loop #02-01,
Jin Xing Distripark, Singapore 129809

John Wiley & Sons Canada Ltd, 22 Worcester Road,
Etobicoke, Ontario, Canada M9W 1L1

Library of Congress Cataloging-in-Publication Data

Substance misuse in psychosis : approaches to treatment and service delivery / edited by
Hermine L. Graham ... [et al.].
       p.   cm.—(The Wiley series in clinical psychology)
    Includes bibliographical references and index.
    ISBN 0-471-49229-9 (cased)
    1. Psychoses—Treatment.   2. Substance abuse—Treatment.   3. Mental health services.
  I. Graham, Hermine L.   II. Series.

  RC512 .S92   2002
  616.89'1—dc21   2002071300

British Library Cataloguing in Publication Data

A catalogue record for this book is available from the British Library

ISBN 0-471-49229-9(hbk)
ISBN 0-470-01361-3(pbk)

Typeset in 10/12 pt Palatino by TechBooks, New Delhi, India
Printed and bound in Great Britain by TJ International Ltd, Padstow, Cornwall
This book is printed on acid-free paper responsibly manufactured from sustainable forestry
in which at least two trees are planted for each one used for paper production.

To Pat S

CONTENTS

ABOUT THE EDITORS

Hermine L. Graham is a consultant clinical psychologist, Head of the Combined Psychosis and Substance Use (COMPASS) Programme in Northern Birmingham, UK, and an Honorary Research Fellow with the School of Psychology, University of Birmingham. In a managerial and clinical research capacity she is developing and evaluating an integrated treatment and service model for people with severe mental health problems who use alcohol/drugs problematically. She has published articles within this area and provides national and international consultancy/advice on service and policy developments for this client group. Her clinical and research interests include the application of cognitive therapy for people with combined psychosis and substance use. A publication that reflects this is her paper, "The Role of Dysfunctional Beliefs in Individuals Who Experience Psychosis and Use Substances: Implications for Cognitive Therapy and Medication Adherence" (1998), *Behavioural and Cognitive Psychotherapy*, **26**, 193–208.

Alex Copello is a consultant clinical psychologist, Head of the Psychology Addiction Speciality within Northern Birmingham Mental Health Trust, and Lecturer in Clinical Psychology at the School of Psychology, University of Birmingham. He is a practising clinician and the lead professional for the Addiction Research and Development Programme for the Trust. In addition, he is one of the principal investigators on an MRC-funded UK multisite study evaluating alcohol treatment. He has been involved in developing a social network-based treatment that will be evaluated in this study. His research and clinical interests include the impact of addiction upon families; the evaluation of services for alcohol and drug users, both in primary care and specialist settings; and the use of qualitative research methods. He has also been involved in international cross-cultural research assessing the impact of addiction on families in Mexico and Australia. He publishes extensively in a number of scientific journals and has co-authored the book *Living with Drink: Women Who Live with Problem Drinkers* (1998).

Max J. Birchwood is Director of the Early Intervention Service and Director of Research and Development for Northern Birmingham Mental

Health Trust, and Professor of Mental Health at the University of Birmingham, UK. His clinical and research interests have centred around the development of methods of promoting individuals' control over their psychotic symptoms, including the application of cognitive therapy to psychotic symptoms, as in acute psychosis, and the recognition and control of early warning signs of relapse. He has published widely in these areas and is a prominent figure within this field. His books include *Psychological Management of Schizophrenia* (1994), *Cognitive Therapy for Hallucinations, Delusions and Paranoia* (1996), *Early Intervention in Psychosis* (2000) and *Schizophrenia* (2001). He is currently involved in the development of community-based early intervention for people with psychosis across the UK and is patron to the National Schizophrenia Fellowship in the UK.

Kim T. Mueser is a Professor in the Departments of Psychiatry and Community and Family Medicine at the Dartmouth Medical School in New Hampshire, USA. He is an active contributor to research and the development of clinical methods for the treatment of comorbid severe mental illness and substance use, has published numerous articles within this area, and provides research consultancy/advice to a number of services. His clinical and research interests include research on the treatment of persons with severe mental illness, and substance use disorders, family treatment and social skills training for severe mental illness, and other aspects of psychiatric rehabilitation. He has co-authored several books, including *Social Skills Training for Psychiatric Patients* (1989), *Coping With Schizophrenia: A Guide for Families* (1994), *Behavioural Family Therapy for Psychiatric Disorders*, 2nd edn, 1999), and *Social Skills Training for Schizophrenia* (1997).

LIST OF CONTRIBUTORS

Jean Addington

Department of Psychiatry, Foothills Hospital, 1403 29th Street NW, Calgary, Alberta, T2N 2T9, Canada

Olympia Athanasopoulos

EPPIC, Locked Bag 10, Parkville, Victoria 3052, Australia

Michael Banghart

UIC Mental Health Services Research Program, 104 South Michigan Avenue, Suite 900, Chicago, IL 60603, USA

Christine Barrowclough

Academic Department of Clinical Psychology, Mental Health Unit, Tameside General Hospital, Fountain Street, Ashton-under-Lyne OL6 9RW, UK

Alison Beck

Chartered Clinical Psychologist, CLAMHS Out of Borough, South London and the Maudsley NHS Trust, 392 Brixton Road, London SW9 7AW, UK

Max J. Birchwood

Director, Early Intervention Service, Harry Watton House, 97 Church Lane, Aston, Birmingham B6 5UG, UK

Tom Burns

Department of General Psychiatry, St Georges Hospital Medical School, University of London, Section of Community Psychiatry, Jenner Wing, Cranmer Terrace, London SW17 ORE, UK

Anne Clair

Senior Clinical Psychologist, Wolston Park Hospital, Wacol, 4076 Qld, Australia

Martin J. Commander

Northern Birmingham Mental Health NHS Trust, Northcroft Site, 71 Fentham Road, Erdington, Birmingham B23 6AL, UK

Judith A. Cook	*UIC Mental Health Services Research Program, 104 South Michigan Avenue, Suite 900, Chicago, IL 60603, USA*
Alex Copello	*Consultant Clinical Psychologist, School of Psychology, University of Birmingham, Edgbaston, Birmingham B15 2TT, UK*
Ilana Crome	*Academic Suite, Harplands Hospital, Hilton Road, Stoke-on-Trent ST46TH, UK*
Ed Day	*Addictive Behaviours Centre, Northern Birmingham Mental Health NHS Trust, 120–122 Corporation Street, Birmingham B4 6SX, UK*
Robert E. Drake	*New Hampshire—Dartmouth Psychiatric Research Center, 105 Pleasant Street, Concord, NH 03301, USA*
Jane Edwards	*EPPIC, Locked Bag 10, Parkville, Victoria 3052, Australia*
Kathryn Elkins	*EPPIC, Locked Bag 10, Parkville, Victoria 3052, Australia*
George Georgiou	*Addictive Behaviours Centre, Northern Birmingham Mental Health NHS Trust, 120–122 Corporation Street, Birmingham B4 6SX, UK*
Hermine L. Graham	*Head of COMPASS Programme, Northern Birmingham NHS Trust, 12–13 Greenfield Crescent, Edgbaston, Birmingham B15 3AU, UK*
Shelly F. Greenfield	*Proctor House, Building 329, McLean Hospital, 115 Mill Street, Belmont, MA 02178-9106, USA*
Professor Heinz Häfner	*Head, Schizophrenia Research Unit, Central Institute of Mental Health, P.O. Box 122120, 68072 Mannheim, Germany*
Martin Hambrecht	*Klinik für Psychiatrie und Psychotherapie, Evang Krankenhaus Elisabethenstift GmbH, Landgraf-Georg-str. 100, 64287 Darmstadt, Germany*

Mark Hinton	*EPPIC, Locked Bag 10, Parkville, Victoria 3052, Australia*
Tim Hunt	*c/o Shaftesbury Clinic, Springfield Hospital, 61 Glenburnie Road, Tooting SW17 7DJ, UK*
David Jeffery	*Consultant Clinical Psychologist, South Devon Healthcare, Kitson Hall, Torbay Hospital, Lawes Bridge, Torquay, South Devon TQ2 7AA, UK*
David J. Kavanagh	*Department of Psychiatry, University of Queensland, K Floor, Mental Health Centre, Royal Brisbane Hospital, Herston, 4029 Qld, Australia*
Ann Ley	*Research Psychologist, Psychology Department, 1st Floor, Hengrave House, Torbay Hospital, Torquay, Devon, TQ2 7AA, UK*
Jenny Maslin	*Doctor of Clinical Psychology Training Course, Psychology Department, University of Hertfordshire, College Lane, Hatfield, Herts, AL10 9AB, UK*
Dermot McGovern	*Consultant Psychiatrist, Early Intervention Service, Harry Watton House, 97 Church Lane, Aston, Birmingham B6 5UG, UK*
Debra V. McQuade	*Department of Psychiatry, Dartmouth Hitchcock Medical Center, 1 Medical Center Drive, Lebanon, NH 03756, USA*
Kim T. Mueser	*New Hampshire—Dartmouth Psychiatric Research Center, Main Building, 105 Pleasant Street, Concord, NH 03301, USA*
Douglas L. Noordsy	*1555 Elm Street, Manchester, NH 03101, USA*
Grace O'Leary	*Proctor House, Building 329, McLean Hospital, 115 Mill Street, Belmont, MA 02178-9106, USA*
Jim Orford	*Professor of Clinical and Community Psychology, School of Psychology, University of Birmingham, Edgbaston, Birmingham B15 2TT, UK*

Susan A. Pickett-Schenk   *UIC Mental Health Services Research Program, 104 South Michigan Avenue, Suite 900, Chicago, IL 60603, USA*

Lisa Razzano   *Assistant Professor of Psychology in Psychiatry, UIC Mental Health Services Research Program, Department of Psychiatry, 104 South Michigan Avenue, Suite 900, Chicago, IL 6063, USA*

Richard N. Rosenthal   *Professor of Clinical Psychiatry, Columbia University College of Physicians and Surgeons Chairman, Department of Psychiatry, St Luke's Roosevelt Hospital Center, 1090 Amsterdam Avenue, 16th Floor, New York, NY 10025, USA*

John B. Saunders   *Department of Psychiatry, University of Queensland, K Floor, Mental Health Centre, Royal Brisbane Hospital, Herston, 4029 Qld, Australia*

Natalie Shockley   *Department of Psychiatry, University of Queensland, K Floor, Mental Health Centre, Royal Brisbane Hospital, Herston, 4029 Qld, Australia*

Jeff Wallis   *Department of Psychiatry, University of Queensland, K Floor, Mental Health Centre, Royal Brisbane Hospital, Herston, 4029 Qld, Australia*

Roger D. Weiss   *Clinical Director, Alcohol and Drug Abuse Program, McLean Hospital, 115 Mill Street, Belmont, MA 02178-9106, USA*

Angela White   *Department of Psychiatry, University of Queensland, K Floor, Mental Health Centre, Royal Brisbane Hospital, Herston, 4029 Qld, Australia*

Ross Young   *Department of Psychiatry, University of Queensland, K Floor, Mental Health Centre, Royal Brisbane Hospital, Herston, 4029 Qld, Australia*

PREFACE

Drug and alcohol misuse among the general population and particularly the young is common. It is therefore not surprising that within the last decade epidemiological studies in the community and treatment settings have noted substance misuse among those with severe mental health problems. However, they have revealed prevalence rates of substance abuse/dependence in this client group as generally higher than in the general population.

Clinicians working in mental health and addiction settings have long been aware of the coexistence of severe mental health and drug/alcohol problems and the difficulties and frustrations that have emerged at an organizational/service level and treatment level when attempting to address the problems these clients and their families experience. It has been said that those with a severe mental health problem who use substances problematically have "fallen between" mental health and addiction services, which have traditionally been separated not only geographically and structurally but also by treatment philosophies. Over the past 10 years there has emerged from this great conceptual divide a view that substance misuse and severe mental health problems now more commonly coexist, and that parallel or serial treatment methods have failed to improve adequately outcomes for such individuals and their families. The resultant research, predominantly from the USA, has promoted what has been referred to as an "integrated treatment" approach as a more effective model of intervention for such individuals. This model of intervention is now widely accepted and used, particularly in the USA. However, there is tremendous variation in the operationalization of "integrated treatment", and the social and contextual factors that have shaped this model in that country. Furthermore, research and service developments are now taking place in this area in Europe, Australia and New Zealand, and some of this work is profiled in this book.

This book provides an opportunity for clinicians, researchers and service providers to become informed about the most important clinical and research issues related to persons with psychosis and substance misuse, and to be exposed to the developments occurring internationally. It will outline practical treatment interventions and approaches that can be used with these comorbid individuals and their families. Part I provides an introduction to the issue of substance misuse among those with psychosis by exploration of different models and levels of conceptual frameworks within which substance misuse among those with severe mental health problems can be understood. Explanations will be offered from biomedical, psychological and socio-cultural perspectives. The focus of part II is to introduce and describe a range of integrated service models that have been developed and implemented at an organizational level, within the social and cultural context of a number of countries. Part III starts with a chapter raising important issues related to the assessment of this client group. The following chapters describe a range of treatment approaches that are typically used within integrated service contexts that have been tailored to address the specific treatment needs of this population. Part IV looks at the needs of special populations of those with substance misuse in psychosis who experience higher levels of substance misuse and other concomitant difficulties. It attempts to outline the specific issues for these special populations and will help those working with these groups to think about the delivery of appropriate and effectively tailored services. Part V examines a number of treatment outcome studies and the evolving evidence base, and seeks to set the stage for the way forward.

Finally, a word on terminology—we feel that the term "dual diagnosis" is not helpful in describing this group. First, the term is not specific, as it could potentially refer to a whole range of coexisting problems, not just severe mental health and substance misuse. Secondly, we are aware that sometimes low levels of substance use (not enough to merit a dependence or abuse diagnosis) could have a significant negative effect for those with severe mental health problems and therefore the emphasis on diagnosis is not always accurate. With this in mind, we have chosen to use the term "substance misuse in psychosis" to refer to those people with severe mental health problems who misuse drugs and or alcohol.

Throughout the text, illustrative case material is used. The names and details of clients have been changed to ensure confidentiality.

Hermine L. Graham, Alex Copello,
Max J. Birchwood, Kim T. Mueser
2003

ACKNOWLEDGEMENTS

The other editors and I would like to thank a number of people who worked hard to make this book possible, including Michael Coombs for his support of this project, and the contributors for their patience and willingness to share their developments in this area.

I particularly thank Jacqui Tame for her calming words during the preparation of this book; Derek Tobin, Mike Preece, and Emma Godfrey in the COMPASS Programme Team; and everyone in HAOR for giving me a chance to learn from them; and my family for their unfailing support and belief in me.

Hermine L. Graham

Part I

SOCIAL AND PSYCHOLOGICAL PERSPECTIVES OF PROBLEM SUBSTANCE USE AMONG THOSE WITH PSYCHOSIS

INTRODUCTION

Max J. Birchwood

In this section we consider the context and the theoretical frameworks which govern our understanding of the problem of substance misuse among people with a severe mental illness. In Chapter 1, Jenny Maslin presents a comprehensive review and synthesis of the epidemiological studies from the USA and the UK concerning the data on the incidence of combined problems. She also summarizes the studies which reveal the domains of functioning that are affected by the joint impact of psychosis and substance misuse. Chapter 2 by Martin Hambrecht and Heinz Häfner unpacks the nature of the complex temporal relationship between substance misuse and psychosis: which one comes first?; are they both the result of a common underlying process? In Chapters 3, 4 and 5, family, social and cognitive conceptualizations are presented by Alex Copello, Martin J. Commander and Hermine L. Graham, respectively. Alex Copello discusses the importance of clients' social network, including their families and informal networks, in the development and maintenance of substance misuse problems. The impact that psychosis and substance misuse has upon the family is discussed, but also, critically, how the presence of substance misuse is constructed by families and how this is linked to the concept of expressed emotion. Martin J. Commander draws upon a sociological perspective, examining the social factors that are involved in both the recognition of substance misuse as a social problem, but also the development of these problems and the stigma they can create. Finally, Hermine L. Graham in Chapter 5 presents a cognitive framework in which individuals' beliefs about the function that drugs may serve in dealing with psychotic experience and their beliefs about change and control can become a target for therapy.

Chapter 1

SUBSTANCE MISUSE IN PSYCHOSIS: CONTEXTUAL ISSUES

Jenny Maslin

Jake's story

At around 15 years of age Jake began using drugs occasionally with his friends. During his late teenage years, he wanted to become a DJ and spent a lot of time at clubs, where he used amphetamine and ecstasy. His use of alcohol and cannabis also increased at this time, as he found these substances would "calm his nerves" and help him "chill out". When Jake was 21, his parents started to put pressure on him to get a "proper job", and he moved out of their home to live with his girlfriend, who occasionally used crack-cocaine. Eventually Jake tried crack-cocaine himself. Substance use was very common among Jake's friends, and he enjoyed the way it made him feel. His drug and alcohol use continued to increase to the point where, at the age of 22, Jake was spending all his money on alcohol/drugs, and his use was causing arguments with his girlfriend. Around this time, Jake began to experience auditory hallucinations. He noticed that following a period of intense drug use the voices became "worse" and more "intense" but found that if he continued to use the drugs he felt good again. He was admitted to an acute psychiatric inpatient unit, and on his discharge the voices had stopped. A few months later he began using crack-cocaine again, and whenever he had the money or could get credit from dealers, he would spend about £60 over one or two days on this. He was also spending about £30 per week on cannabis and drinking up to three cans of extra-strong lager every day. Simultaneously, Jake's auditory hallucinations became more intense and commanding, telling him that his next-door neighbour was "evil". Acting on the instructions of the voices, Jake tried to set fire to his next-door neighbour's flat. As a result of this, Jake was admitted to hospital for a second time.

Substance Misuse in Psychosis: Approaches to Treatment and Service Delivery.
Edited by Hermine L. Graham, Alex Copello, Max J. Birchwood and Kim T. Mueser.
© 2003 John Wiley & Sons, Ltd.

Since the early 1980s, the high rate of co-occurring severe mental health and substance use problems, such as those experienced by Jake, and the range and number of problems associated with these joint difficulties have been increasingly recognized. This chapter attempts to provide some context for the rest of the book by discussing definitions of severe mental health and substance use problems, prevalence rates of substance use problems among those with severe mental health problems and the difficulties associated with the experience of these joint problems.

DEFINITIONS

Despite several attempts to designate a single label for the phenomenon of co-occurring severe mental health and substance use problems (e.g., comorbidity, dual disorders), no consensus has emerged around a single term. The term *"dual diagnosis"* is most commonly used, although it is not officially recognized in either DSM or ICD nomenclature (First and Gladis, 1993). It has been suggested that the term "dual diagnosis" is inadequate for a number of reasons. First, it could apply to any two coinciding difficulties; indeed, the term has been used for a number of years in relation to mental health problems and learning difficulties before its current definition became popular. Secondly, the term focuses too narrowly on medical problems when the client group often have a number of other needs, such as housing, social, physical, psychological and financial (Barker, 1998; Bean, 1998). Some authors argue that our lack of understanding of this client group is related to our "tendency to medicalize human problems" (Hodge and Thomas, 1998: 13), an approach which may be particularly inappropriate for substance use and mental health problems. Thirdly, definitions of dual diagnosis vary considerably in terms of both the type and severity of mental health problems and the type and pattern of substance use problems. Lehman et al (1994), for example, argue that "the range of definitions for dual diagnosis includes persons with addictions who have some psychiatric symptoms, persons with serious mental illness who use psychoactive substances, persons with co-occurrent psychiatric (either Axis I or Axis II) and substance use diagnosis, as well as persons who have experienced both types of disorders during their lifetime, but not necessarily concurrently" (p. 106). Many researchers and clinicians now argue that a collective term for all clients with combined severe mental health and substance use problems may obscure considerable clinical heterogeneity among those it is intended to help. Indeed, Weiss (1992) refers to the typical dual diagnosis patient as a "mythical creature", and states that even those using the same substance and with the same mental health diagnosis do not constitute a homogeneous group due to the many other risk factors present within such subgroups.

Those experiencing combined severe mental health and substance use problems are frequently classified as having either a primary mental health problem and a secondary substance use problem or vice versa. The terms *"primary"* and *"secondary"*, however, have multiple variations with either meaning that are often dependent on the perception of the user. Primary may mean "to cause", i.e., determining, or "to be central", i.e., overriding a secondary condition that is a direct or indirect consequence (Miller, 1993). While one condition may precede another, there is no direct or obligatory causal relationship (see Chapter 2). More recently clinicians have suggested that many individuals meet criteria for both a primary mental health and a primary substance use problem (Barker, 1998). Ultimately, adapting a biopsychosocial model to the understanding of combined severe mental health and substance use problems is likely to provide the most helpful basis for building treatment programmes. This approach avoids setting one problem against another in terms of primacy, and its explanation of causality in terms of multiple factors provides the basis for an integrated, flexible and targeted approach to treatment that is more likely to meet the varied needs of each individual (Manley, 1998).

The terminology adopted throughout this book is "substance misuse" and "psychosis". For the purposes of this chapter, the term *"psychosis"* is replaced by the term *"severe mental health problems"*, which covers the full range of psychotic disorders and major mood disorders as defined by the American Psychiatric Association's *Diagnostic and Statistical Manual of the Mental Disorders* (DSM-IV) (APA, 1994) and the World Health Organization's *International Classification of Diseases* (ICD-10) (WHO, 1994). The term *"substance misuse"* is replaced by the term *"substance use problems"*, which encompasses not just DSM-IV/ICD-10 classifications of substance use disorders, but any experience of problems (social, psychological or physical) associated with the use of substances. The word *"substance"* is used in reference to any drug that alters thoughts, moods or behaviours, whether legal or illegal.

It has been suggested that those with certain severe mental health problems may show a preference for particular types of substances. If this were the case, it might be expected that alcohol, for example, would be preferred by those experiencing anxiety and cocaine by those experiencing depression, but no such patterns appear. In a survey of 263 briefly hospitalized psychiatric inpatients with a diagnosis of schizophrenia, schizo-affective disorder, bipolar disorder or major depression, Mueser et al (1992) found little difference in the choice of substances used. Ultimately, choice may be largely determined by availability factors. Some substances, however, are more frequently used than others, specifically alcohol, cannabis, and stimulants (amphetamine, cocaine and crack-cocaine) (Buckley, 1998; Cuffel, 1996). Nevertheless, problematic use across the full range of substances, including over-the-counter medicines, prescribed substances, caffeine and nicotine, does occur, and polydrug use is extremely common. Rates of cigarette consumption among people with severe mental health problems are three to four times that of the general population. Lyons (1999) reports that studies across different mental health populations show those with a diagnosis of schizophrenia to be most likely to be heavy smokers, i.e., to smoke more than one and a half packs a day and to smoke high-tar cigarettes.

PREVALENCE OF SUBSTANCE USE PROBLEMS

To some extent, increased rates of combined mental health and substance use problems in clinical settings are due to enhanced awareness of these difficulties existing jointly. In addition, de-institutionalization and increased social acceptance of and experimentation with substances are two factors that have contributed to a real increase in the prevalence of combined problems among treated populations (Drake et al, 1991). Studies looking at prevalence have now been conducted around the world, but presentation of prevalence rates is not straightforward because of several methodological issues that influence the results of studies and contribute to the diverse range of prevalence rates cited. Osher and Drake (1996), for example, cite prevalence rates across studies ranging from 10% to 65%. Methodological issues include differences in sampling methods, populations, diagnostic systems, definitions of substance use problems and severe mental health problems, assessment tools, time frames, and demographic characteristics, and failure to assess polydrug use (El-Guebaly, 1990; Mueser et al, 1995). These will be discussed in more detail later.

The study most widely cited in relation to prevalence is the National Institute of Mental Health Epidemiological Catchment Area (ECA) study (Regier et al, 1990), which includes 20 291 people spread over five countries, resident in the community, in institutional settings (including mental hospitals, nursing homes, and prisons) and in community treatment settings. This provides an ideal sampling method for studying the prevalence of combined problems. Using a structured diagnostic interview, 1-month, 6-month and lifetime prevalence rates were assessed for a number of disorders. Lifetime prevalence rates of 22.5% were found for mental disorder alone, 13.5% for alcohol disorders alone and 6.1% for other drug disorders. Of those participants with a diagnosis of schizophrenia, however, 47% also had a lifetime prevalence of some form of substance use disorder. Consequently, for those with a diagnosis of schizophrenia, the odds of having an alcohol disorder were three times higher, and the odds of having another drug disorder were six times higher than in the general population. Those participants with a diagnosis of bipolar disorder had a substance use disorder prevalence rate of 56.1%. Consequently, for those with this diagnosis, the odds of having an alcohol disorder were five times higher and the odds of having another drug disorder were eight times higher than in the general population.

Examples of treatment setting studies assessing prevalence rates in different countries are summarized in Table 1.1. Most prevalence research has been conducted in the USA (e.g., Cohen and Henkin, 1993; Mueser et al, 1990, 2000; Rosenthal et al, 1992; Safer, 1987; Test et al, 1989) and findings from treatment settings are largely consistent with those of the ECA study. Mueser et al (2000), for example, examined lifetime substance use prevalence across a range of different diagnostic categories. Alcohol use disorder was most common across the different diagnoses (43% schizophrenia, 61% schizo-affective, 52% bipolar and 48% major depression), followed by cannabis (26% schizophrenia, 29% schizo-affective, 26% bipolar and 16% major depression) and cocaine (12% schizophrenia, 7% schizo-affective, 8% bipolar and 12% major depression). Concurrent alcohol and drug use disorders were also common within the group (23% schizophrenia, 26% schizo-affective, 27% bipolar and 23% major depression).

In Australia, Fowler et al (1998) found 6-month and lifetime prevalences of substance abuse/dependence to be 26.8% and 59.8%, respectively, with alcohol (18.1%), cannabis (12.9%) and amphetamines (2%) being the most commonly abused substances over the previous 6 months. Participants were divided into those with no current or past history of abuse/dependence, those reporting a history but no current abuse/dependence and those with current abuse/dependence. The groups with either current or past history of abuse/dependence were younger, more likely to be male, less likely to have been married and more likely to be smokers than the no-abuse/dependence group. Studies of prevalence rates have also been conducted in Taiwan (Lin et al, 1998), France (Launay et al, 1998) and Germany (Krausz et al, 1996; Soyka et al, 1993). Soyka et al (1993) assessed prevalence rates of substance use among patients with a diagnosis of schizophrenia admitted to two psychiatric facilities in Munich, over a 6-month period. Lifetime prevalence for substance abuse was estimated at 42.9% at the mental state hospital, where participants were considered to be a more "chronic" group (in terms of higher rates of past psychiatric admissions and longer duration of psychosis), and 21.8% in the university hospital. Alcohol was the substance most commonly abused with prevalence estimates of 34.6% and 17.4%, respectively, across facilities. Cannabis, amphetamines and cocaine were the most frequently abused illegal drugs, followed by opiates and hallucinogens.

UK studies (Bernadt and Murray, 1986; Brown, 1998; Duke et al, 1994; Glass and Jackson, 1988; Graham et al, 2001 Menezes et al, 1996; Smith et al, 1994; Virgo et al, 1998; Wheatley, 1998) show lower prevalence rates than

Table 1.1 Examples of prevalence rate studies

Authors (listed alphabetically)	n	Population and location	Mental health diagnosis	Substance use criteria/screen	Time frame for substance use problems	Results
Brown, 1998	185	Rehabilitation Psychiatry Service, Southampton, UK	Chronic psychosis (schizophrenia, affective illness, other)	Abuse/dependence rating by keyworker interview using Barry et al, 1995. Lifetime use identified from case notes	6-month and lifetime	6-month = 22% any substance, 18% alcohol, 10% illicit drugs, 15% prescribed drugs. Lifetime = 29% alcohol, 17% drugs
Fowler et al, 1998	194	Community mental health service, New South Wales, Australia	Schizophrenia	Participant assessment for abuse/dependence DSM-III-R criteria, case manager ratings (Drake et al, 1990) plus urine analysis	6-month and lifetime	6 month = 26.8% any substance, 18.1% alcohol, 12.9% cannabis, 2% amphetamine, 0% cocaine. Lifetime = 59.8% any substance
Graham et al (2001)	1369	Community mental health and substance misuse services, Birmingham, UK	Psychotic disorders, bipolar and major depression	Abuse/dependence rating by keyworker using CRS (Drake et al, 1996)	12 months	24% any substance
Krausz et al, 1996	99	Psychiatric clinic, Hamburg, Germany	Schizophrenia spectrum	Participant assessment for abuse/dependence ICD-9 criteria plus other methods	Lifetime	47.5% any substance

Study	N	Setting	Diagnosis	Assessment	Timeframe	Prevalence
Menezes et al, 1996	171	Inpatient, outpatient and community mental health services, London, UK	Any form of functional psychosis	Participant assessment using Duke et al. 1994, DAST (Skinner, 1982) and abuse/dependence rating by keyworker using Drake et al (1989)	12 months	31.6% alcohol, 15.8% other drugs
Mueser et al, 1990	149	Psychiatric inpatients, Pennsylvania, USA	Schizophrenia spectrum	Participant assessment for abuse/dependence DSM-III-R criteria	Lifetime	47% alcohol, 42% cannabis, 25% stimulants, 18% hallucinogens, 7% sedatives, 4% narcotics
Mueser et al, 2000	325	Psychiatric inpatients, New Hampshire, USA	Schizophrenia (SZ), schizo-affective (SA), bipolar (BP) and major depression (MD), and other	Participant assessment for abuse/dependence DSM-III-R criteria plus case manager ratings using CRS (Drake et al, 1996)	Lifetime	Alcohol = 43% SZ, 61% SA, 52% BP, 48% MD. Cannabis = 26% SZ, 29% SA, 26% BP, 16% MD. Cocaine = 12% SZ, 7% SA, 8% BP, 23% MD
Soyka et al, 1993	a) 183 b) 447	Psychiatric inpatients, Munich, Germany	Schizophrenia spectrum	Participant assessment for abuse/dependence ICD-9 criteria	Lifetime	a) 21.8% any substance and 17.4% alcohol b) 42.9% any substance and 34.6% alcohol

Notes: CRS: Clinician Rating Scales; DAST: Drug Abuse Screening Test.

those cited in US studies. Menezes et al, (1996), for example found 1-year prevalence rates of 36.3% for any substance use problem (31.6% for alcohol problems and 15.8% for drug problems, with cannabis, amphetamines and LSD being the most frequently used substances) among psychosis patients in London. The study by Graham et al (2001) assessing prevalence across both community mental health and substance misuse services in Birmingham, UK, found that 24% of clients with a diagnosis of severe mental illness were identified by their keyworkers as having used substances problematically in the previous 12 months. Problem use among the identified group was mainly of alcohol (61%), cannabis (43%), stimulants (21%) and opiates (9%), with 30% of the sample being polydrug users.

A number of demographic characteristics appear to correlate with substance use problems among those with severe mental health problems, specifically being male, young, single, less educated and having a family history of substance use problems (Menezes, 1996; Mueser et al, 1995). Other studies conducted in mental health settings report mixed findings in relation to the rates of men and women experiencing combined problems (Alexander, 1996). While some studies show significantly more men than women with combined problems (e.g., Cuffel et al, 1993; Westreich et al, 1997), others find no significant differences between the sexes (e.g., Dixon et al, 1991; Watkins et al, 1999). Demographic profiles may also vary, however, according to the type of substance used (Mueser et al, 1990; 1992).

Racial/cultural group has also been related to differences in prevalence rates, although the number of relevant studies that include data on or analysis of these factors is very small (Westermeyer, 1995). Westermeyer (1995) points out that racial and cultural groups may differ in their rates of problem substance use and severe mental health problems for many reasons, which include the type of substances and pattern of use that are prescribed, approved of or permitted by the group; behavioural norms in the group regarding types of psychoactive substances and approved patterns of use; availability of psychoactive substances in the community; access of people in the community to the substance; symbolic meaning of the substance in the group, as related to the group's identity, world view and values; and the economic role of the substance to the group. In addition, treatment access and efficacy for either problem can differ across ethnic and cultural groups, a delay in which could affect the prevalence of combined problems.

As mentioned previously and as highlighted in Table 1.1, differences between studies in diagnostic criteria for mental health and substance use problems make results difficult to compare. Some studies, for example, focus on substance use, abuse, dependence or alternative definitions of problem use. The methods used to determine diagnosis, whether by self-report ratings, structured/non-structured clinical interviews or examination of medical records, also influence findings. In addition, establishing diagnosis may be problematic because the symptoms of substance use and withdrawal may mimic those of the severe mental health problem. In a review of 14 papers citing prevalence rates of combined severe mental health and substance use problems, where participants were diagnosed as a result of standardized interviews, Weiss et al (1992) found a substantial degree of variability in three areas. These were the timing of the participant interviews, how the diagnoses were made and what abstinence criteria were utilized. The location from which samples are drawn also has a bearing on prevalence rates. Those with severe mental health problems who are homeless, in jail, or in emergency or acute care settings are more likely to have substance use problems than others (Galanter, 1988). Mueser et al (1998) note that most estimates of combined problems are probably inflated by sampling bias because samples are usually drawn from treatment settings, and having either disorder increases the likelihood of receiving treatment.

A number of methodological refinements that would enable comparisons between prevalence studies have been suggested by Mueser et al (1990). These include the use of standardized instruments to diagnose mental health and substance use problems, information to assess problem substance use gathered from multiple sources, evaluation of both history of substance use and current use, assessment of problem substance use prevalence in more than one diagnostic group, matching of patient and non-patient groups on demographic variables and assessment of the problematic use of specific types of substances. Multiple methods of assessment of substance use problems may also increase the reliability of prevalence study results. One difficulty with relying on self-report information alone is that clients with severe mental health problems may deny substance-related problems or the use of any substances at all, for a number of reasons, including "psychological defences, neuropsychological impairments that decrease their ability to perceive the relationships between drinking and adjustment difficulties, and the tendency to provide socially desirable answers" (Drake et al, 1990: 64). They may also be concerned about how an admission of substance use might affect the support they receive. A combination of urine screening, and interviews with clients, their service providers and family members is reported to provide the most accurate and usually the highest estimates of substance use (Ananth et al. 1989).

In summary, prevalence studies show a range of rates depending on the type of methodology adopted. However, substance use problems are clearly common among those with severe mental health problems and appear to occur more frequently in this group than within the general population. Research suggests that approximately 50% of people with severe mental health problems have experienced problems related to their substance use at some time in their lives, and between a quarter and a third are experiencing current substance use problems.

CORRELATES OF SUBSTANCE USE

Many studies have shown additional consequences, specific to those with severe mental health problems, over and above the usual adverse social, health, economic and psychological consequences associated with problem substance use. Mueser et al (1998) argue that there is some evidence to suggest that substance use simply exacerbates all the negative outcomes that frequently occur among those with severe mental health problems. An early study by Drake et al (1989) examined patterns of alcohol use among 115 participants diagnosed with schizophrenia who were participating in an aftercare programme. Heavy alcohol use (meeting DSM criteria for abuse/dependence) was related to medication non-adherence, homelessness, financial problems and not eating regular meals. In terms of mental health symptoms, hostile, threatening behaviour and disorganized, incoherent speech were the symptoms most strongly related to heavy alcohol use. Rehospitalization was associated with alcohol use with 27% of abstainers, 48% of mild users and 68% of heavy users being rehospitalized during the 1-year course of the study. Table 1.2 summarizes difficulties as they occur within three broad areas: social functioning, mental and physical health and treatment outcome. In spite of a substantial number of negative associations, however, many substance users report positive effects from their use, and these will be discussed in relation to each area.

Table 1.2   Correlates of substance use

Social functioning
- Reduced social contact/competence (Drake et al, 1998)
- Housing instability/homelessness (Drake et al, 1991; Koegel and Burnam, 1988; Soyka et al, 1993)
- Increased family conflict (Clark, 1996; Dixon et al, 1995; Mueser and Gingerich, 1994)
- Violent behaviour (Cuffel et al, 1994; Scott et al, 1998; Smith et al, 1994)
- Financial difficulties (Drake et al, 1989)

Mental and physical health
- Earlier onset of mental health problems (Kovasznay et al, 1997)
- Psychotic relapse (Linzsen et al, 1994)
- Exacerbation of mental health symptoms (Noordsy et al, 1991; Shumway et al, 1994)
- Increased risk of HIV (Carey et al, 1995; Mahler, 1995)
- Risk of sexual and physical abuse (Alexander, 1996; Bellack and Gearon, 1998)

Treatment outcome
- Increased hospitalization (Cuffel and Chase, 1994; Drake and Wallach, 1989)
- Medication adherence problems (Owen et al, 1996)
- Reduced effect of antipsychotics (Lyons, 1999; Ziedonis et al, 1994)
- Increased use of services (Bartels et al, 1993; Hipwell et al, 2000)

Effects on social functioning

In general, the literature supports the view that those with combined problems, at least before their substance use becomes too chronic, tend to have
better social competence and more social contacts than those who have
severe mental health problems alone (Drake et al, 1998). It is possible that
those who are more socially competent and active are at increased risk of
developing problems with their substance use, perhaps due to their increased exposure to substances through social relationships. The use of
alcohol is reported to reduce social anxiety (e.g., Noordsy et al, 1991), and
alcohol, cannabis and cocaine have all been associated with the relief of
depression (e.g., Dixon et al, 1991). Thus, the use of substances may be
driven by a desire to reduce anxiety and depression and improve social
facilitation (Mueser et al, 1995). Drake et al, (1998) state that "there appears
to be a reciprocal relationship between social functioning and substance
abuse in schizophrenia. More socially active patients with schizophrenia
use substances, and substance use in turn promotes greater social activity
by virtue of the social context in which substances are used" (p. 283). As
substance use progresses, however, social competence and social networks
can be destroyed as relationships diminish and the possibility of housing
instability or homelessness emerges.

People with combined problems appear particularly vulnerable to housing
instability and homelessness (Drake et al, 1991; Soyka et al, 1993). Koegel
and Burnam (1988), for example, found that the rate of schizophrenia
was nine times higher in homeless alcohol-dependent persons than in a
household sample of alcohol-dependent persons in the ECA study (Regier
et al, 1990). Similarly, bipolar disorder was seven times more prevalent
in homeless alcohol-dependent individuals than in their housed counterparts. Homeless persons with combined problems are more likely to be
older, to be male, to be unemployed, to have greater health difficulties and
to receive more services than homeless persons with one or no diagnosis (Fischer, 1990). They are also more likely than other homeless groups
to suffer from psychological distress and demoralization, to grant sexual
favours for food and money, and to be picked up by the police and im-
prisoned; are less likely to receive help from their families; and are highly
prone to victimization (Koegel and Burnam, 1987).

Homelessness may occur as a direct result of family conflict, which is a common experience in this group (Clark, 1996; Mueser and Gingerich, 1994).
As Clark (1996) notes, those with combined problems often rely heavily on
their families for assistance because of difficulties in managing the tasks
of daily living. Indeed, a study by Clark (1994) showed that the parents
of adult children with combined problems spent significantly more time
caring for them (e.g., cooking, cleaning, providing transport, interacting
with health-care workers, and creating structured leisure activities) and

gave them significantly more financial support than parents of children who had no such problems. Although living with a relative who has combined problems does not always lead to conflict or burden, it can lead to increased levels of stress, and family members may find themselves feeling frustrated, anxious, fearful, angry, helpless and desperate (Mueser and Gingerich, 1994). Those with combined problems themselves report feeling significantly worse about their families than clients with severe mental health problems alone, in spite of no differences in objective indicators of family contact (Dixon et al, 1995). A stressful family atmosphere can in turn lead to increased relapse rates (Kavanagh, 1992), weakened family ties, increased possibilities of homelessness and increased rates of substance use for those with combined problems.

Substance use has also been associated with an increased risk of violence among those with severe mental health problems. Smith et al (1994) looked at 33 consecutive admissions for predominantly violent behaviour to a regional secure unit in the UK. They found that in 54% of admissions, drug or alcohol abuse was implicated, but that among those with a diagnosis of schizophrenia, 73% had such a history. A study by Cuffel et al (1994) of 103 patients with a diagnosis of schizophrenia reviewed substance use and violent behaviour through medical records. The use of alcohol and drugs was associated with increased odds of concurrent and future violent behaviour (e.g., verbal and non-verbal threats to harm others, physical assaults or altercations, brandishing a weapon or starting fires), and there was an increased likelihood of violence among those who were polysubstance users. Smith and Hucker (1994) found strong links between psychotic disorders and problem substance use leading to increased rates of violence. It has been speculated that intoxication accounts for increased rates of violence, but, as studies have shown violence frequently occurring without intoxication, other factors need to be considered. Social factors may account for the apparent association, particularly as severe mental health problems and substance use problems can often lead to considerable social disadvantage (Smith and Hucker, 1994).

Effects on mental and physical health

Problem substance use has been associated with an earlier onset of schizophrenia and poor clinical functioning (Kovasznay et al, 1997). In a prospective study comparing those with a diagnosis of schizophrenia or a related disorder, divided according to whether they were cannabis abusers or non-abusers, Linszen et al (1994) found that significantly more and earlier psychotic relapses occurred in the cannabis-abusing group. The association became stronger when mild and heavy cannabis use was distinguished. Not only has alcohol been shown to exacerbate psychosis but it may also accelerate the appearance of tardive dyskinesia (Dixon et al, 1992).

Although numerous studies report negative effects of substance use on clinical symptoms, Dixon et al (1990) review a number of experimental, clinical and self-report studies that show positive effects on clinical symptoms. All substances appear to have the potential to exacerbate psychosis, but reductions of depression levels, anxiety and negative symptoms have been observed in subgroups of experimentally medicated schizophrenic patients. Clinical studies have also produced a varied pattern of results, and it appears that drug response is heterogeneous among those with a diagnosis of schizophrenia, with both favourable and unfavourable subjective effects reported. In a study by Dixon et al (1989), 83 consecutively admitted inpatients with a diagnosis within the schizophrenia spectrum and a lifetime diagnosis of drug or alcohol abuse were asked to indicate the direction in which selected symptoms and effects changed during acute drug intoxication. The results focused on alcohol, cannabis and cocaine, and the majority of participants reported that all three drugs decreased levels of depression. Reported effects on anxiety, energy levels and psychotic symptoms differed for the three drugs. For example, participants reported that cannabis and alcohol reduced feelings of anxiety, but cocaine increased them.

A common self-reported reason for substance use among those with severe mental health problems is to cope with symptoms and the effects of medication (Mueser et al, 1995). It is possible, however, that the use of substances might cause the difficulty that the person is using substances to cope with. In a study of 75 outpatients with a diagnosis of schizophrenia by Noordsy et al (1991), over half the sample reported that alcohol reduced social anxiety, tension, dysphoria, apathy, anhedonia and sleep difficulties. Participants were also asked to state whether they had experienced each of nine common psychotic symptoms (such as auditory hallucinations and paranoia) and whether alcohol reduced or increased that symptom. The rate of reported symptom relief was between 5% and 30% for individual symptoms, but 7% to 32% of participants reported that alcohol increased psychotic symptoms. Improvements in negative symptoms have also been demonstrated among cigarette smokers who report feeling more relaxed and less anxious after smoking (Ziedonis et al, 1994).

In addition to exacerbation of mental health symptoms, those with combined problems may also be at increased risk of other physical health problems, including HIV (Mahler, 1995). Carey et al (1995) reviewed nine studies, nearly all conducted in New York City, which assessed the prevalence of HIV infection among those with severe mental health problems. Prevalence rates ranged from 4% to 23%, and collapsing data across all studies yielded an overall rate of 8%. The authors state that this rate exceeds the rate found in the US general population, which is estimated to be between 0.3% and 0.5% (Steele, 1994).

For women with combined problems, additional risks have been reported, specifically in relation to sexual and physical abuse (Alexander, 1996; Bellack and Gearon, 1998). Alexander (1996) reports studies showing that women with combined problems are more likely to have experienced childhood physical and sexual abuse than women with severe mental health problems alone (e.g., Brown and Anderson, 1991). Women are also more likely than men to report having been victims of crime (e.g., Brunette and Drake, 1997; Westreich et al, 1997).

Effects on treatment outcome

A number of studies have shown increased hospitalization rates among those with combined problems (e.g., Cuffel and Chase, 1994; Drake and Wallach, 1989; Graham et al, 2001), although other studies have found no such differences (e.g., Fowler, 1998). It has been suggested that increased hospitalization may be directly related to the type of substance used (Mueser et al, 1990; 1992). In addition, medication adherence problems have been highlighted as a factor in rehospitalization and as being common among those using substances. In a study by Owen et al (1996), for example, participants with a diagnosis of schizophrenia were interviewed during their hospital stay and 6 months later to obtain information on demographic characteristics, medication non-adherence, substance abuse, symptom severity and medication side effects. Participants were asked about their medication adherence within the 30 days before hospital admission and the 30 days before the follow-up interview. Those with current substance abuse were substantially more likely to report medication non-adherence. A combination of current substance abuse, medication non-adherence and no outpatient contact was associated with significantly worse symptom severity at follow-up. There are a number of reasons that might account for medication adherence problems. Some clients stop taking medication because they have been told it should not be combined with other substances. In other cases, the effects of using substances lead clients to neglect their medication. Even when medication is taken, its effects might be compromised by the use of substances. For example, cigarette smokers metabolize antipsychotics faster than non-smokers (Lyons, 1999), and smoking has been shown to lower the blood levels of some antipsychotics by up to 50% (e.g., Ziedonis et al, 1994).

As a consequence of the clinical and social effects of combined severe mental health and substance use problems, clients appear to utilize more services than those with severe mental health problems alone. Bartels et al (1993) prospectively examined service utilization and costs across a range of institutional and outpatient services, including psychiatric and substance abuse hospitalization, incarceration, psychosocial rehabilitation, emergency services, case management, other outpatient services and housing support. They studied three groups of schizophrenic patients: current substance abusers, past substance abusers and those with no history of substance abuse. Current substance abusers accounted for all episodes of incarceration and substance abuse hospitalization and had a greater rate of psychiatric hospitalization. They were also approximately twice as likely to use emergency services over the study period than past abusers or those who had never abused. Otherwise, there were no significant differences in the use of non-institutional services, including psychosocial rehabilitation, outpatient treatment (case management, psychotherapy and psychiatric visits) and residential support services. An estimate of total economic costs between the three groups showed a trend toward greater total costs for current abusers, followed by past abusers and those who had never abused, due to greater use of hospital and emergency services. A study by Hipwell et al (2000), among attendees at a community mental health day centre in the UK, compared 16 clients with a diagnosis of schizophrenia/schizo-affective illness and problem substance use and 16 clients with a diagnosis of schizophrenia/schizo-affective illness alone. Clients with combined problems were more likely to miss appointments at the day centre and to fail to attend on the days they had been expected. They had also been admitted to an inpatient facility significantly more times in the previous year because of psychotic relapse and were more likely to have had multiple inpatient stays.

CONCLUSION

In spite of many adverse consequences of substance use among those with severe mental health problems, it is clear that many do make positive changes to their substance use patterns (Bartels et al, 1995; Cuffel and Chase, 1994), and that substance use does not necessarily impair functioning (Shumway et al, 1994). Bartels et al (1995) followed a cohort of participants with severe mental health problems over 7 years, and over this period their substance use behaviour was rated by their case managers. Rates of substance use in the cohort as a whole were consistent over time, but there was considerable variation in the substance use behaviour of individuals. Although 41% of those meeting criteria for alcohol dependence at baseline remained dependent at the 7-year follow-up, there were also a number of participants who made positive changes to their substance use patterns. The remission rates for alcohol abuse and alcohol dependence were 67% and 33%, respectively. The remission rates for drug abuse (other than alcohol) and drug dependence were 54% and 31%, respectively. Risk status for the negative outcomes associated with substance use problems has been shown to reduce when use stabilizes in terms of both symptoms and service utilization (Bartels et al, 1993; Dixon et al, 1991; Zisook et al, 1992).

The high prevalence, significant risk factors and high use of resources associated with combined severe mental health and substance use problems logically means that this client group merit the degree of attention paid to them over the last two decades. Clinicians and researchers now face the challenge of developing and evaluating appropriate treatment and services for this client group, and a number of innovative approaches from around the world are presented in subsequent chapters.

REFERENCES

Alexander, M.J. (1996) Women and co-occurring addictive and mental disorders: an emerging profile of vulnerability. *American Journal of Orthopsychiatry*, **66**: 61–70.
American Psychiatric Association (1994) *Diagnostic and Statistical Manual of Mental Disorders*, 4th edn. Washington, DC, APA.
Ananth, J., Vandewater, S., Kamai, M., Brodsky, A., Gamal, R. and Miller, M. (1989) Missed diagnosis of substance abuse in psychiatric patients. *Hospital and Community Psychiatry*, **40**: 297–299.
Barker, I. (1998) Mental illness and substance misuse. *Mental Health Review*, **3**: 6–13.
Barry, K., Fleming, M., Greenly, J., Widlak, P., Kropp, S. and McKee, D. (1995) Assessment of alcohol and other drug disorder in the seriously mentally ill. *Schizophrenia Bulletin*, **21**: 313–321.
Bartels, S.J., Drake, R.E. and Wallach, M.A. (1995) Long term course of substance use disorders among patients with severe mental illness. *Psychiatric Services*, **46**: 248–251.
Bartels, S.J., Teague, G., Drake, R.E., Clark, R.E., Bush, P.W. and Noordsy, D.L. (1993) Substance abuse in schizophrenia: service utilization and costs. *Journal of Nervous and Mental Disease*, **181**: 81–85.
Bean, P. (1998) Dual diagnosis and beyond. *Alcohol Update*, **Oct**, 2–3.
Bellack, A.S. and Gearon, J.S. (1998) Substance abuse treatment for people with schizophrenia. *Addictive Behaviours*, **23**: 749–766.
Bernadt, M.W. and Murray, R.M. (1986) Psychiatric disorder, drinking and alcoholism. *British Journal of Psychiatry*, **148**: 393–400.
Brown, S. (1998) Substance misuse in a chronic psychosis population. *Psychiatric Bulletin*, **22**: 595–598.
Brown, G.R. and Anderson, B. (1991) Psychiatric comorbidity in adult inpatients with childhood histories of sexual and physical abuse. *American Journal of Psychiatry*, **148**: 55–61.
Brunette, M.F. and Drake, R.E. (1997) Gender differences in patients with schizophrenia and substance abuse. *Comprehensive Psychiatry*, **38**: 109–116.
Buckley, B.F. (1998) Substance abuse in schizophrenia: A review. *Journal of Clinical Psychiatry*, **59**: 26–30.

Carey, M.P., Weindhardt, L.S. and Carey, K.B. (1995) Prevalence of infection with HIV among the seriously mentally ill: review of research and implications for practice. *Professional Psychology: Research and Practice*, **26**: 262–268.

Clark, R.E. (1994) Family costs associated with severe mental illness and substance use. *Hospital and Community Psychiatry*, **45**: 808–813.

Clark, R.E. (1996) Family support for persons with dual disorders. In R. E. Drake and K.T. Mueser (Eds), *Dual Diagnosis of Major Mental Illness and Substance Use Volume 2: Recent Research and Clinical Implications*. New Directions for Mental Health Services, No. 70. San Francisco, Jossey-Bass.

Cohen, E. and Henkin, I. (1993) Prevalence of substance abuse by seriously mentally ill patients in a partial hospital program. *Hospital and Community Psychiatry*, **44**: 178–180.

Cuffel, B.J. (1996) Comorbid substance use disorder: prevalence, patterns of use and course. *New Directions for Mental Health Services*, **70**: 93–105.

Cuffel, B.J. and Chase, P.C. (1994) Remission and relapse of substance use disorders in schizophrenia. *Journal of Nervous and Mental Disease*, 182: 342–348.

Cuffel, B.J., Heithoff, K.A., and Lawson, W. (1993) Correlates of patterns of substance abuse among patients with schizophrenia. *Hospital and Community Psychiatry*, **44**: 247–251.

Cuffel, B.J., Shumway, M., Choulhan, T.L. and MacDonald, T. (1994) A longitudinal study of substance use and community violence in schizophrenia. *Journal of Nervous and Mental Disease*, **182**: 704–708.

Dixon, L., Haas, G., Weiden, P., Sweeney, J. and Frances, A. (1990) Acute effects of drug abuse in schizophrenic patients: clinical observations and patients self-report. *Schizophrenia Bulletin*, **16**: 69–79.

Dixon, L., Haas, G., Weiden, P., Sweeney, J. and Frances, A.J. (1991) Drug abuse in schizophrenic patients: clinical correlates and reasons for use. *American Journal of Psychiatry*, **148**: 224–230.

Dixon, L., McNary, S. and Lehman, A. (1995) Substance abuse and family relationships of persons with severe mental illness. *American Journal of Psychiatry*, **152**: 456–458.

Dixon, L., Haas, G.H., Dulit, R.A., Weiden, P.J., Sweeney, J. and Hien, D. (1989) Substance abuse in schizophrenia: preferences, predictors and psychopathology. *Schizophrenia Research*, **2**: 6.

Dixon, L., Weiden, P.J., Haas, G., Sweeney, J. and Frances, A.J. (1992) Increased tardive dyskinesia in alcohol abusing schizophrenic patients. *Comprehensive Psychiatry*, **33**: 121–122.

Drake, R.E. and Wallach, M.A. (1989) Substance abuse among the chronic mentally ill. *Hospital and Community Psychiatry*, **40**: 1041–1046.

Drake, R.E., Mueser, K.T. and McHugo, G.J. (1996) Clinician Rating Scales: Alcohol Use Scale (AUS), Drug Use Scale (DUS) and Substance Abuse Treatment Scale (SATS). In L. Sederer and B. Dickey (Eds), *Outcomes Assessment in Clinical Practice*. Baltimore, MD, Williams and Wilkins.

Drake, R.E., Osher, F.C. and Wallach, M.A. (1989) Alcohol use and abuse in schizophrenia: a prospective community study. *Journal of Nervous and Mental Disease*, **77**: 408–414.

Drake, R.E., Osher, F.C. and Wallach, M.A. (1991) Homelessness and dual diagnosis. *American Psychologist*, **46**: 1149–1158.

Drake, R.E., McLaughlin, P., Pepper, B. and Minkoff, K. (1991) Dual diagnosis of major mental illness and substance disorder: an overview. In K. Minkoff and R.E. Drake (Eds.), *Dual Diagnosis of Major Mental Illness and Substance Disorder*. San Francisco, Josey-Bass.

Drake, R.E., Mercer-McFadden, C., Mueser, K.T., McHugo, G.J. and Bond, G.R. (1998) Review of mental health and substance abuse treatment for patients with dual disorders. *Schizophrenia Bulletin*, **24**: 589–608.

Drake, R.E., Osher, F.C., Noordsy, D.L., Hurlbut, S.C., Teague, G.B. and Beaudett, M.S. (1990) Diagnosis of alcohol use disorders in schizophrenia. *Schizophrenia Bulletin*, **16**: 57–67.

Duke, P., Pantelis, C. and Barnes, T. (1994) South Westminster schizophrenia survey: alcohol use and its relationship to symptoms tardive dyskinesia and illness onset. *British Journal of Psychiatry*, **164**: 630–636.

El-Guebaly, N. (1990) Substance abuse and mental disorders: The dual diagnoses concept. *Canadian Journal of Psychiatry*, **35**: 261–267.

Endicott, J., Spitzer, R.L., Fleiss, J.L., and Cohen, J. (1976) The Global Assessment Scale: a procedure for measuring overall severity of psychiatric disturbance. *Archives of General Psychiatry*, **33**: 766–771.

First, M.B. and Gladis, M.M. (1993) Diagnosis and differential diagnosis of psychiatric and substance use disorders. In J. Solomon, S. Zimberg and E. Shollar (Eds.), *Dual Diagnosis: Evaluation, Treatment, Training and Program Development*. New York, Plenum.

Fischer, P.J. (1990) *Alcohol and Drug Abuse and Mental Health Problems Among Homeless Persons: A Review of the Literature, 1980–1990*. Rockville, MD, National Institute on Alcohol Abuse and Alcoholism and National Institute of Mental Health.

Fowler, I.L., Carr, V.J., Carr, N.T., and Lewin, T.J. (1998) Patterns of current and lifetime substance use in schizophrenia. *Schizophrenia Bulletin*, **24**, 443–455.

Galanter, M., Castenada, R. and Ferman, J. (1988) Substance abuse among general psychiatric patients. *American Journal of Drug and Alcohol Abuse*, **14**, 211–235.

Glass, I.B. and Jackson, P. (1988) Maudsley Hospital Survey: prevalence of alcohol problems and other psychiatric disorders in a hospital population. *British Journal of Addiction*, **83**: 1105–1111.

Graham, H.L., Maslin, J., Copello, A., Birchwood, M., Mueser, K.T., McGovern, D. and Georgiou, G. (2001). Drug and alcohol problems amongst individuals with severe mental health problems in an inner city area of the UK. *Social Psychiatry and Psychiatric Epidemiology*, **36**: 448–455.

Hipwell, A.E., Singh, K. and Clark, A. (2000) Substance misuse among clients with severe and enduring mental illness: service utilisation and implications for clinical management *Journal of Mental Health*, **9**: 37–50.

Hodge, J. and Thomas, G. (1998) Clients with complex needs. *Alcohol Update*, Oct, 13–15.

Kavanagh, D.J. (1992) Recent developments in expressed emotion and schizophrenia. *British Journal of Psychiatry*, **160**: 601–620.

Koegel, P. and Burnam, M.A. (1987) *The Epidemiology of Alcohol Abuse and Dependence among the Homeless: Findings from the Inner City of Los Angeles*. Rockville, MD, National Institute on Alcohol Abuse and Alcoholism.

Koegel, P. and Burnam, M.A. (1988) Alcoholism among homeless adults in the inner city of Los Angeles. *Archives of General Psychiatry*, **45**: 1011–1018.

Kovasznay, B., Fleischer, J. and Tanenberg-Karant, M. (1997) Substance use disorder and the early course of illness in schizophrenia and affective psychosis. *Schizophrenia Bulletin*, **23**: 195–201.

Krausz, M., Haasen, C., Mass, R., Wagner, H.-B., Peter, H. and Freyberger, H.J. (1996) Harmful use of psychotropic substances by schizophrenics: coincidence, patterns of use and motivation. *European Addiction Research*, **2**: 11–16.

Launay, C., Petitjean, F., Perdereau, F. and Antoine, D. (1998) Addictive behaviour in mental disorders: a survey in the Paris area. *Annales Medico-Psychologiques*, **156**: 482–485.

Lehman, A.F., Myers, C.P., Corty, E. and Thompson, J.W. (1994) Prevalence and patterns of "dual diagnosis" among psychiatric inpatients. *Comprehensive Psychiatry*, **35**: 106–112.

Lin, C.C., Bal, Y.M., Hu, P.G. and Yeh, H.S. (1998) Substance use among inpatients with bipolar and major depressive disorder in a general hospital. *General Hospital Psychiatry*, **20**: 98–101.

Linszen, D.H., Dingemans, P.M. and Lenior, M.E. (1994) Cannabis abuse and the ⊔⊔⊔⊔ ⊔⊔ ⊔⊔⊔ ⊔⊔⊔⊔ ⊔⊔⊔⊔⊔⊔ ⊔⊔⊔⊔⊔⊔⊔⊔⊔⊔⊔⊔ ⊔⊔⊔⊔⊔⊔⊔⊔⊔. *Archives of General Psychiatry*, **51**: 273–279.

Lyons, R. (1999) A review of the effects of nicotine on schizophrenia and antipsychotic medications. *Psychiatric Service*, **50**: 1346–1350.

Mahler, J.C. (1995) HIV, substance abuse and mental illness. In A.F. Lehman and L.B. Dixon (Eds), *Double Jeopardy, Chronic Mental Illness and Substance Use Disorders*. London, Harwood Academic.

Manley, D. (1998) Dual diagnosis: approaches to the treatment of people with dual mental health and drug abuse problems. *Mental Health Care*, **1**: 190–192.

Menezes, P.O., Johnson, S., Thornicroft, G., Marshall, J., Prosser, D., Bebbington, P. and Kuipers, E. (1996) Drug and alcohol problems among individuals with severe mental illness in South London. *British Journal of Psychiatry*, **168**: 612–619.

Miller, N.S. (1993) Comorbidity of psychiatric and alcohol/drug disorders: interactions and independent status. *Journal of Addictive Diseases*, **12**: 5–16.

Mueser, K.T. and Gingerich, S. (1994) *Coping with Schizophrenia: A Guide for Families*. Oakland, CA, New Harbinger.

Mueser, K.T., Bennett, M. and Kushner, M.G. (1995) Epidemiology of substance use disorders among persons with chronic mental illness. In A.F. Lehman and L.B. Dixon (Eds), *Double Jeopardy: Chronic Mental Illness and Substance Use Disorders*. London, Harwood Academic Publishers.

Mueser, K.T., Drake, R.E. and Noordsy, D.L. (1998) Integrated mental health and substance abuse treatment for severe psychiatric disorders. *Journal of Practical Psychiatry and Behavioral Health*, May: 129–139.

Mueser, K.T., Yarnold, P.R. and Bellack, A.S. (1992) Diagnostic and demographic correlates of substance abuse in schizophrenia and major affective disorder. *Acta Psychiatrica Scandinavica*, **85**: 48–55.

Mueser, K.T., Nishith, P., Tracy, J.I., DeGirolamo, J., and Molinaro, M. (1995) Expectations and motives for substance use in schizophrenia. *Schizophrenia Bulletin*, **21**: 367–378.

Mueser, K.T., Yarnold, P.R., Rosenberg, S.D., Swett, C., Miles, K.M. and Hill, D. (2000) Substance use disorder in hospitalized severely mentally ill psychiatric patients: prevalence, correlates and subgroups. *Schizophrenia Bulletin*, **26**: 179–192.

Mueser, K.T., Yarnold, P.R., Levinson, D.F., Singh, H., Bellack, A.S., Kee, K., Morrison, R.L., and Yadalam, K.G. (1990) Prevalence of substance abuse in schizophrenia: demographic and clinical correlates. *Schizophrenia Bulletin*, **16**: 31–56.

Noordsy, D.L., Drake, R.E., Teague, G.B., Osher, F., Hurlbut, S.C., Beaudett, M.S. and Paskus, T.S. (1991) Subjective experiences related to alcohol use among schizophrenics. *Journal of Nervous and Mental Disease*, **179**: 410–414.

Osher, F.C. and Drake, R.E. (1996) Reversing a history of unmet needs: approaches to care for persons with co-occurring addictive and mental disorders. *American Journal of Orthopsychiatry*, **66**: 4–11.

Owen, R.R., Fischer, E.P., Booth, B.M., and Cuffel, B.J. (1996) Medication noncompliance and substance abuse among patients with schizophrenia. *Psychiatric Services*, **47**: 853–858.

Regier, D.A., Farmer, M.E., Rae, D.S., Locke, B.Z., Keith, S.J., Judd, L.L. and Goodwin, F.K. (1990) Co-morbidity of mental disorders with alcohol and other drug abuse: results from the Epidemiologic Catchment Area (ECA) Study. *Journal of the American Medical Association*, **264**: 2511–2518.

Rosenthal, R.N., Hellerstien, D.J., and Miner, C.R. (1992) Integrated services for treatment of schizophrenic substance abusers: demographics, symptoms and substance abuse patterns. *Psychiatric Quarterly*, **63**: 3–26.

Safer, D.J. (1987) Substance abuse by young adult chronic patients. *Hospital and Community Psychiatry*, **38**: 511–514.

Scott, H., Johnson, S., Menezes, P., Thornicroft, G., Marshall, J., Bindman, J., Bebbington, P. and Kuipers, E. (1998) Substance misuse and risk of aggression and offending among the severely mentally ill. *British Journal of Psychiatry*, **172**: 345–350.

Shumay, M., Chouljian, T.L. and Hargreaves, W.A. (1994) Patterns of substance use in schizophrenia: a Markov modelling approach. *Journal of Psychiatric Research*, **28**: 277–287.

Skinner, H.A. (1982) The Drug Abuse Screening Test. *Addictive Behaviors*, **7**: 363–371.

Smith, J., Frazer, S., and Boer, H. (1994) Dangerous dual diagnosis patients. *Hospital and Community Psychiatry*, **45**: 280–281.

Smith, J. and Hucker, S. (1994) Schizophrenia and substance abuse. *British Journal of Psychiatry*, **165**: 13–21.

Soyka, M., Albus, M., Kathmann, N., Finelli, A., Hofstetter, S., Holzbach, R., Immler, B. and Sand, P. (1993) Prevalence of alcohol and drug abuse in schizophrenic inpatients. *European Archives of Psychiatry and Clinical Neuroscience*, **242**: 362–372.

Steele, F.R. (1994) A moving target: CDC still trying to estimate HIV prevalence. *Journal of NIH Research*, **6**: 25–26.

Test, M.A., Wallisch, L.S., Allness, D.J. and Ripp, K. (1989) Substance use in young adults with schizophrenic disorders. *Schizophrenia Bulletin*, **15**: 465–476.

Virgo, N., Bennett, G., Bennett, L., Higgins, D. and Thomas, P. (1998) *The Prevalence of Co-occurring Severe Mental Illness and Problematic Substance Misuse (Dual Diagnosis) in the Patients of Mental Health and Addiction Services in East Dorset*. Poster presented at Addictions '98 Conference, Newcastle-upon-Tyne, 25–27 September.

Watkins, K.E., Shaner, A. and Sullivan, G. (1999) The role of gender in engaging the dually diagnosed in treatment. *Community Mental Health Journal*, **35**: 115–126.

Weiss, R.D. (1992) The myth of the typical dual diagnosis patient. *Hospital and Community Psychiatry*, **43**: 107–108.

Weiss, R.D., Mirin, S.M. and Griffin, M.L. (1992) Methodological considerations in the diagnosis of coexisting psychiatric disorders in substance abusers. *British Journal of Addiction*, **87**: 179–187.

Westermeyer, J. (1995) Ethnic and cultural factors in dual disorders. In A.F. Lehman and L.B. Dixon (Eds.), *Double Jeopardy: Chronic Mental Illness and Substance use Disorders*. London, Harwood Academic.

Westreich, L., Guedj, P., Galanter, M. and Baird, D. (1997) Differences between men and women in dual diagnosis treatment. *American Journal on Addictions*, **6**: 311–317.

Wheatley, M. (1998) The prevalence and relevance of substance use in detained schizophrenic patients. *Journal of Forensic Psychiatry*, **9**: 114–129.

World Health Organization (1994) *Classification of Mental and Behavioural Disorders. Clinical Descriptions and Diagnostic Guidelines (10th Revision)*. Geneva, World Health Organization.

Ziedonis, D.M., Kosten, T.R., Glazer, W.M. and Frances, R.J. (1994) Nicotine dependence and schizophrenia. *Hospital and Community Psychiatry*, **45**: 204–206.

Zisook, S., Heaton, R., Mornaville, J., Kuck, J., Jernigan, T. and Braff, D. (1992) Past substance abuse and clinical course of schizophrenia. *American Journal of Psychiatry*, **149**: 552–553.

Chapter 2

TEMPORAL ORDER AND AETIOLOGY

Martin Hambrecht and Heinz Häfner

Despite methodological differences, the majority of clinical and epidemiological studies found significantly increased rates of substance misuse in persons with severe mental illness, particularly schizophrenia (see Chapter 1). For decades, this comorbidity has raised the question of a causal relationship between schizophrenia and substance abuse. The hypotheses that have been proposed can be classified in to four logical groups (cf. Thornicroft, 1990; Silver and Abboud, 1994; Mueser et al, 1998):

1. Substance misuse is a precipitating if not causal factor for schizophrenia.
2. Substance misuse is a consequence of a pre-existing severe mental disorder.
3. A third common factor causes both disorders.
4. Comorbidity is nothing but an incidental association.

The last hypothesis of mere coincidence may appear plausible given the similiar demographic distribution of onsets and first incidences of schizophrenia and substance misuse, namely, adolescence and young adulthood in males. In addition, it is more likely to diagnose a second disorder when someone presents with a psychiatric disorder in the first place (cf. Schuckit, 1994). An association purely by chance, however, and without any causal interrelationship is unlikely. If this were true, substance abuse should have about the same prevalence among patients suffering from schizophrenia and in the general population of the same age and sex. Not only clinical but also population-based studies (Chapter 1) show

Substance Misuse in Psychosis: Approaches to Treatment and Service Delivery.
Edited by Hermine L. Graham, Alex Copello, Max J. Birchwood and Kim T. Mueser.
© 2003 John Wiley & Sons, Ltd.

consistently a 2–4 times higher relative risk of substance abuse in patients with severe mental disorder. Comorbidity rates vary between studies, but these variations can be attributed to methodological and similar differences. These findings suggest a causal relationship between the two disorders.

SCHIZOPHRENIA AS A SECONDARY DISORDER

Causation models state that substance abuse precipitates or causes schizophrenia, at least in vulnerable individuals (e.g., Mueser et al, 1990, 1992; McGuire et al, 1995). This hypothesis received its strongest support from a wide range of clinical observations and systematic studies on the acute psychotic effects of hallucinogens, amphetamines, cocaine, and higher dosages of other stimulants (cf. Schuckit, 1994). In very high (toxic) dosages, cannabis may lead to schizophrenia-like psychoses. The pharmacological basis for these acute states appears to be a dramatic increase in dopaminergic neurotransmission, but glutamatergic mechanisms as in phencyclidine (PCP), which elicits positive and negative symptoms very similar to genuine schizophrenia, may also be involved. The strongest argument against secondary psychosis refers to the duration of substance-induced acute psychotic states. The longer these states persist beyond the intake of the drug, the more likely an independent psychotic disorder appears to be. Psychotic states beyond a duration of 3 weeks after cessation of drug intake cannot be considered to be only a drug psychosis. In addition, these transient psychotic states show differences in psychopathology, e.g., predominating agitation or confusion, and lower prevalence of Schneiderian first-rank symptoms.

The concept that drugs precipitate schizophrenia in vulnerable individuals represents a weaker form of a causation model. Relapse and first-episode studies provide ample support for this concept, at least with regard to cannabis. Cannabis misuse appears to be a very strong predictor of psychotic symptoms, hospitalizations, and relapses, even when concomitant misuse of alcohol, stimulants, or hallucinogen is controlled for (Linszen et al, 1994). In addition, treatment of substance abuse in comorbid patients was found to decrease the risk of psychotic relapses. The precipitation of relapses was less convincingly demonstrated for other substances, particularly for alcohol (e.g., Swofford et al, 1996), and it should be considered that the aetiology of relapses and first episodes might be quite different.

The precipitation model is supported indirectly by numerous studies with strong evidence for an earlier age of onset of schizophrenia in comorbid cases (cf. Hambrecht and Häfner, 1996)—an argument already pointing to the issue of temporal order of onsets that will be discussed later. In some studies (e.g., Barbee et al, 1989; Bowers et al, 1990), this difference did not reach statistical significance, often due to small sample sizes. Studies that challenged the general finding of an earlier psychotic illness with comorbid substance misuse are rare and point to matters of gender and of diagnostic accuracy. According to Pulver et al (1989), males with schizophrenia and comorbid alcoholism were younger at first hospitalization than non-alcoholic patients with schizophrenia. For female patients, this effect was reversed. Duke et al (1994) reported an average 4-year delay of the onset of schizophrenia with comorbid alcohol abuse, and speculated that, in fact, accurate diagnosis of schizophrenia may have been delayed because drinking may have masked its onset. This may also explain Zisook et al's finding (1992), as they had defined age at first psychiatric contact as age at onset of psychosis. In a large study by Kovasznay et al (1993), age at onset of first psychotic symptoms did not vary with substance abuse status, and in a later study by the same group (Rabinowitz et al, 1998), an earlier age of onset of psychosis was associated with prior substance abuse only in females. Diagnostic heterogeneity, however, impedes the comparability of these results, because only 35% of the cases had a schizophrenia-like psychosis.

SUBSTANCE MISUSE AS A SECONDARY DISORDER

Alternative models of causality posit that persons with schizophrenia have an increased risk of substance misuse. Self-medication models are most prominent among these concepts, but social factors have also been put forth. Some authors argue that patients are more vulnerable to peer-group pressure and find a more acceptable self-concept and social identity for themselves as drug addicts than as persons with severe mental illness (Baigent et al, 1995). Indeed, comorbid cases with polysubstance abuse often belong to specific subcultures (e.g., the "surf scene"). Another more sociological approach holds that the social decline associated with schizophrenia results in unemployment, poor housing, and living in drug-exposed, deprived, inner-city neighbourhoods. These conditions then result in an increase of substance misuse. While these concepts certainly apply to a subgroup of comorbid cases, they have not been tested broadly enough for substance misuse in general.

The majority of empirical studies with regard to secondary substance misuse in persons with psychotic disorders circle around the issue of self-medication (cf. Schneier and Siris, 1987). There is, indeed, much evidence from clinical experience that patients use alcohol or non-prescribed drugs to counter distressing symptoms of the illness or side effects of treatment, but clinicians as well as empirical research mostly rely on self-reports (e.g., Test et al, 1989; Dixon et al, 1991; Noordsy et al, 1991; Warner et al, 1994).

Many studies attempted to distinguish the self-observed effects of various non-prescribed substances. *Alcohol* was reported to relax and improve depression (Dixon et al, 1991), but also to worsen depression (Addington and Duchak, 1997); to decrease anxiety (Noordsy et al, 1991); to improve sleep (Noordsy et al, 1991; Pristach and Smith, 1996); to worsen hallucinations (Sokolski et al, 1994); to worsen psychotic symptoms in general (Pristach and Smith, 1996); to alleviate psychotic symptoms (Baigent et al, 1995; Addington and Duchak, 1997); and to worsen and to improve psychotic symptoms in about the same degree (Noordsy et al, 1991). The effects were usually reported by some, but not by all comorbid patients, and there were always some patients who experienced nothing or the opposite. *Cannabis*-misusing patients with schizophrenia tended to report an improvement of anxiety and energy (Dixon et al, 1991; Warner et al, 1994), improved social integration (Warner et al, 1994; Baigent et al, 1995), more happiness, more relaxation, and less slowing-down, a probable side effect of the medication (Addington and Duchak, 1997). At the same time, a substantial portion of patients reported an increase of suspiciousness (Dixon et al, 1991), positive and negative symptoms (Baigent et al, 1995), psychotic symptoms (Lambert et al, 1997), confusion, delusions, strange thoughts, and, in some cases, even more depression (Addington and Duchak, 1997). With *cocaine*, comorbid patient's reported feeling more energetic but more anxious, too (Dixon et al, 1991), and to see more symptoms worsened than improved (Castaneda et al, 1991). *Amphetamine* misuse was also reported to increase energy, more than alcohol or cannabis, to elevate mood, and to improve negative symptoms (Baigent et al, 1995).

Since many of these self-reported effects of the various drugs appear to be interchangeable, substance misuse in persons with an established psychotic illness is now seen to be less deterministic. An increasing number of authors underline the general effects of misused substances, regardless of the specific substance (cf. Mueser et al, 1998)—for example, Test et al (1989), who collected evidence for generally more positive than negative changes in symptoms after recent use of any substance. Misuse of any substance is now increasingly seen as an attempt to counter negative symptoms or find relief from unpleasant affective states, particularly dysphoria (Lambert et al, 1997).

The limitations of self-report studies are obvious; patients, for instance, were found to underreport substance abuse (Test et al, 1989; Shaner et al, 1993). The reliability and validity of self-reports is challenged by memory deficits, limited insight, and the subjects' perceptions of the most desirable response. With regard to aetiology, post-hoc attribution is the major problem of all self-report studies. Very easily, just by asking, patients are directed to link their substance intake to symptoms. In addition, most of the self-report studies comprised chronic samples, but the reasons for and effects of substance misuse may change over the years. Baigent et al (1995), separated the reasons for starting substance misuse (when mostly peer pressure and, to a lesser degree, relief of depression, dysphoria, and anxiety were reported) from the reasons for its continuation (relief from depression, dysphoria, or anxiety in the large majority; improved social interaction in only one-fifth).

Besides the methodological limitations of self-reports, the self-medication hypothesis is also challenged by the relative stability of consumption patterns over the years, often unaffected by variations of the clinical status (Bartels et al, 1995). Consumption may be linked more to dimensions of personality or temperament, e.g., Cloninger's novelty seeking, than to clinical variables (Van Ammers et al, 1997). Drug-abuse patterns in persons with schizophrenia and with other major mental illnesses were found to be similar, and persons with schizophrenia apparently do not choose specific drugs to ameliorate specific negative states, although they know about these different effects (Dixon, 1999; Lambert et al, 1997). Availability and affordability become the most important factors in the choice of substance— more than drug-specific effects. This observation can explain variations in the geographical distribution of substance misuse in schizophrenia, with a preponderance of polysubstance abuse in urban areas and a predominant misuse of alcohol and cannabis in rural settings (Dixon, 1999). The self-medication hypothesis was directly tested by Hamera et al (1995), who detected no association of symptom level and consumption of alcohol or cannabis in a pooled time series analysis with daily protocols by 17 subjects with schizophrenia and comorbid alcohol and/or cannabis misuse. Small sample size, serious level of misuse (mean of 6 drinks or 5 joints per day), and the counterintuitive finding of a decrease in smoking at the emergence of prodromal symptoms, however, necessitate a replication of this elegant study.

Overall, these results contradict a specific typology of substance misuse of persons with psychotic disorders. It became apparent that persons with psychotic disorders have similar patterns of substance misuse to non-psychiatric groups (cf. Mueser et al, 1998). Seriously mentally ill persons, however, have a higher risk of substance misuse in general, and self-medication with whatever relaxes and improves mood remains one plausible reason for comorbidity.

CAUSATION BY A THIRD COMMON FACTOR

The issue of a third factor leading to both disorders is intriguing but still speculative. This third factor might be a common genetic risk, a common fetal brain lesion, common social stressors, or common personality factors.

Mueser et al (1998) found poor evidence for a shared genetic vulnerability. They argue for antisocial personality disorder as a third factor that independently increases patients' vulnerability to both psychiatric and substance use disorders. This association, however, is not schizophrenia-specific, and studies of selected inpatient samples with high rates of involuntary admission that showed an association of psychosis, substance misuse, and antisocial personality need to be replicated in broader settings (Mueser et al, 1999). The relevance of personality factors (i.e., relatively stable patterns of individual behaviour) is underlined by the results of birth cohort studies (cf. Jones, 1997). Among childhood precursors of schizophrenic disorders in later life, two typical patterns of social-emotional behaviour were over-represented: "schizoid habits" (shyness, lack of emotional responsiveness, etc.) and "antisocial tendencies" (naughtiness, aggressive overreactions, etc.). Both typologies of childhood behaviour contributed to the (quite accurate) predictions made by schoolteachers regarding the later development of schizophrenia (Olin et al, 1998). The antisocial type, in particular, is associated with substance misuse, and personality factors thus seem to link the risk of psychosis and the risk of substance misuse—at least in a subgroup of patients. Whether personality is indeed causal as a third common factor, whether it is just an intervening variable of something behind, whether it is only a result of correlation or a result of diagnostic uncertainty (e.g., schizophrenia versus spectrum disorders)—these questions require further investigation, preferably with a prospective longitudinal design.

CLARIFICATION THROUGH ASSESSMENT OF THE TEMPORAL SEQUENCE

As posited by Aristotelian logic, the exploration of the causality between two events includes the determination of their temporal order—in everyday life as well as in science. If event B preceded event A, event A cannot be the cause of event B. Temporal relation should be of great importance in comorbidity research (Thornicroft, 1990), and temporal analyses have already been applied to this issue long ago. In 1911, Eugen Bleuler, the Zurich psychiatrist who coined the term "schizophrenia", wrote:

> The unstable schizophrenic easily becomes a drinker. About 10% of our drunkards are schizophrenics as well. In these cases alcoholism should probably be considered as a symptom of schizophrenia. I have never seen the latter appear in an alcoholic afterwards. (1911: 219, translation by M.H.)

In spite of this historical dimension, the temporal approach has apparently been often neglected. A recent review on comorbidity (Dixon, 1999) does not mention temporal order at all. Something similar happens in clinical practice. In 198 medical records of patients with schizophrenia, for instance, Boutros et al (1996) always found information about the presence or absence of a drug abuse history, but none of the records attempted to relate drug use to the onset of psychotic symptoms.

The reason for this neglect might be that clinicians as well as researchers encounter a number of difficulties as they investigate the temporal sequence of substance misuse and psychosis in their patients. These difficulties include reliability and validity issues as well as general logical and methodological questions of research.

- In many psychiatric disorders, onset is an ill-defined process over time which can be quite heterogeneous. The onset of psychosis may be rapid, but more often it is insidious, and prodromal symptoms may stretch back 5–10 years. Schizophrenia, in particular, emerges gradually over months and even years in the majority of cases. This process often coincides roughly with the development of substance use disorders (cf. Mueser et al, 1998).
- Multiple-substance misuse is frequent in comorbid cases, making temporal analyses and the determination of the most relevant factor even more difficult. Cocaine misuse, for example, often coincides with cannabis misuse, and comparisons of schizophrenia patients with and without cocaine misuse are difficult to interpret when these groups also differ significantly with regard to cannabis misuse (Sevy et al, 1990).
- The temporal order cannot be assessed cross-sectionally, and longitudinal data are necessary. Prospective studies would be most appropriate, but they encounter considerable difficulties—in particular, the low incidence of schizophrenia that forces one to begin with large numbers of vulnerable persons. To avoid this problem, relapse studies follow-up remitted first-episode cases with known increased vulnerability to investigate the temporal order (see above). These studies indeed found higher relapse rates in cannabis consumers, but the comparability of first episodes and relapses, i.e., different stages of the illness, is unclear.
- Longitudinal studies, however, have to consider secular trends in the consumption of different substances. Drug abuse patterns in the general population and in psychiatric patients are specific for time and place. From 1990 to 1992, for instance, the rates for cannabis and stimulant abuse were found to decrease in US patients with schizophrenia, while the rate of cocaine abuse increased (Mueser et al, 1990; 1992).
- Finally, logic teaches that determining the sequence of two events can falsify, but not verify, a hypothesized causal relationship. Temporal order does not prove causality.

In spite of these difficulties, a small number of studies attempted to investigate systematically the temporal sequence of the onsets of schizophrenia

and substance misuse. The studies employed different materials and definitions, particularly more or less heterogeneous samples with regard to
chronicity and misused substances; various operationalizations of onset;
and reliance on self-report, relatives' reports, charts, or case registers.

From an Israeli inpatient sample with multiple readmissions, Silver and
Abboud (1994) reported that 60% started to use illicit drugs before and
40% started to use them after the first hospitalization for schizophrenia—a
reliable but very crude measure of onset. A more sophisticated but long
reliable definition of onset of schizophrenia was used in a retrospective
study in Munich (Soyka et al, 1993). In this predominantly chronic sample,
secondary substance misuse was more frequent: 55% of the patients reported that the first positive or negative symptom of schizophrenia had
appeared before and 40% said that it had appeared after the onset of substance abuse. Barbee et al (1989) assessed ages of onset in emergency-room
schizophrenia patients with and without comorbid alcohol abuse and/or
alcohol dependency. They found schizophrenia to be more often secondary
in patients who were diagnosed with a combination of alcohol abuse and
alcohol dependency. A primary schizophrenic disorder was more often
seen with alcohol abuse, and patients with alcohol dependence but without alcohol abuse had an onset at about the same time as schizophrenia.
This classification of alcohol-related disorders, however, is implausible,
and the high rate of comorbidity with cannabis misuse in this sample was
not taken into account.

Without specifying their definitions of onset, Lambert et al (1997) reported
that in a chronic sample in Hamburg the mean age of onset of substance
misuse was always earlier than the mean age at first manifestation of psychotic illness, namely, by 3.7 years (alcohol misuse), 6.0 years (alcohol dependency), 3.2 years (cannabis misuse), and 3.1 years (multiple substance
misuse). This indicates a higher prevalence of primary substance misuse
for all four misuse patterns. In a large sample with affective, schizophrenia-
like psychosis and other psychoses, Kovasznay et al (1993) found median
ages of onset of substance abuse and of psychotic symptoms of 17 years
and 24 years, respectively. The same group later confirmed that the diagnosis of substance abuse almost always predated the onset of psychosis
(Rabinowitz et al, 1998).

The self-reports of rather severely disabled Australian patients point in
the same direction. Baigent et al (1995) reported that alcohol or cannabis
misuse had started on average about 5 years before schizophrenia, and
78% of their sample was convinced that alcohol or cannabis abuse had
preceded their schizophrenic disorder, while 57% thought that abuse had
caused or exacerbated it. Taylor and Warner (1994) based their study of 32
chronic patients on retrospective interviews with relatives and on charts.

In more than 75% of the comorbid cases, the onset of alcohol use preceded the onset of illness by 1 year or more, and in more than 60% of the comorbid cases, cannabis use preceded the onset of illness by more than 1 year.

Narrowing the scope to cannabis, Eikmeier et al (1991) investigated the medical records of 45 comorbid cases. In 71% of these cases, cannabis use had started more than 1 year before the onset of DSM-IIIR prodromal symptoms or clear symptoms of schizophrenia, compared to 13% of cases with onsets within the same year and only 4% with an onset of schizophrenia after the onset of cannabis use. This finding was replicated by Caspari (1999) in a retrospective study of 39 cannabis-abusing patients with schizophrenia (23 of them with a first psychotic episode). The mean delay between onset of cannabis abuse and first psychotic episode was 4.4 years. Only one patient had started to misuse cannabis after the onset of schizophrenia. Strictly limiting the sample to recent onset cases, a Dutch study (Linszen et al, 1994) found that in 23 out of 24 cannabis-abusing patients the abuse preceded the onset of first psychotic symptoms by at least 1 year. A systematic survey of the Stockholm psychiatric register (Allebeck et al, 1993) identified 112 patients with a diagnosis of schizophrenia and comorbid cannabis dependence. In 69% of these cases, heavy cannabis abuse had occurred at least 1 year before the onset of psychotic symptoms. The reverse order was seen in only 11% of the sample, and the authors concluded that cannabis abuse might be a risk factor for schizophrenia.

More representative findings (but only small numbers) can be expected from case register and from population studies, such as the Edmonton study. Among 2144 adults in a defined catchment area, Bland et al (1987) detected 20 persons with a lifetime diagnosis of schizophrenia and a lifetime comorbidity with a substance misuse disorder in 12 of these cases. In four cases, substance misuse had started before and in eight cases it had started after the onset of schizophrenia. However, because in four of these cases the onset of schizophrenia was reported to be as early as age 6–10, the validity of this temporal order remains doubtful. On the basis of data from the Epidemiologic Catchment Area Program, Tien and Anthony (1990) prospectively analysed the association of self-reported substance use and consecutive psychotic experiences, i.e., any positive response to 12 questions regarding psychotic experiences. With this broad definition, daily cannabis use resulted in a significantly increased twofold risk of psychotic experiences, daily cocaine use in a 3.5 times increased risk, and alcohol disorder (only in males) in an almost eightfold risk. Diagnostic accuracy is certainly a problem in this kind of household survey carried out by lay interviewers, but a broad, unselected database may outweigh this disadvantage.

Since truly prospective studies starting prior to first episodes are almost impossible, case register linkage was employed in a "quasi-prospective" approach. The best known of these studies with regard to comorbidity was based on the combination of self-reported cannabis use at conscription and psychiatric hospitalization records 15 years later (Andreasson et al, 1987). The relative risk of receiving a diagnosis of schizophrenia was 2.4 times higher among those who had tried cannabis by age 18 than those who had not. In addition, Andreasson et al found a dose-response relationship between the number of cannabis consumptions and the risk of developing schizophrenia later. This study remains important—in spite of several critical points against its design, e.g., the large temporal gap, the reliance on self-reports and on case-register diagnoses, and the lack of information about the use of cannabis or other drugs in the interval. Some of these criticisms were addressed in a later paper by Andreasson et al (1989), although it remains open whether an emerging psychiatric disorder (of which cannabis use might have been a prodromal sign) could indeed have been excluded at conscription.

To summarize these studies, there is converging evidence that cannabis misuse precedes the "onset of schizophrenia" in the majority of patients—usually for a number of years. The temporal relation of alcohol misuse to the onset of schizophrenic symptoms was less often studied, and the results are less convincing. This applies even more to the misuse of stimulants, cocaine, hallucinogens, opiates, and other illicit drugs, for which the few results are not generalizable.

To a greater or lesser degree, these sophisticated and important studies have shortcomings, e.g., lack of representativeness, reliance on unvalidated self-reports, doubtful diagnostic validity, or, in particular, the operationalization of the onset of schizophrenia. First hospitalization and even the onset of psychotic symptoms are definitions that oversimplify the onset of schizophrenia. The large majority of schizophrenic disorders begin insidiously. Stage models (cf. Docherty et al, 1978) conceptualize psychotic symptoms as the last step in the development of the disorder. The onset of schizophrenia, therefore, should be seen as a gradual process rather than as a single point in time, as empirically and representatively demonstrated by the ABC Schizophrenia Study (Häfner et al, 1992; 1993).

TEMPORAL ORDER IN A REPRESENTATIVE FIRST-EPISODE SAMPLE

Careful operationalization of the different stages in early psychosis was a major focus of the ABC (*Age, Beginning,* and *Course*) Schizophrenia

Study (Häfner et al, 1992; 1993). In a defined catchment area of 1.5 million inhabitants, the ABC Study investigated a representative sample of 232 first admissions with a first episode of schizophrenia or paranoid disorder according to ICD-9. The presence of a first psychotic episode was identified by means of a structured clinical assessment. The previous history of any sign or symptom of mental disturbance was carefully investigated with special emphasis on the exact timing of the first appearance of the symptoms. This was accomplished with the "Interview for the Retrospective Assessment of the Onset of Schizophrenia—IRAOS", which retrospectively assesses the presence, onset, and course of 66 symptoms during the early course of schizophrenia (Häfner et al, 1992). The IRAOS determines the points in time when the first symptom of schizophrenia, the first positive and the first negative symptom had emerged. The definition of the *"first symptom of schizophrenia"* took the differing specificity of symptoms for schizophrenia into account. Non-specific symptoms were only considered as "first symptoms" if they persisted continuously into the psychotic episode; negative symptoms were considered if they continued or recurred until the first psychotic episode; positive symptoms were always considered as "first symptoms" if they appeared earliest. The agreement between patients' and relatives' reports on these "milestones" during the early course of schizophrenia was significant (e.g., Pearson correlations of 0.77 for the first symptom, 0.93 for the first positive symptom, 0.73 for the first negative symptom), and this congruence demonstrated the validity of the data (Häfner et al, 1993).

Within the IRAOS, a special section addresses substance misuse, differentiating substances and the frequency of their consumption during various intervals. Drug misuse was defined as consumption of illegal drugs more than once a week over at least 1 month. The onset of drug misuse was defined as the first month in which the criteria for misuse were fulfilled. If the patient quit substance misuse for at least 1 month and then started again, two separate episodes of substance misuse were rated. Of the sample, 24% had a history of alcohol misuse and 14% had a history of illicit drug misuse, i.e., twice the rates of population controls matched according to age, sex, and place of residence (Hambrecht and Häfner, 1996). Male sex and early symptom onset were major risk factors. Cannabis played a prominent role among the illicit drugs; 88% of the drug misusers had abused cannabis at some time, usually as the first illicit drug, but only 37% had taken only cannabis in their substance abuse history. Other relevant drugs were hallucinogens, cocaine, and stimulants (in about 30% of the misusing patients). Multiple substance abuse was frequent, particularly concomitant alcohol abuse by cannabis-abusing patients.

Again, the comparison of patients' and relatives' reports on the patients' substance abuse history corroborated the validity of this information. Their

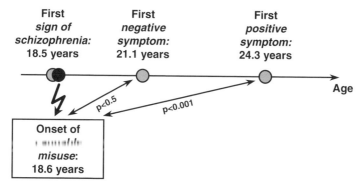

Figure 2.1 Comparison of mean ages of onset in patients with cannabis misuse ($n=29$)

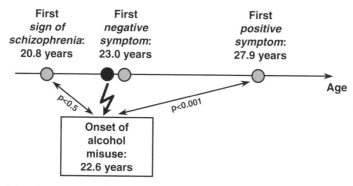

Figure 2.2 Comparison of mean ages of onset in patients with alcohol misuse ($n=55$)

reports on alcohol abuse showed a high concordance (kappa $= 0.65$) and a highly significant Pearson correlation of 0.62 of the reported time of onset of alcohol abuse. Drug abuse was also reported quite congruently by patients and relatives, as demonstrated by a kappa of 0.52 and a Pearson correlation for first occurrence of 0.69 (Hambrecht et al, 1994).

The temporal sequence of the first occurrence of signs and symptoms of schizophrenia and of the onset of substance misuse was compared group-wise for all comorbid cases (t-test for paired samples). The comparison of the group means (Figures 2.1 and 2.2) indicated that the age of onset of alcohol abuse was later than the first symptom of schizophrenia, not significantly different from the onset of negative symptoms, but significantly earlier than the first positive symptom with a long interval in between. The mean age of onset of drug abuse did not differ from the mean age at the first symptom of schizophrenia, but occurred significantly earlier than the first negative symptom and earlier than the first positive symptom.

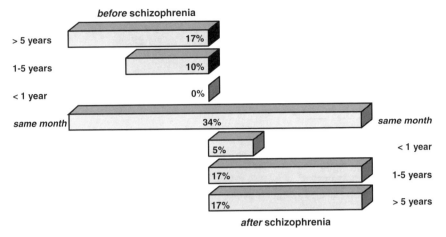

Figure 2.3 Temporal order of onset of drug misuse and the first sign of schizophrenia ($n=29$)

The comparison of group means shows the general trends, but may blur the temporal order in individual cases. This necessitates inspection of the numbers of patients with onsets of substance abuse before, within the same month, and after the described "milestones" during the early course of schizophrenia. The analysis of the sequence of illicit drug misuse and of the first symptom of schizophrenia was particularly interesting, since the group means for these two events did not differ significantly. As shown in Figure 2.3, drug-misusing, first-episode schizophrenia patients can be subdivided into three groups of almost equal size: 27.5% had a drug problem more than 1 year (often more than 5 years) before the first sign of schizophrenia. In 34.6%, the first signs of schizophrenia and drug abuse started at almost the same time. In 37.9%, drug abuse began after the first symptoms of schizophrenia.

With regard to alcohol abuse, the analyses of the individual sequences (not shown here) corroborated the findings from the group analysis. Alcohol misuse most often starts after the first signs of schizophrenia and has a particular temporal relation to negative symptoms. Obviously, Bleuler is still right: alcohol abuse does not precipitate schizophrenia. With regard to illicit drug misuse, particularly cannabis, Hambrecht and Häfner (2000) interpreted the results in the light of the vulnerability-stress-(coping-) model of schizophrenia (Zubin and Spring, 1977; Nuechterlein, 1987). This model provides a useful framework for communication between researchers and clinicians from the diverse backgrounds of neurobiological and psychosocial approaches to schizophrenia. It suggests the following possible interpretations of the ABC Study's findings on subgroups of comorbid patients:

- Group 1 with an onset of cannabis abuse years before the onset of the first signs of the disease may be called the *"vulnerability group"*. These patients might suffer from a chronic deterioration by cannabis that reduces the vulnerability threshold and/or their coping resources. The linear relationship between the frequency of cannabis use and the risk of a subsequent schizophrenic disorder found by Andreassen et al (1987) reflects this process of deterioration, which could be of a biological, psychological, and/or social nature. Neurobiological studies (cf. Castle and Ames, 1996) have demonstrated the effects of cannabis on the brain. Regular heavy ingestion of cannabis may cause subacute encephalopathy, resulting in cognitive, motivational, and affective changes (cf. Lundquist, 1995). Repetitive exposure to cannabis and even more to stimulants and hallucinogens with their "psychotomimetic effects" was hypothesized to result in an increased sensitivity of response. Post et al (1984) had put forward the concept of "behavioral sensitization and kindling", which then was applied by Lieberman et al (1990) to explain the precipitation of psychosis by drug abuse (cf. Mueser et al, 1998).
- Group 2 with an onset of both disorders at about the same time may be called the *"stress group"*. This group comprises individuals already vulnerable to schizophrenia due to genetic, pre- or perinatal influences. Cannabis consumption then acts as the dopaminergic stress factor and precipitates the onset of the disease (cf. Gardner and Lowinson, 1991).
- Group 3 with an onset of cannabis abuse after the first symptoms of schizophrenia may be called the *"coping group"*: These patients consume cannabis predominantly for self-medication against (or for coping with) symptoms of schizophrenia, particularly negative and depressive symptoms (Schneier and Siris, 1987; Test et al, 1989; Dixon et al, 1991; Noordsy et al, 1991). The patients learn to counterbalance an unpleasant hypodopaminergic prefrontal state by the dopaminergic effects of cannabis.

Mueser et al (1998) rightly stated that in many patients the closeness of the onsets of both disorders precludes conclusive findings regarding aetiology at the present state of knowledge. Further research is needed to validate this preliminary proposal for a differentiation of comorbid cases, and the following aspects should be kept in mind. Confounding variables, such as subtle cognitive, perceptual, affective, and social deficiencies preceding schizophrenia, may also contribute to an increased risk of pre-schizophrenic substance abuse. They are difficult to assess in retrospect and cannot be ruled out. A third risk factor, that is, neurodevelopmental and morphological brain anomalies, frequently preceding both the onset of schizophrenia and substance abuse, remains possible.

Neurobiological variables will contribute to characterize further the three groups, whose actual size has to be determined in larger samples. It is most likely that a patient can belong to more than one group—longitudinally as well as cross-sectionally. During the course of the illness, a patient may shift from one group to another, and even at a given point in time, all three relations of cannabis to psychosis may converge to produce comorbidity. Prospective studies and sophisticated case studies should explore this issue further.

Several fields of psychiatric research, including biological, psychopathological, or epidemiological studies, contribute to a better understanding of the role of psychotropic substances in the aetiology of psychoses. Biological studies in animals and man have been able to illuminate the pathogenetic action of psychotropic drugs. Epidemiological studies in first-episode patients, such as the ABC Study, can test whether these experimentally derived models are applicable to the natural course of schizophrenia, particularly, the order of onset of substance abuse and schizophrenic symptoms. The differentiation of important steps during the early course of schizophrenia (namely, the appearance of the first sign, the first negative symptom, and the first positive symptom) is necessary for a sophisticated analysis of the temporality of onsets. Of course, the determination of the temporal sequence of events cannot prove, but only falsify, causal hypotheses. While Rosenthal (1998) rightly summarized that "no compelling evidence to date has been presented for causality" (p. 45), the ABC Study suggests that causal links between schizophrenia and cannabis may go in both directions, and that the vulnerability-stress-coping model of schizophrenia is a helpful framework for the interpretation of these findings.

REFERENCES

Addington, J. and Addington, D. (1998) Effect of substance misuse in early psychosis. *British Journal of Psychiatry*, **172** (Suppl 33): 134–136.

Addington, J. and Duchak, V. (1997) Reasons for substance abuse in schizophrenia. *Acta Psychiatrica Scandinavica*, **96**: 329–333.

Allebeck, P., Adamsson, C. and Engstrom, A. (1993) Cannabis and schizophrenia: a longitudinal study of cases treated in Stockholm County. *Acta Psychiatrica Scandinavica*, **88**: 21–24.

Andreasson, S., Allebeck, P., Engstrom, A. and Rydberg, U. (1987) Cannabis and schizophrenia: a longitudinal study of Swedish conscripts. *Lancet*, **26**: 1483–1486.

Andreasson, S., Allebeck, P. and Rydberg, U. (1989) Schizophrenia in users and nonusers of cannabis. *Acta Psychiatrica Scandinavica*, **79**: 505–510.

Arndt, S., Tyrrell, G., Flaum, M. and Andreasen, N.C. (1992) Comorbidity of substance abuse and schizophrenia: the role of premorbid adjustment. *Psychological Medicine*, **22**: 379–388.

Baigent, M., Holme, G. and Hafner, R.J. (1995) Self reports of the interaction between substance abuse and schizophrenia. *Australian and New Zealand Journal of Psychiatry*, **29**: 69–74.

Barbee, J.G., Clark, D.C., Crapanzano, M.S., Heintz, G.C. and Kehoe, C.E. (1989) Alcohol and substance abuse among schizophrenic patients presenting to an emergency psychiatric service. *Journal of Nervous and Mental Disease*, **177**, 400–407.

Bartels, S.J., Drake, R.E. and Wallach, M.A. (1995) Long term course of substance use disorders among patients with severe mental illness. *Psychiatric Services*, **46**: 248–251.

Bleuler, E. (1911) *Dementia praecox oder Gruppe der Schizophrenien*. Leipzig, Franz Deuticke.

Boutros, N., Bonnet, K. and Mak, T. (1996) Drug abuse: a significant variable in schizophrenia research. *Biological Psychiatry*, **39**: 1053–1054.

Bowers, M.B., Mazure, C.M., Nelson, J.C. and Jatlow, P.I. (1990) Psychotogenic drug use and neuroleptic response. *Schizophrenia Bulletin*, **16**: 81–85.

Caspari, D. (1999) Cannabis and schizophrenia: results of a follow-up study. *European Archives of Psychiatry and Clinical Neuroscience*, **249**: 45–49.

Castle, D.J. and Ames, F.R. (1996) Cannabis and the brain. *Australian and New Zealand Journal of Psychiatry*, **30**: 179–183.

Cleghorn, J.M., Kaplan, R.D., Sczechtman, B., Sczechtman, H., Brown, G.M. and Franco, S. (1991) Substance abuse and schizophrenia: effect on symptoms but not on neurocognitive function. *Journal of Clinical Psychiatry*, **52**: 26–30.

Dixon, L. (1999) Dual diagnosis of substance abuse in schizophrenia: prevalence and impact on outcomes. *Schizophrenia Research*, **35**: S93–S100.

Dixon, L., Haas, G., Weiden, P.J., Sweeney, J. and Frances, A.J. (1991) Drug abuse in schizophrenic patients: clinical correlates and reasons for use. *American Journal of Psychiatry*, **148**: 224–230.

Docherty, J.P., van Kammen, D.P., Siris, S.G. and Marder, S.R. (1978) Stages of onset of schizophrenic psychosis. *American Journal of Psychiatry*, **135**: 420–426.

Done, J., Crow, T., Johnstone, E.C. and Sacker, A. (1994) Childhood antecedents of schizophrenia and affective illness: social adjustment at ages 7 and 11. *Lancet*, **309**: 699–703.

Duke, P., Pantelis, C. and Barnes, T. (1994) South Westminster schizophrenia survey: alcohol use and its relationship to symptoms tardive dyskinesia and illness onset. *British Journal of Psychiatry*, **164**: 630–636.

Eikmeier, G., Lodemann, E., Pieper, L. and Gastpar, M. (1991) Cannabis use and the course of schizophrenia. *Sucht*, **37**: 377–382.

Gardner, E.L. and Lowinson, J.H. (1991) Marijuana's interaction with brain reward systems: update 1991. *Pharmacology and Biochemistry of Behavior*, **40**, 571–580.

Häfner, H., Riecher-Rössler, A., Maurer, K., Fätkenheuer, B. and Löffler, W. (1992) First onset and early symptomatology of schizophrenia. A chapter of epidemiological and neurobiological research into age and sex differences. *European Archives of Psychiatry and Clinical Neuroscience*, **242**: 109–118.

Häfner, H., Maurer, K., Löffler, W. and Riecher-Rössler, A. (1993) The influence of age and sex on the onset and early course of schizophrenia. *British Journal of Psychiatry*, **162**: 80–86.

Häfner, H., Riecher-Rössler, A., Hambrecht, M., Maurer, K., Meissner, S., Schmidtke, A., Fätkenheuer, B., Löffler, W. and an der Heiden, W. (1992) IRAOS: an instrument for the retrospective assessment of the onset of schizophrenia. *Schizophrenia Research*, **6**: 209–223.

Hambrecht, M. and Häfner, H. (1996) Substance abuse and the onset of schizophrenia. *Biological Psychiatry*, **40**: 1155–1163.

Hambrecht, M. and Häfner, H. (2000) Cannabis, vulnerability, and the onset of schizophrenia—an epidemiological perspective. *Australian and New Zealand Journal of Psychiatry*, **34**: 468–475.

Hambrecht, M., Häfner, H. and Löffler, W. (1994) Beginning schizophrenia observed by significant others. *Social Psychiatry and Psychiatric Epidemiology*, **29**: 53–60.

Hamera, E., Schneider, J.K. and Deviney, S. (1995) Alcohol, cannabis, nicotine, and caffeine use and symptom distress in schizophrenia. *Journal of Nervous and Mental Disease*, **183**: 559–565.

Hurlbut, K.M. (1991) Drug induced psychosis. *Emergency Medicine Clinics of North America*, **9**: 31–52.

Jones, P. (1997) The early origins of schizophrenia. *British Medical Bulletin*, **53**: 135–155.

Kovasznay, B., Bromet, E., Schwartz, J.E., Ram, R., Lavelle, J. and Brandon, L. (1993) Substance abuse and onset of psychotic illness. *Hospital and Community Psychiatry*, **44**: 567–571.

Lambert, M., Haasen, C., Maß, R. and Krausz, M. (1997) Konsummuster und Konsummotivation des Suchtmittelgebrauchs bei schizophrenen Patienten. *Psychiatrische Praxis*, **24**: 185–189.

Lieberman, J.A., Kinon, B.J. and Loebel, A.C. (1990) Dopaminergic mechanisms in idiopathic and drug-induced psychoses. *Schizophrenia Bulletin*, **16**: 97–110.

Linszen, D.H., Dingemans, P.M. and Lenior, M.E. (1994) Cannabis abuse and the course of recent-onset schizophrenic disorders. *Archives of General Psychiatry*, **51**: 273–279.

Lundquist, T. (1995) *Cognitive Dysfunctions in Chronic Cannabis Users*. Stockholm, Almquist & Wiksell International.

McGuire, P.K., Jones, P., Harvey, I., Williams, M., McGuffin, P. and Murray, R.M. (1995) Morbid risk of schizophrenia for relatives of patients with cannabis-associated psychosis. *Schizophrenia Research*, **15**: 277–281.

Mueser, K.T., Yarnold, P.R., Levinson, D.F., Singh, H., Bellack, A.S., Kee, K., Morrison, R.L. and Yadalam, K.G. (1990) Prevalence of substance abuse in schizophrenia: demographic and clinical correlates. *Schizophrenia Bulletin*, **16**: 31–56.

Mueser, K.T., Yarnold, P.R. and Bellack, A.S. (1992) Diagnostic and demographic correlates of substance abuse in schizophrenia and major affective disorder. *Acta Psychiatrica Scandinavica*, **85**: 48–55.

Mueser, K.T., Drake, R.E. and Wallach, M.A. (1998) Dual diagnosis: a review of etiological theories. *Addictive Behaviors*, **23**: 717–734.

Mueser, K.T., Rosenberg, S.D., Drake, R.E., Miles, K.M., Wolford, G., Vidaver, R. and Carrieri, K. (1999) Conduct disorder, antisocial personality disorder and substance use disorders in schizophrenia and major affective disorders. *Journal of Studies of Alcohol*, **60**: 278–284.

Mueser, K.T., Nishith, P., Tracy, J.I., DeGirolamo, J. and Molinaro, M. (1995) Expectations and motives for substance use in schizophrenia. *Schizophrenia Bulletin*, **21**: 367–378.

Noordsy, D.L., Drake, R.E., Teague, G.B., Osher, F., Hurlbut, S.C., Beaudett, M.S. and Paskus, T.S. (1991) Subjective experiences related to alcohol use among schizophrenics. *Journal of Nervous and Mental Diseases*, **179**: 410–414.

Nuechterlein, K. (1987) Vulnerability models for schizophrenia: state of the art. In H. Häfner, W, Janzarik (Eds), *Search for the Causes of Schizophrenia*, pp. 297–316. Berlin, Springer.

Olin, S.S., Mednick, S.A., Cannon, T., Jacobsen, B., Parnas, J., Schulsinger, F. and Schulsinger, H. (1998) School teacher ratings predictive of psychiatric outcome 25 years later. *British Journal of Psychiatry*, **172**: (Suppl 33): 7–13.

Pristach, C.A. and Smith, C.M. (1996) Self-reported effects of alcohol use on symptoms of schizophrenia. *Psychiatric Services*, **47**: 421–423.

Pulver, A.E., Wolyniec, P.S., Wagner, M.G., Moorman, C.C. and McGrath, J.A. (1989) An epidemiologic investigation of alcohol-dependent schizophrenics. *Acta Psychiatrica Scandinavica*, **79**: 603–612.

Rabinowitz, J., Bromet, E.J., Lavelle, J., Carlson, G., Kovasznay, B. and Schwartz, J.E. (1998) Prevalence and severity of substance use disorders and onset of psychosis in first admission psychotic patients. *Psychological Medicine*, **28**: 1411–1419.

Rosenthal, R.N. (1998) Is schizophrenia addiction prone? *Current Opinion in Psychiatry*, **11**: 45–48.

Schneier, F.R. and Siris, S.G. (1987) A review of psychoactive substance use and abuse in schizophrenia. Patterns of drug choice. *Journal of Nervous and Mental Disease*, **175**: 641–652.

Schuckit, M.A. (1994) The relationship between alcohol problems, substance abuse, and psychiatric syndromes. In American Psychiatric Association Task Force on DSM-IV (Eds.), *DSM-IV Sourcebook*, pp. 45–66. Washington, DC, APA.

Sevy, S., Kay, S.R., Opler, L.A. and van Praag, H.M. (1990) Significance of cocaine history in schizophrenia. *Journal of Nervous and Mental Disease*, **178**: 642–648.

Shaner, A., Khalsea, M.E., Roberts, L., Wilkins, J., Anglin, D. and Hsieh, S.C. (1993) Unrecognized cocaine use among schizophrenic patients. *American Journal Psychiatry*, **150**: 758–762.

Silver, H. and Abboud, E. (1994) Drug abuse in schizophrenia: comparison of patients who began drug abuse before their first admission with those who began abusing drugs after their first admission. *Schizophrenia Research*, **13**: 57–63.

Sokolski, K.N., Cummings, J.L., Abrams, B.I., DeMet, E.M., Katz, L.S. and Costa, J.F. (1994) Effects of substance abuse on hallucination rates and treatment responses in chronic psychiatric patients. *Journal of Clinical Psychiatry*, **55**: 380–387.

Soyka, M., Albus, M., Kathmann, N., Finelli, A., Hofstetter, S., Holzbach, R., Immler, B. and Sand, P. (1993) Prevalence of alcohol and drug abuse in schizophrenic inpatients. *European Archives of Psychiatry and Clinical Neuroscience*, **242**: 362–372.

Swofford, C.D., Kasckow, J.W., Scheller-Gilkey, G. and Inderbitzin, L.B. (1996) Substance use: a powerful predictor of relapse in schizophrenia. *Schizophrenia Research*, **20**: 145–151.

Taylor, D. and Warner, R. (1994) Does substance use precipitate the onset of functional psychosis? *Social Work and Social Reviews*, **5**: 64–75.

Test, M.A., Wallach, L., Allness, D.J. and Ripp, K. (1989) Substance use in young adults with schizophrenic disorders. *Schizophrenia Bulletin*, **15**: 465–476.

Thornicroft, G. (1990) Cannabis and psychosis. Is there epidemiological evidence for an association? *British Journal of Psychiatry*, **157**: 25–33.

Tien, A.Y. and Anthony, J.C. (1990) Epidemiological analysis of alcohol and drug use as risk factors for psychotic experiences. *Journal of Nervous and Mental Disease*, **178**: 473–480.

Tien, A.Y. and Eaton, W.W. (1992) Psychopathologic precursors and sociodemographic risk factors for the schizophrenia syndrome. *Archives of General Psychiatry*, **49**: 37–46.

Van Ammers, E.C., Sellman, J.D. and Mulder, R.T. (1997) Temperament and substance abuse in schizophrenia: Is there a relationship? *Journal of Nervous and Mental Disease*, **185**: 283–288.

Warner, R., Taylor, D., Wright, J., Sloat, A., Springett, G., Arnold, S. and Weinberg, H. (1994) Substance use among the mentally ill: prevalence, reasons for use, and effects on illness. *American Journal of Orthopsychiatry*, **63**: 30–39.

Zisook, S., Heaton, R., Mornaville, J., Kuck, J., Jernigan, T. and Braff, D. (1992) Past substance abuse and clinical course of schizophrenia. *American Journal of Psychiatry*, **149**: 552–553.

Zubin, J. and Spring, B. (1977) Vulnerability—a new view of schizophrenia. *Journal of Abnormal Psychology*, **86**: 103–126.

Chapter 3

SUBSTANCE MISUSE AND PSYCHOSIS IN CONTEXT: THE INFLUENCES OF FAMILIES AND SOCIAL NETWORKS

Alex Copello

Traditionally, with a few exceptions, the majority of theories and resulting interventions within the areas of substance misuse and mental health have focused on the individual rather than the social context. On the whole, the focus has been on variables or characteristics within the individual that are seen as affecting the development and course of addiction and/or mental health problems. This chapter stands in contrast with this trend by taking a wider perspective that incorporates the important role that families and social networks can play in the course and maintenance of both substance misuse and mental health problems.

Historically, there have been a number of attempts at understanding the role of families in both substance misuse and psychosis. The latter two areas have mostly developed in parallel with few attempts at integration (for an exception, see Orford, 1987: "Coping with Disorder in the Family"). Given that the fields of substance use and severe mental health had shown little in the way of integration until comparatively recently, it is not surprising that the work on families and social networks in both areas developed on the whole as two separate enterprises.

This chapter will start by discussing some of the ideas and research findings in both the substance use and psychosis areas separately and move towards an attempt to integrate what we know into a coherent view of the role and

Substance Misuse in Psychosis: Approaches to Treatment and Service Delivery.
Edited by Hermine L. Graham, Alex Copello, Max J. Birchwood and Kim T. Mueser.
© 2003 John Wiley & Sons, Ltd.

potential influence of the social environment in those people experiencing combined substance misuse and psychosis (SMP).

In order to explore the social environment, the chapter will first focus on the most immediate social unit, the family, and then move on to consider wider social networks. Finally, implications for intervention strategies will be briefly considered.

THE ROLE OF FAMILIES IN SUBSTANCE MISUSE

Some of the early theories of families and addiction focused on spouses of people with drinking problems. These theories tended to be concerned with two questions: why did partners marry problem drinkers? and why did partners stay in these marriages in the face of continuing problems? (for a fuller discussion, see Hurcom et al, 2000; Copello, 2001). Much of the focus was then on the presumed pathology of the partners without the drinking problem—e.g., the spouses' disturbed personality hypothesis (Whalen, 1953)—and the decompensation hypothesis (Futterman, 1953) that postulated that wives would develop significant psychological problems if the husbands stopped drinking. In the absence of any supporting evidence, some of these ideas remained speculative, and in time different models emerged. In relation to drug problems other than alcohol, early models tended to focus on the deficits of family members, mainly parents. These deficits were seen as giving rise to "addiction" within the family setting. Early theories were therefore mostly preoccupied with the causal role that families or particular family members played in relation to addiction.

Later theories focused on stress and coping (Moos et al, 1990; Orford, 1998). According to the stress-coping paradigm, alcohol and drug problems were seen as resulting in stress for the whole family with family members other than the user of alcohol and/or drugs trying to respond by a variety of coping behaviours. As defined in general psychology, coping behaviours include cognitive and behavioural responses used by those who perceive that the environment poses demands that exceed individual resources (Lazarus and Folkman, 1980).

One of the strengths of the stress-coping paradigm, as applied to addiction and the family, is that it draws on general principles of psychology and can accommodate the experiences of the wide range of families experiencing addiction problems, which are also varied in nature. In contrast to some of the other approaches, the stress-coping model is not concerned with the cause of the addiction problem. Addiction problems are seen to occur for a range of reasons that may include both environmental and individual factors.

GENERAL WAYS OF COPING

SPECIFIC WAYS OF COPING
WITH EXAMPLES

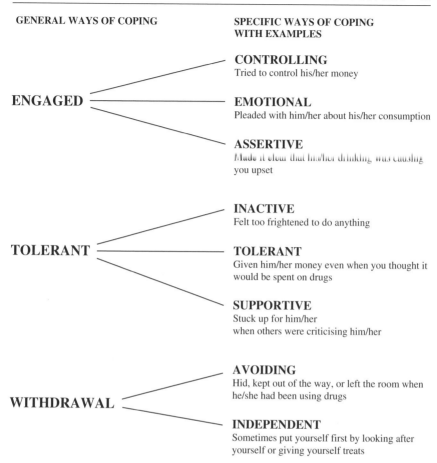

CONTROLLING
Tried to control his/her money

ENGAGED

EMOTIONAL
Pleaded with him/her about his/her consumption

ASSERTIVE
Made it clear that him/her drinking was causing
you upset

INACTIVE
Felt too frightened to do anything

TOLERANT

TOLERANT
Given him/her money even when you thought it
would be spent on drugs

SUPPORTIVE
Stuck up for him/her
when others were criticising him/her

AVOIDING
Hid, kept out of the way, or left the room when
he/she had been using drugs

WITHDRAWAL

INDEPENDENT
Sometimes put yourself first by looking after
yourself or giving yourself treats

Figure 3.1   Three general and eight specific ways of coping (Adapted from Orford, 1998 by permission of Longmans)

In brief, the stress-coping model suggests that when addiction problems occur in the family setting, those family members other than the user experience stress that can be severe and long-lasting. Stress includes experiences such as finding the user difficult to live with, concern about the user's whereabouts and health, financial difficulties, and arguments and conflict with the user but also with other family members (Orford et al, 1998a). Faced with these stressors, family members try a range of coping responses. Work based on the stress-coping model has led to the development of a coping typology (Orford et al, 1998b), as illustrated in Figure 3.1. The figure shows three broad ways of responding when faced with alcohol and drug problems: tolerating substance misuse, engaging in trying to change the problem, or withdrawing from the user. Figure 3.1 also shows eight more specific ways of coping that have been identified. These ways of coping show similarities to general ways of coping with stress, but they have been developed through careful study of families facing and responding to alcohol and drug problems and are therefore specific to addiction.

Research using this typology has focused on the interactions between family members and the substance user, and has also led to the development of intervention strategies (e.g., Copello et al, 2000a; b). Coping responses are seen as consisting of behaviours, thoughts, and attitudes, and as being associated with advantages and disadvantages depending on family circumstances. Figure 3.2 illustrates examples of common thoughts and emotions as well as the advantages and disadvantages associated with the three broad types of coping.

In essence, the stress-coping model is a transactional one; that is, the interactions between the substance misuser and the family member at a particular point in time are affected by previous interactions and in turn influence future interactions. The family is therefore seen as an interacting group attempting to adapt and respond to highly stressful circumstances. The responses in turn are believed to influence the course of addiction.

THE ROLE OF FAMILIES IN PSYCHOSIS

When reviewing the literature on families and schizophrenia, one is struck by the similarity between early ideas in the schizophrenia literature and those in the addiction literature, and the parallels that can be drawn between the two areas in the way in which different models developed over time. Perhaps this is not surprising given that most theories of alcohol, drugs and the family have originated in the mental health field (Orford, 1998; Orford et al, 2001).

Early theories of schizophrenia and the family focused on the potential role of the family environment in the aetiology of schizophrenia. As Barrowclough and Tarrier (1992) describe:

> A number of workers identified the family as an important cause of the illness. Such writers as Bateson, Lidz, Wynne and Laing described various patterns of family structure, interactions and communications, which they proposed were responsible for causing schizophrenia (Hirsch and Leff 1975). Some writers such as Laing suggested that schizophrenia was a family illness. (p. 17)

Barrowclough and Tarrier continue:

> Although these ideas were influential, there was little if any evidence to substantiate them: most of the speculations resulted from a few clinical observations rather than rigorous scientific investigation. (p. 17)

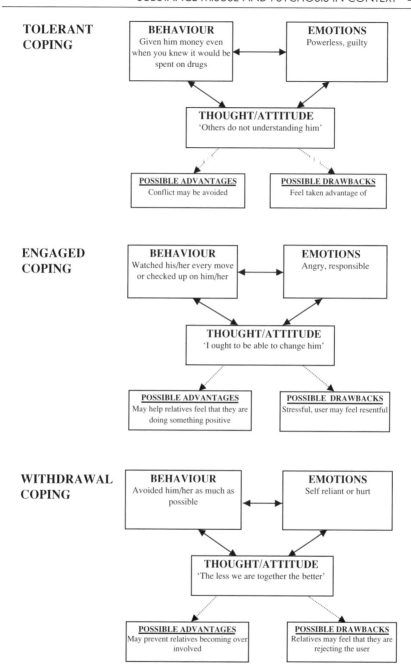

Figure 3.2   Examples of behaviours, emotions and thoughts associated with three coping positions (adapted from Copello et al, 2000 by permission of *Journal of Mental Health*)

The parallels between the two areas during the early stages of theory development are so strong that in fact, with minor alterations (changing the names of the authors quoted and substituting schizophrenia), the two paragraphs just quoted could also be used to describe early theories of addiction and the family.

The development of ideas in substance misuse and schizophrenia followed a similar trend. The focus moved away from seeking a cause for schizophrenia within the family to study factors that may contribute to the maintenance of the problem. Since the late 1950s, the finding that people with schizophrenia who returned to live with the family following treatment tended to show higher relapse rates than those who did not (Brown et al, 1958) gave impetus to research into the area of "expressed emotion" (EE) in schizophrenia (Birchwood and Jackson, 2001). These findings led to the hypothesis that "emotional overinvolvement" is the key factor increasing risk within family environments. Brown et al (1962) operationalized this in terms of the positive and negative emotion and hostility rated during the course of a factual interview about the patient (Birchwood and Jackson, 2001). The finding that patients returning to families with relatives rated "high in EE" showed higher rates of relapse was replicated by Vaughan and Leff (1976). EE has been refined and developed to include aspects of interpersonal behaviour measuring criticism, hostility, warmth, positive comments and overinvolvement (Wearnden et al, 2000). EE has been researched extensively since the initial findings. A meta-analysis carried out by Bebbington and Kuipers (1994) looked at data from 1346 patients and established that the relapse rate in high-EE families was 50%, while in low-EE families it was 21%. Despite criticisms about the lack of theoretical basis for the EE concept, these findings are very robust and suggest that the family environment can significantly influence the short-term course of schizophrenia.

Two important themes related to EE and discussed by Birchwood and Jackson (2001) include coping difficulties and attributions, and they are described below. These are of particular importance when considering families facing coexisting psychosis and substance misuse, as will be discussed later.

Based on results from a number of studies, Birchwood and Jackson suggest that difficulty in coping may be prominent in high-EE relatives. Coping difficulty may arise as a result of greater burden, the presence of more behavioural problems to cope with, having less options available for coping, and being more isolated and hence having less social support. This has important implications for the development of intervention strategies.

The second theme is that of attribution. Attribution here refers to the belief that relatives hold about the cause of the symptoms of their offspring/spouse. Those relatives that view symptoms as within the control of the individual tend to show more critical comments (high EE), as opposed to those relatives who perceive the symptoms as part of the illness and not within the individual's control (Weisman et al, 1998). Using content analysis based on interviews with 40 family members of people with schizophrenia, Weisman and colleagues showed that symptoms related to behavioural deficits (e.g., poor hygiene) were criticized more often that symptoms reflecting behavioural excesses (e.g., hallucinations). In line with an "attribution-affect" model, this was interpreted as evidence that behaviours seen as intentional are target of criticism more commonly than those seen as core symptoms of mental illness.

Finally, it is important to note the position put forward by some authors (e.g., Birchwood and Smith, 1987) that EE should be viewed as a result of interactions between carer and patient over time, as opposed to a set of enduring characteristics of relatives that cause relapse. This focus on the interaction between the person with schizophrenia and the relative (Birchwood and Cochrane, 1990) finds commonality with the stress-coping model described for addiction, which is essentially a model of interaction over time between the persons using substances and members of their families. In the case of EE, the key dimension is one of emotional involvement and criticism that at high levels can increase the risk or psychotic relapse.

Work using the stress-coping paradigm to understand addiction and the family and the work on EE in schizophrenia provide a good platform from which to attempt to understand the process that can arise when substance misuse and psychosis co-occur in the family setting. This will be discussed after considering the role of wider social networks.

SUBSTANCE MISUSE AND THE WIDER SOCIAL ENVIRONMENT

Widening the focus, it is worth extending the social environment to consider the role of other members of the user's social network. A finding from longitudinal studies of young people and drug use is that peer influence is important in determining both onset and course of alcohol, marihuana and tobacco use (e.g., Duncan et al, 1995), the first two being the most common substances used by those with psychosis (Graham et al, 2001). Furthermore, the influence of the substance misuser's environment has been evident in research that has led to models of relapse to substances (e.g., Marlatt and Gordon, 1985) where interpersonal conflict and social pressure are two of the three main precursors to relapse.

More recently, further impetus to the important role that social networks can play in relation to addiction problems has emerged following the findings from Project MATCH (Matching Alcohol Treatment to Client Heterogeneity), the largest randomized trial of treatments for alcohol problems ever conducted (Project MATCH, 1998). The study involved comparing three treatments for alcohol problems, namely, motivational enhancement therapy, cognitive behaviour therapy, and 12-step facilitation therapy, in a randomized design with 1726 patients attending a range of services for alcohol problems. The main aim of the study was to explore treatment matching—the idea that, according to certain characteristics, some people with alcohol problems would fare better with certain types of treatments (for example, people with religious beliefs would do better in treatments, such as 12-step facilitation therapy, that involve a spiritual dimension). The overall results of Project MATCH were disappointing in terms of supporting this type of matching hypotheses. Few matching effects were evident from the results (Project MATCH, 1998). One of the strongest matching effects found, however, involved social networks and the role of these networks in supporting drinking behaviour. The findings suggested that people who had social networks supportive of drinking behaviour prior to treatment did less well overall whatever treatment they received. Furthermore, people who started treatment with social networks supportive of drinking but, during and after treatment, changed the composition of these networks to include people who were supportive of abstinence from alcohol had better outcomes. The changes in the networks were more evident in one of the treatments, namely, 12-step facilitation therapy, and resulted from continued involvement in self-help groups following the treatment episode. Self-help groups provide a network supportive of abstinence.

The above evidence points to a consistent picture supporting the notion that the social context of people who misuse substances is central to the maintenance and resolution of the substance-related problem. There appear to be two important ways in which social networks influence substance misuse. First, in terms of peer influence, modelling and introduction to substances, and, second, in terms of maintenance; that is, once substance use takes place, the social network can either support and encourage continued use or support efforts to change the substance-using behaviour. There is some evidence, including that from Project MATCH, that the network response to the substance misuse can influence treatment outcome. More specifically, changes in network composition that involve reductions in the number of those supporting substance misuse and an increase of those supportive of change are associated with better substance-related outcomes.

THE WIDER SOCIAL ENVIRONMENT OF PEOPLE WITH SUBSTANCE MISUSE AND PSYCHOSIS (SMP)

There are studies, albeit a small number, that help to develop a picture of the networks of those experiencing SMP, and these have been reviewed by Drake et al (1998). The first interesting finding is that those with schizophrenia who also use substances tend to be more socially competent and active when compared to those who do not. This evidence comes from a small number of comparative studies reviewed by Drake et al (1998). The second finding of interest is that early on, when substance use starts to develop, people with SMP tend to experience a deterioration or loss of familial relationships (e.g., Test et al, 1989). The third finding relates to the fact that, away from the family, a large number of people with SMP have contact with a substance-misusing network of peers that provide both social contacts and social reinforcement. The networks include both other people with SMP and substance misusers without psychosis. A significant amount of the interaction within the network centres on the use of substances. The network appears to be important in terms of providing support and friendship, and one of the difficult issues faced by those with SMP is that giving up substance misuse involves also giving up the network and hence an important source of social contact.

When considered together, the findings in these three areas support the view that the wider social environment of those with SMP is an important arena within which the use of substances and other substance-related social interactions (e.g., provision of drugs) act to support and maintain problematic substance use. A further important development, though, is that when substance misuse becomes severe, the social networks may collapse, leaving individuals vulnerable to further deterioration (Drake et al, 1998).

TOWARDS AN INTEGRATION

Overall, the material presented so far supports the idea that the social environment is inextricably linked to SMP. It seems clear that SMP poses a significant number of challenges given that the two sets of problems can interact in a number of complex ways. The impact on families and wider networks is therefore influenced not only by the substance misuse and the psychosis independently but also by the complex interaction of the two sets of problems (e.g., substance misuse increasing the risk of psychotic relapse, and the use of substances to control the symptoms of psychosis). In turn, the social environment exerts a powerful influence on the use of substances in people with SMP. Having discussed the different strands of work, this section will attempt to integrate the findings and discuss how they may apply to those with SMP.

In focusing on the more immediate environment, the family, it seems clear that the combined presence of substance misuse and psychosis creates the potential to expose families to a wider range of stressors than either problem alone. It is also clear that the interactions between family members and those with SMP are important. The potential for conflict, however, is high.

When trying to respond, families are faced with difficult dilemmas. In view of the findings from both the literature on family coping with addiction and that related to EE in schizophrenia, the following tentative conclusions can be put forward. High levels of emotional expression and criticism increase the risk of psychotic relapse, and there is some evidence, although so far limited to one study, to suggest that this is also the case in relation to relapse to alcohol use (O'Farrell et al, 1998). Furthermore, interpersonal conflict can lead to relapse to substance misuse (Marlatt, 1985). Supportive family responses, however, may be helpful, although they may risk being perceived as tolerant if the substance misuse is not discussed. We know from the addiction literature that tolerant-inaction responses are bad for relatives' health and tend to be seen as unhelpful, as they are perceived as condoning substance use (Orford et al, 2001). Families have the option to withdraw, but this strategy may lead to disengagement and the person with SMP moving away from the family and gravitating towards substance-using networks (Drake et al, 1998). Each one of these options may be seen as having advantages and disadvantages that are influenced by the particular family circumstances of each case. It is also worth considering the evidence discussed by Birchwood and Jackson (2001) that families experiencing difficulty in coping may be predisposed to high EE. This suggests that an important task for those working with families facing SMP is to explore the coping responses of family members, discussing those behaviours that are already being used and attempting to enlarge the repertoire of coping behaviours by increasing awareness of those not used, and, if necessary, developing specific coping skills. This work needs to be guided by the fact that the resulting family environment can play a key role in the maintenance of both the substance misuse and the psychosis.

However, a range of factors can influence the ability of family members to adopt constructive coping responses. Orford (1987), in his analysis of coping with a range of disorders in the family setting, discusses the influence of interpretation of behaviour as important in determining coping responses. This is akin to the issue of attribution and its influence on EE. In relation to attributions, it is of interest to consider the additive influence of substance misuse on the attributions made by family members about those with psychosis. One could predict that SMP can influence attributions in two ways.

First, it is possible that family members perceive the psychosis to result from the use of substances and hence be within the person's control. A second possible scenario can occur in which the family member perceives the psychosis to be outside the person's control and yet perceives the substance use to be volitional and hence an appropriate focus for criticism. Both scenarios may predispose family members to high EE. In the context of addiction in the family, the issue of blame is usually present, and there is no reason to expect this to be different in families facing SMP. Blame in turn can also increase the tendency to be critical within the family setting.

Other beliefs may also be important determinants of coping behaviour. A study by Hurcom et al (1999), using multiple regression analyses to explore the predictors of coping in female partners of problem drinkers, found that "engaged" coping responses were best predicted by a single cognitive variable (self-demands). "Tolerant" coping, in contrast, was best predicted by a combination of the partner's beliefs about her ability to withdraw from the drinker and the degree of drink-related hardship experienced within the family unit. Finally, beliefs about the need to withdraw and the length of time that partners had been coping with excessive drinking were the two best predictors of "withdrawal" coping. Hence, to give an example, tolerant-type responses may be influenced by the belief that "If I take a firm stance in response to his alcohol use, he may leave me and I will not survive on my own."

The importance of the social environment beyond the immediate family is becoming increasingly clear from the evidence emerging from substance misuse, psychosis, and the more limited number of studies focused on those with SMP. People with SMP may, by virtue of their increased social competence compared to those with psychosis who do not use substances (Drake et al, 1998), have access to mixed networks (i.e., networks including also others who misuse substances but do not have psychosis), and hence some of the findings from the general addiction literature are of relevance. Social networks are therefore influential in terms of introducing people to substances and modelling substance-using behaviour (Ginsberg and Greenley, 1978; Duncan et al, 1995). Once substance misuse occurs, network support for continued use of substances can contribute to maintenance of the problem (Project MATCH, 1998). A particular problem for those with SMP is that even though the social networks that support continued use of substances are problematic, they may at the same time constitute the main source of social support and friendship, and therefore it may be difficult to cease contact (Drake et al, 1998) or replace them with non-substance-using networks. Whether this is different for people with SMP when compared to people without psychosis remains speculative. A study by Leonard et al (2000), for example, found that the social networks of heavy drinkers differed from those of infrequent drinkers in that drinking buddies accounted for most of the network. Heavy drinkers, however, appeared to experience a similar level of emotional, financial and practical support from their peer network. One potential difference, however, is that certain behaviours that may be part of the psychosis and perceived as unusual by others may be less salient within substance-misusing networks, hence providing a strong attachment and a sense of belonging for people with SMP.

The tendency reported by Drake et al (1998) for the relationships between those with SMP and the immediate family to weaken early on in the development of the substance misuse, with an increased move towards substance-using networks, is important and needs to be taken into account in intervention strategies.

A final issue to consider is the role of the wider social networks in terms of providing support for the family as a whole, and, in particular, family members attempting to respond to the problems arising from SMP. Findings from qualitative and quantitative interviews with family members facing alcohol and drug problems suggest that access to social support and more specific support for coping can be hampered by a range of factors. These include disagreements with others (including other family members) about how to cope, lack of knowledge on the part of others, shame surrounding disclosure, and other people encouraging use of substances (Orford et al (1998c). Given societal attitudes towards both substance misuse and psychosis, one could predict that these difficulties will apply at least equally to families facing SMP.

In summary, it can be seen that there is a bidirectional interaction between people with SMP and the multiple levels of their social environment. The results of these interactions have some bearing on the maintenance/resolution of substance misuse and thereby influence the psychosis itself. Supportive environments with lower levels of conflict and high levels of support for change in substance use are associated with improvements, whereas the opposite occurs within environments high in conflict and supportive of continued substance use.

IMPLICATIONS FOR TREATMENT

Given that the social environment is highly influential, interventions geared to help people with SMP need to include this dimension. Ignoring the social context may hamper progress and lead to repeated relapse to both substance misuse and psychosis.

When one considers the attention paid to the social environment within already existing intervention strategies used with either substance misuse or psychosis, it becomes evident that family interventions have been more widely developed than other social network approaches. We know that family interventions for schizophrenia are superior to routine care (Mari and Streiner, 1997). Fadden (1998) discusses the findings from the literature on family interventions, stating that positive results are robust to the point that it is ethically indefensible for services for schizophrenia not to include a family element, although Fadden also notes that there is no evidence that family approaches are offered on a global scale in mental health services, and this is a major cause for concern (Fadden, 1997).

Once again, a similar parallel exists within addiction services. Despite accumulating evidence from recent treatment overviews that alcohol interventions with social components (both family and community dimensions) have been shown to lead to better outcomes than other treatment approaches (Hodgson, 1994; Miller et al, 1995), a paradox is evident in services where the focus remains on individually focused approaches, and families are not, in general, involved in the treatment process. A recent national survey in the USA of 398 randomly chosen addiction services found that only 27% of programmes surveyed provided some form of couple-based treatments, and none used behavioural couples therapy, for which there is strong evidence of effectiveness (Fals-Stewart and Bichler, 2001).

Overall, the literature from the addiction and psychosis fields has consistently shown that inclusion of the family in the treatment process leads to improved outcomes, although there is still some way to go in order to achieve routine implementation.

Social network interventions are still mostly experimental and in need of further rigorous evaluation. Examples include attempts to restructure social support networks for the seriously mentally ill (e.g., Bebout, 1993), network therapy for substance misuse (Galanter, 1999) and social behaviour and network therapy (Copello et al, 2001), the last currently under evaluation in the UK Alcohol Treatment Trial for people with alcohol problems (UKATT Research Team, 2001).

While a number of questions remain unanswered and further research is necessary to test some of the hypotheses that emerge in relation to the interaction between the social environment and people with SMP, the following points could be proposed with relevance to treatment.

The wider social environment needs to be included in the assessment process. Family relationships and available social networks need to be identified and the influence of these on the maintenance of SMP needs to be established (see "Assessment of psychosocial adjustment" in Chapter 10). The social environment of people with SMP can then influence the process in a number of ways, including the potential for early detection of problems, the potential to reduce risk of relapse, the potential to support the maintenance of change, and the potential to create change even when the patient with SMP is not ready to recognize and/or tackle substance misuse or psychosis.

Interventions for clients with SMP can include the family in the following ways:

- Providing information to families on both psychosis and substance misuse. This is important in terms of addressing the area of attributions and hence EE and in order to reduce uncertainty. The information needs to cover both the impact of substances and psychosis and the important interactions between the two problem areas.
- Exploring the coping responses already used by family members and attempting to enlarge the available repertoire of coping behaviours through both discussion and skill development. It is important that this work is conducted in a non-judgemental way and with a positive attitude towards the whole family. The discussion needs to be guided by the principle that family members experience possible responses as dilemmas associated with advantages and drawbacks. A full understanding of these dilemmas is necessary as well as an exploration of attributions and beliefs that may influence coping responses.

The family can also help early in the process. There is accumulating evidence in the substance misuse field that working directly with family members other than the user of substances often results in the latter (who up to that point had been resistant and denying the problem) approaching services for help (Barber and Crisp, 1995; Meyers and Smith, 1995; Miller et al, 1999). There are also a number of approaches under the name of "unilateral family therapy" that influence the family environment by working with those family members available for treatment sessions even if the substance user is not present (Thomas and Ager, 1993). This potential for the family to influence the process can be used positively with people with SMP, either to generate change within the family system or gradually to influence those with SMP in order to facilitate seeking help for substance misuse.

Overall, the approach needs to be a flexible one in which the interactions between members of the family, including the person with SMP, can be influenced in a way that leads to less stressful environments that are supportive of change. Families should have access to services at different stages of the treatment process. Clearly, some of the difficulties associated with confidentiality and the need to obtain permission from the person with SMP in order to involve families and members of the wider social network need to be considered. A clear discussion of the parameters of confidentiality, both at the beginning of treatment and throughout the intervention process, with everyone involved and a positive orientation towards the benefits of working with the social environment can reduce some of the potential problems that may arise. (For a good example of family work with people with SMP, see Chapter 14.)

In relation to the wider social network, the potential exists to restructure the network in a way that maximizes support for change and reduces support for substance misuse. If conducted concurrently, these changes would result in no overall loss to general social support. How to achieve this in practice remains a challenge for treatment interventions, although there is strong evidence to suggest that self-help groups such as Alcoholics Anonymous and Narcotics Anonymous can go some way in fulfilling this function (Drake et al, 1998; Trumbetta et al, 1999). A potential problem is that not everyone with SMP finds it easy to join such groups; hence, other alternatives need to be developed.

Finally, even when the main focus of the approach is cognitive or motivational, the social dimension can be included by, for example, considering thoughts related to the social environment (e.g., "Everyone I know uses substances so it is normal to use them") or exploring the role of important people as motivators for change (e.g., "Our relationship will improve if I stop drinking alcohol").

The impact of SMP on the sufferer and the social cost associated with these problems are high. Addressing SMP in context can help not only people with psychosis who misuse substances but also those people close to them who are concerned and affected by the problems, and are usually eager to help. The results can lead to an overall reduction in the level of personal and social harm.

REFERENCES

Barber, J.G. and Crisp, B.R. (1995) The "pressures to change" approach to working with the partners of heavy drinkers. *Addiction*, **90**: 269–276.

Barrowclough, C. and Tarrier, N. (1992) *Families of Schizophrenic Patients: Cognitive Behavioural Intervention.* London, Chapman and Hall.

Bebbington, P. and Kuipers, L. (1994) The predictive utility of expressed emotion in schizophrenia: an aggregate analysis. *Psychological Medicine*, **24**: 707–718.

Bebout, R.R. (1993) Restructuring the social support networks of seriously mentally ill adults. In M. Harris and H.C. Bergman (Eds), *Case Management for Mentally Ill Patients: Theory and Practice*, pp. 59–82. Harwood.

Birchwood, M. and Jackson, C. (2001) *Schizophrenia.* Sussex, Psychology Press.

Birchwood, M.J. and Smith, J. (1987) Expressed emotion and first episodes of schizophrenia. *British Journal of Psychiatry*, **151**, 859–860.

Birchwood, M. and Cochrane, R. (1990) Families coping with schizophrenia: coping styles, their origins and correlates. *Psychological Medicine*, **20**: 857–865.

Brown, G.W., Carstairs, G.M. and Topping G. (1958) Post hospital adjustment of chronic mental patients. *Lancet*, **ii**: 685–689.

Brown, G.W., Monck, E.M. and Carstairs, A.M. (1962) Influence of family life on the course of schizophrenic illness. *British Journal of Preventative Social Medicine*, **16**: 55–68.

Copello, A. (2002, in press) Is codependency real? In B. Saunders and S. Helfgcott (Eds), *Drug Problems: Understanding the Issues*. Harwood Academic.

Copello, A., Orford, J., Velleman, R., Templeton, L. and Krishnan, M. (2000a) Methods for reducing alcohol and drug related family norm in non-specialist settings. *Journal of Mental Health*, **9**: 319–333.

Copello, A., Templeton, L., Krishnan, M., Orford, J. and Velleman, R. (2000b) A treatment package to improve primary care services for relatives of people with alcohol and drug problems. *Addiction Research*, **8**: 471–484.

Copello, A., Orford, J., Hodgson, R., Tober, G. and Barrett, C. on behalf of the UKATT research team. (2002). Social behaviour and network therapy: key principles and early experiences. *Addictive Behaviors*, **26**, 345–366.

Drake, R.E., Bebout, R.R. and Roach, J.P. (1998) A research evaluation of social network case management for homeless persons with dual disorders. *Social Network Research*, **5**: 83–98.

Duncan, T.E., Tildesley, E., Duncan, S.C. and Hops, H. (1995) The consistency of family and peer influences on the development of substance use in adolescence. *Addiction*, **90**: 1647–1660.

Fadden, G. (1997) Implementation of family interventions in routine clinical practice following staff training programs: a major cause for concern. *Journal of Mental Health*, **6**: 599–612.

Fadden, G. (1998) Research update: psychoeducational family interventions. *Journal of Family Therapy*, **20**: 293–309.

Fals-Stewart, W. and Birchler, G. (2001) A national survey of the use of couples therapy in substance abuse treatment. *Journal of Substance Abuse Treatment*, **20**: 277–283.

Futterman, S. (1953) Personality trends in wives of alcoholics. *Journal of Psychiatric Social Work*, **23**: 37–41.

Galanter, M. (1999) *Network Therapy for Alcohol and Drug Abuse* (2nd edn). New York, Guilford.

Ginsberg, I.J. and Greenley, J.R. (1978) Competing theories of marijuana use: a longitudinal study. *Journal of Health and Social Behaviour*, **19**: 22–34.

Graham, H., Maslin, J., Copello, A., Birchwood, M., Mueser, K., McGovern, D. and Georgiou, G. (2001) Drug and alcohol problems amongst individuals with severe mental health problems in an inner city area of the UK. *Social Psychiatry and Psychiatric Epidemiology*, **36**: 448–455.

Hirsch, S.R. and Leff, J.P. (1975) *Abnormalities in Parents of Schizophrenics*. Maudsley Monography No. 22. London, Oxford University Press.

Hodgson, R. (1994) The treatment of alcohol problems. *Addiction*, **89**: 1529–1534.

Hurcom, C.A., Copello, A., Orford, J. (2000) The family and alcohol: effects of excessive drinking and conceptualisation of spouses over recent decades. *Journal of Substance Use and Misuse*, **35**: 473–502.

Hurcom, C., Copello, A. and Orford, J. (1999) An exploratory study of the predictors of coping and psychological well being in female partners of excessive drinkers. *Behavioural and Cognitive Psychotherapy*, **27**: 311–327.

Lazarus, R. and Folkman, S. (1984) *Stress, Appraisal and Coping*. New York, Springer-Verlag.

Leonard, K.E., Kearns, J. and Mudar, P. (2000) Peer networks among heavy, regular and infrequent drinkers prior to marriage. *Journal of Studies on Alcohol*, **61**: 669–673.

Marlatt, A. and Gordon, J. (1985) *Relapse Prevention: Maintenance Strategies in the Treatment of Addictive Behaviours.* New York, Guilford Press.

Mari, J. and Streiner, D.L. (1997) Family intervention for those with schizophrenia. In C. Adams, J. Anderson, J.J. Mari (Eds), *Schizophrenia Module of the Cochrane Database of Systematic Reviews.* Available in the Cochrane Library. The Cochrane Collaboration, Issue 3, Oxford: Update Software. London, BMJ Publishing Group.

Meyers, R.J., Dominguez, T.P. and Smith, J.E. (1996) Community reinforcement training with concerned others. In V.B. Van Hasselt and R.K. Hersen (Eds), *Sourcebook of Psychological Treatment Manual for Adult Disorders.* New York, Plenum Press.

Miller, W.R., Brown, J.M., Simpson, T.L., Handmaker, N.S., Bien, T.H., Luckie, L.F., Montgomery, H.A., Hester, R.K., Tonigan, J.S. (1995) What works? A methodological analysis of the alcohol treatment outcome literature. In R.K. Hester and W.R. Miller (Eds), *Handbook of Alcoholism Treatment Approaches—Effective Alternatives* (2nd edn). Boston, Allyn and Bacon.

Miller, W.R., Meyers, R.J., Tonigan, J.S. (1999) Engaging the unmotivated in treatment for alcohol problems: a comparison of three strategies for intervention through family members. *Journal of Consulting and Clinical Psychology*, **67**, 688–697.

Moos, R.H., Finney, J.W. and Cronkite, R.C. (1990) *Alcoholism Treatment: Context, Process and Outcome.* New York, Oxford University Press.

O'Farrell, T.J., Hooley, J., Fals-Stewart, W. and Cutter, H.S.G. (1998) Expressed emotion and relapse in alcoholic patients. *Journal of Consulting and Clinical Psychology*, **66**: 744–752.

Orford, J. (1987) *Coping with Disorder in the Family.* London, Croom Helm.

Orford, J. (1994) Empowering family and friends: a new approach to the secondary prevention of addiction. *Drug and Alcohol Review*, **13**: 417–429.

Orford, J. (1998) The coping perspective. In R. Vellman, A. Copello and J. Maslin (Eds), *Living with Drink: Women Who Live with Problem Drinkers.* London, Longman.

Orford, J., Natera, G., Davies, J., Nava, A., Mora, J., Rigby, K., Bradbury, C., Copello, A., and Velleman, R. (1998a) Stresses and strains for family members living with drinking or drug problems in England and Mexico. *Salud Mental (Mexico)*, **21**: 1–13.

Orford, J., Natera, G., Davies, J., Nava, A., Mora, J., Rigby, K., Bradbury, C., Bowie, N., Copello, A., and Velleman, R. (1998b) Tolerate, engage or withdraw: a study of the structure of families coping with alcohol and drug problems in South-West England and Mexico City. *Addiction*, **93**: 1799–1813.

Orford, J., Natera, G., Davies, J., Nava, A., Mora, J., Rigby, K., Bradbury, C., Copello, A., and Velleman, R. (1998c) Social support in coping with alcohol and drug problems at home: findings from Mexican and English families. *Addiction Research*, **6**: 395–420.

Orford, J., Natera, G., Velleman, R., Copello, A., Bowie, N., Bradbury, C., Davies, J., Mora, J., Nava, A., Rigby, K. and Tiburcio, M. (2001) Ways of coping and the health of relatives facing drug and alcohol problems in Mexico and England. *Addiction*, **96**: 761–774.

Project MATCH Research Group (1998) Matching alcoholism treatment to client heterogeneity: Project MATCH three-year drinking outcomes. *Alcoholism: Experimental and Clinical Research*, **22**: 1300–1311.

Test, M.A., Wallish, L., Allness, D. and Ripp, K. (1989) Substance use in young adults with schizophrenic disorders. *Schizophrenia Bulletin*, **15**: 465–476.

Thomas, E.J. and Ager, R.D. (1993) Unilateral family therapy with the spouses of uncooperative alcohol abusers. In T.J. O'Farrell (Ed.), *Marital and Family Therapy in Alcoholism Treatment*, pp. 3–33. New York, Guilford Press.

Trumbetta, S.L., Mueser, K.T., Quimby, E., Bebout, R. and Teague, G.B. (1999) Social networks and clinical outcomes of dually diagnosed homeless persons. *Behavior Therapy*, **30**: 407–430.

UKATT Research Team (2001) United Kingdom Alcohol Treatment Trial: hypotheses, design and methods. *Alcohol and Alcoholism*, **36**: 11–21.

Vaughan, C.E. and Leff, J.P. (1976) The influence of family and social factors on the course of psychiatric illness: a comparison of schizophrenic and depressed neurotic patients. *British Journal of Psychiatry*, **129**: 125–137.

Wearnden, A.J., Tarrier, N. and Barrowclough, C. (2000) A review of expressed emotion research in health care. *Clinical Psychology Review*, **20**: 633–666.

Weisman, A.G., Neuchterlein, K.H., Goldstein, M.J. and Snyder, K.S. (1998) Expressed emotion, attributions, and schizophrenia symptom dimensions. *Journal of Abnormal Psychology*, **2**: 355–359.

Whalen, T. (1953) Wives of alcoholics: four types observed in a family service agency. *Quarterly Journal of Studies on Alcohol*, **39**: 632–641.

Chapter 4

SOCIOLOGICAL ASPECTS OF SUBSTANCE MISUSE AMONG PEOPLE WITH SEVERE MENTAL ILLNESS

Martin J. Commander

INTRODUCTION

Health and illness is a complex topic, the comprehension of which necessitates the deployment of a range of theories and methodologies. To date, research into substance misuse among people with severe mental illness has primarily adopted a positivist agenda and focused on individualistic explanatory models. This chapter deliberately adopts a sociological stance in an attempt to offer a fresh perspective on familiar themes and to reframe issues relating to service provision in this expanding area of clinical practice. Three levels of analysis warrant consideration (Turner, 1995: 4). First, sociology furnishes descriptions of the experience of illness as conveyed by the individual. Secondly, it explores the social construction of disease and the processes by which people are categorized and managed by institutions. Finally, sociology concerns itself with the politics of health and problems of social inequality. A failure to distinguish and subsequently to synthesize findings at each of these levels risks fracturing the fragile knowledge base relating to substance misuse among people with severe mental illness. To paraphrase Mills (1959: 248), is it a personal trouble embedded in the make-up of the individual and forged by intimate past and current circumstances, or is it a public issue traceable to the origins and workings of our institutions and attitudes in society at large? This chapter

Substance Misuse in Psychosis: Approaches to Treatment and Service Delivery.
Edited by Hermine L. Graham, Alex Copello, Max J. Birchwood and Kim T. Mueser.
© 2003 John Wiley & Sons, Ltd.

begins by looking at the biographical nature of illness. There then follows an examination of the sick role and, finally, the medicalization thesis. In conclusion, it is suggested that these themes can be integrated through the pivotal relationship between service user and provider.

INDIVIDUALS AND THE ILLNESS EXPERIENCE

In a seminal sociological work, Bury (1982) conceptualizes the experience of the person with chronic illness as a biographical disruption. While acknowledging the vicissitudes of chronic illness, he establishes a temporal perspective to the illness experience. This includes an onset phase characterized by the emergence of the health problem and its recognition (what is going on here?), a second phase, one of explanation and legitimation (why has this happened to me and why now?), and a final phase, adaptation, concerned with mobilizing assistance and developing suitable responses (what can I do about it?). Kelly and Field (1996) point to the centrality of the concept of self ("a cognitive construct expressed in accounts offered by the individual in self-presentation") and identity ("public and shared aspects of the individual") in this phasic model. They argue that bodies change in chronic illness, and as they do so, the persons, as known to themselves and others, undergo transformation. Both the idea of persons passing through a sequence of illness stages and of their rebuilding a sense of self recur throughout the emergent recovery literature relating to both substance misuse (McIntosh and McKeganey, 2000) and severe mental illness (Young and Ensing, 1999). As in Bury's (1982) biographical framework, the initial step in the recovery pathway is the capacity to acknowledge some awareness of having a problem:

> Until I was able to overcome my own denial regarding my substance abuse, I was not able to seek the help I needed.... The only person who could alter my course was me.... I learned the importance of personal responsibility in maintaining my own good health. (Green, 1996: 12)

This step is inherently threatening, and the presence of both substance misuse and psychosis makes it especially so. As Green (1996) elaborates in her autobiographical account, there is a difficulty in disentangling different problems (in her case, alcoholism, drug addiction and manic depression) while at the same time recognizing that they are interconnected. This is particularly bewildering when both professionals and the significant people in their lives experience similar confusion; is this a result of alcohol or drug abuse, is this bad behaviour, or is this mental illness? Addiction and mental health services often contest their respective roles and have been culpable of shuttling people from one service to another (O'Neill, 1993). Until a clear explanatory framework is achieved, it is impossible for people to proceed effectively to address their problems. An integrated substance misuse and mental illness programme which is able to negotiate a coherent narrative early on in the help-seeking process may accelerate progress and avoid the hindrances which arise when the initial formulation is questioned.

The theme of empowerment is central to the concept of recovery (Fisher, 1994); consistent with this, Green (1996) emphasizes the need for the person to take control. In an ethnographic study of people with substance misuse and psychosis who were homeless, Quimby (1995) found that many complained of being treated like children by service providers. People wanted responsibility for making their own decisions, including any mistakes. Yet there is a clinical dilemma when people are not considered ready or able to take on this responsibility. The competence of a person with substance misuse and severe mental illness to make adult, rational choices is open to challenge:

> They rant and rail about taking control, about not being able to be self-reliant. Yet many eventually realise their lack of self reliance is not fundamentally caused by their case manager or their relationship to treatment structures and cultures. Retrospectively and occasionally during periods of spiralling acts of degeneration there is acknowledgement that help is needed. There is awareness that addiction, coupled with irrational thinking, propelled them into self-destruction. (Quimby, 1995: 287)

The diagnosis of a psychotic disorder is inextricably tied to notions of irrationality (Ingleby, 1982). On the contrary, substance misuse is strongly linked with individual accountability and even culpability. The balance between demands for independence and an acceptance of a degree of assistance must be continually negotiated as people move through the different stages of their illness experience and as various aspects of their condition predominate. An appreciation of a temporal component to interventions has necessarily been incorporated into combined substance misuse and psychosis treatment programmes, ensuring that services are delivered in phase with each person's progress towards recovery (Drake et al, 1997).

Another facet of the recovery process prominent in the literature is that of rebuilding a sense of self. Quimby (1995: 275) confirms the requirement for people with substance misuse and severe mental illness to generate a "definable, defendable, and presentable sense of self". As well as being challenged by their new illness experiences and by comparisons between their former and present selves, people's responses are complicated and undermined by the reactions of those around them. Illness changes the ways in which other people construct the identity of a person. These transformations may be not only significant but, as with mental illness and substance misuse, also highly stigmatizing. The diagnosis of a severe mental illness threatens to bar people from citizenship and to deny them the rights and obligations attached to that status (Anspach, 1979). Identification as a "drug abuser" or "alcoholic" may mark people as weak, sinful or criminal

(Conrad and Schneider, 1982). It is evident why people might reject these spoiling labels and express ambivalence about their involvement with the health-care providers who wield them. Quimby (1995) found that while there was irritation at a deficit of services for people with combined substance misuse and psychosis, this was coupled with resentment at the threat to their identity and the loss of autonomy that was involved when people did make contact with services. People were frustrated at the dependency relationships that developed, with staff monitoring their health, checking their finances, scrutinizing their medication and randomly checking their urine:

> When you're used and abused and battered for a hundred years, it's hard to trust and not think that people are taking advantage of you. When you're not treated with respect and trust, it's taking away from being a person, from being myself. (Quimby, 1995: 284)

Service users have identified a trusting and respectful relationship with mental health professionals as a crucial feature of successful assertive community treatment teams (McGrew et al, 1996). The ability to forge effective alliances is likely to be a critical attribute for staff working with people with combined substance misuse and psychosis and should inform recruitment and training strategies.

INSTITUTIONS AND THE SICK ROLE

Medical practice was first conceptualized as a form of social control by Parsons (1951) in his classic writing on the "sick role". The latter allows people two exemptions; firstly from normal social roles (such as working) and secondly from responsibility for their condition and associated (possibly antisocial) behaviour. In return for these dispensations, the person is required to fulfil two obligations; firstly, to recognize the sick/deviant state as undesirable and to want to recover/change, and, secondly, to co-operate with the relevant institutions to do so. Bury (1982) challenges the relevance of this structural-functionalist paradigm to chronic illness. The responsibilities and allowances attached to the experience of acute short-lived disorders are ambiguous and fluctuating in chronic illness, while the potentially long-term relationship between the clinician and patient is likely to be less determined. Nevertheless, Parson's model (1951) serves to sensitize us to shifts in responsibility for deviance and sickness. Whereas a humanitarian medical model emphasizes the objective causation of deviance and diminishes the role of the individual, the sick role, with its voluntaristic framework, places the issue of responsibility to the fore. Health professionals occupy a key social control function in legitimizing the sick role. In so doing, they take on a therapeutic responsibility to provide or facilitate access to expert assistance and to return persons to their normal roles. "Bad" patients, who lack motivation to change or fail to comply with recommended interventions, compromise the social control role of staff (Kelly and May, 1982). In addition, they may undermine a worker's therapeutic role if there is little that can be done for them clinically or they demand a level of help that they are not perceived to need. "Good" patients, in contrast, fulfil their sick role obligations and allow staff to practise their therapeutic skills.

As revealed in Brown's (1987; 1989; 1990) ethnographic study of the work of a walk-in psychiatric service in the USA, diagnosis is fundamental to accessing the sick role and lies firmly within the orbit of the clinician. A central tenet of modern psychiatric services is the necessity to target limited resources on those people with the most severe conditions, predominantly those identified as having a psychotic disorder. This diagnostic category ostensibly acts as a gatekeeping device for entry to treatment (Brown, 1990). Psychotic disorders come closest to the conventional model of illness in psychiatry. They are, to some extent, amenable to pharmacological and psychotherapeutic interventions and so legitimize the psychiatric team's therapeutic role. The social control function of services is also reinforced by laws allowing these patients (in the interests of their health or safety, or with a view to the protection of other persons) to be forcibly detained in a psychiatric hospital. Substance misuse alone is explicitly exempt from these legal provisions in the UK. Yet, when people have substance misuse in addition to a psychotic disorder, these relatively clear-cut designations become blurred. In particular, unacceptable or dangerous behaviour becomes less easy to condone within a model of irrationality. Indeed, psychiatric staff may make matters worse by offering people access to an illness label that might inadvertently exempt them from normal social rules and responsibility for their behaviour:

> When one deals with characterological problems, delinquency, psychosomatic conditions...the prescription inherent in the term illness breaks down because...there are many whose very illness consists of unwillingness or an inability to assume responsibility...[and] one is in the position of treating people whose very pathology is that they believe themselves to be passive victims of circumstances....The boundaries of the illness conception therefore become extended to a point at which the prescription it implies is often inappropriate. (Linder, 1965: 1088)

In the context of psychiatry's growing preoccupation with risk management (Szmukler, 2001), staff may also fear recriminations regarding their failure to avert future criminal behaviour. Brown (1987) records how competing agencies use diagnosis to promote or defend their own position when responsibilities are poorly circumscribed. He found that psychiatric professionals downplayed symptoms in troublesome or undesirable clients, especially those considered to be milking the system to get prescribed drugs for abuse, to obtain additional help with benefits and accommodation, or to avoid impending court appearances (1989). O'Neill (1993: 128) identifies similar practices and gives the example of this comment attributed to a social worker in a psychiatric emergency room: "He's manipulative and sociopathic. So what if he's hearing voices, he's an addict" (O'Neill, 1993: 128).

Addiction staff too may seek to place people with substance misuse and psychosis outside their traditional therapeutic domain. This is typified by a counsellor in an alcoholism treatment centre: "They're too sick to be here. They don't respond to what helps other people here. Honestly, they scare me, and I think they scare the other clients" (O'Neill, 1993: 128).

Brown (1989) utilizes the notion of "dirty work" designations to examine the process whereby staff devalue certain work tasks. These typically involve areas of activity where the staff's social control role is prominent, but opportunities for therapeutic work are perceived to be limited. One strategy to overcome this reluctance is to commission teams to target designated populations, such as those with combined substance misuse and psychosis, as has been achieved for people who are homeless and have a severe mental illness (Commander et al, 1997). In addition, it may be possible to train staff to be better able to tackle the clinical dilemmas they face and to raise the prestige of working in certain areas. Innovative treatment approaches to combined substance misuse and psychosis may facilitate this (Graham, et al., unpublished). Even so, contentions surrounding the social control role of staff remain with respect to the difficult and fluctuating negotiation of responsibilities between providers and service users. A more egalitarian relationship, in which professional and patient share equally the responsibility for recovery, has gained currency. However, what is portrayed as negotiation often simply involves the deployment of methods to strengthen a patient's adherence to the clinician's recommendations (Taussig, 1980). An opposite example is "motivational interviewing", a technique developed to attract and retain ambivalent patients in addiction treatment programmes (Rollnick and Miller, 1995). This approach has been adapted and applied to improving medication compliance in patients with psychosis (Buchanan, 1998). In so doing, an explicit tolerance of service users' uncertainty about treatment goals has arguably been supplanted by a dominant clinical view that patients should take their medication as prescribed (Perkins and Repper, 1999). Against the background of an increasingly powerful and vocal consumer movement, a more active role may have to be conceded to the patient (Anspach, 1979). While this is not contentious in the addiction field, it may meet resistance in general psychiatry, where the capacity of patients with severe mental illness to take responsibility for their actions is likely to be questioned. As Lerpiniere states (1998: 10), "There is an accepted tension between treating someone as a patient for a mental health problem whilst offering a harm reduction approach for their alcohol and drug use."

This conflict needs to be acknowledged and a reflective approach to differences in philosophy and therapeutic relationships between addiction and mental health services embraced by staff working with people experiencing both substance misuse and psychosis.

SOCIETY AND MEDICALIZATION

Medicalization is the process by which non-medical problems become defined and treated as medical conditions, usually in terms of illnesses or disorders (Conrad and Schneider, 1982). Typically, this arises where other measures have failed or been deemed unacceptable and some form of medical intervention (commonly founded on a biophysiological rationale) is available. Strong (1979) cites alcoholism as an example but notes that, despite the criteria for medicalization seemingly being met, many clinicians are reticent about offering treatment for this condition:

> In a situation where professionals of very low status are presented with vast numbers of patients with whom they can do little, demedicalisation, not imperialism, is the strategy which serves their interest best. (21)

Likewise, psychiatrists have shown considerable reluctance to embrace the UK government's proposals for compulsory powers to incarcerate "dangerous" people with antisocial personality disorders (Szmukler, 2001). Yet, even where the evidence for interventions is limited and opposition is faced from clinicians, medicalization may remain attractive to planners and politicians. When the only alternative is major societal change, such as the redistribution of wealth, medicalization may effectively serve to deflect attention away from the relevance of wider socio-economic factors. As Quimby (1995: 272) saliently points out,

> One of the serious limitations of treatment for dual disorders is its inability to alter social forces (e.g. housing issues, unemployment, community breakdown) that have shattered social relationships and family structures and functioning.

Despite the UK government's commitment to tackle social exclusion (Department of Health, 1998), it is likely that sections of society will continue to be economically and socially marginalized. Pleace (1998: 49) discusses the fact that:

> As economic uncertainty and insecurity increase in the West the liberal assumption that the market will always provide for all has come into question. At the same time the ability to provide either distributional compensation for not being in the market or ... to attempt to generate social cohesion through a range of supports has also been undermined because the costs of doing so are widely perceived as uncompetitive and perhaps ultimately unsustainable.

In order to digest this unpalatable analysis, it becomes expedient to construe some people as less deserving. A fundamental facet underpinning judgements about the assistance to be given to people who are sick or deviant is the attribution of responsibility. If someone is responsible for their predicament, there is generally less inclination to feel compelled to help them. McHugh (1970) proposes that there are two aspects to assessing responsibility; conventionality and theoreticity. Conventionality refers to behaviour where "someone has failed to follow a rule in a situation when the normal grounds for failure (accident or coercion) are absent" (Jeffrey, 1979: 99). Theoreticity refers to the persons' ability to formulate actions in accord with some rule.

People with psychotic disorders involved in conventional rule breaking are usually considered to be pre-theoretic. By virtue of their inherent irrationality, they are excused their behaviour (O'Neill, 1993), and they secure on-going help from health and social care agencies. If people with substance misuse conventionally breaks rules, they are ordinarily held to be responsible, that is, theoretic. Within society, their behaviour has typically been viewed as criminal or sinful rather than a health issue (O'Neill, 1993). The disease model of alcoholism, endorsed by the self-help movement, has been overtly mobilized in efforts to legitimize the claims of people with alcohol abuse to assistance, and to reject stigmatizing beliefs that they are simply weak-willed or antisocial. Conrad and Schneider (1982) present this as part of a pervasive change in Western society during the twentieth century which saw rehabilitation and treatment displace punishment as the favoured response to deviance. However, Lowenberg and Davis (1994: 584) contend that popular lay opinion increasingly "resists the notion that ... dependent personalities, wife beaters, gamblers, child molesters, alcoholics or for that matter workaholics are sick and stand in need of medical treatment", and they suggest that the limits of medicalization have been reached.

The reluctance of both clinicians and the public to offer assistance to people who display antisocial behaviour or abuse alcohol or drugs invites the question of why people with combined psychosis and substance misuse are the focus of so much interest. Where people have both conditions, often with varying intensity over time, attributions regarding responsibility for their behaviour are likely to be uncertain. This doubt is problematic given that people with severe mental illness who misuse substances have higher rates of violence than those who do not (Smith and Huckler, 1984). Whatever the basis for this increased risk, the need to contain or modify such antisocial behaviour has assumed growing importance. The Secretary of State for Health's foreword to the White Paper, *Modernising Mental Health Services* (Department of Health, 1998) pithily summarizes the perceived shortcomings of care in the community in the UK:

While it improved the treatment of many people who were mentally ill, it left far too many walking the streets often at risk to themselves and a nuisance to others. A small but significant minority have been a threat to others or themselves.

The document outlines a range of measures to ensure "safe, sound and supportive" services. These include proposals to allow compulsory treatment in the community and the introduction of assertive outreach teams to track down people who elude psychiatric services, among whom those with combined substance misuse and psychosis are overrepresented. The momentum to drive these measures to enhance the place of coercion and surveillance within mental health services stems from a flawed analysis of dangerousness. Muijen (1996) recalls that 1988 saw the publication not only of *Community Care: An Agenda for Action* but also of *The Report of the Committee of Enquiry into the Care and Aftercare of Miss Sharon Campbell*. The latter gives an account of the circumstances surrounding Sharon Campbell's killing of her psychiatric social worker. Like other subsequent reports concerning similarly tragic incidents, it received a prominent media profile. Although there is no evidence to link the emergence of community care with an escalating risk of serious violence (Taylor and Gunn, 1999), the coverage of these events has inculcated an atmosphere of fear and alienation in the public and undermined confidence in their personal safety. A discourse has been established around risk which, with alarming rapidity, has become deeply ingrained in the language and practice of psychiatry. Despite the acknowledged inability of psychiatrists to predict dangerousness, and in the face of opposition from an unusual alliance of mental health professionals and service users, there is mounting pressure on psychiatry to eliminate the risk of violence from people with mental illness and to embrace other areas of deviancy, such as severe antisocial personality disorder (Szmukler, 2001). The complexities of assessing individuals' competence to make decisions and to accept responsibility for their behaviour have been expediently set aside. Instead, politicians and the public demand that psychiatry safeguard the community from possibly dangerous individuals, if necessary by compulsory detention, regardless of whether or not they have the capacity to decide what is in their best interests, and whether or not they have yet committed a crime (Szmukler and Holloway, 2000). This agenda may ultimately leave service users, particularly those with combined substance misuse and psychosis, and mental health staff in a relationship that neither wants but society demands.

CONCLUDING COMMENTS

Although this chapter has necessarily been highly selective, it is proposed that the linkage between societal discourse and an individual's lived experience of illness can be most fruitfully explored through the sick role (Turner, 1995). The relationship between people with combined substance misuse and psychosis and service providers reverberates through all three levels of this sociological analysis. In his exposition of the sick role, Parsons (1951) relied heavily on psychoanalysis when describing how clinicians establish a trusting relationship with patients in order to use it as a lever for compelling them to cooperate with treatment and to get well. This paternalistic model of the clinician-patient relationship, focusing on re-repressing dependency, is inherently conservative. It is unable to embrace the tension that now exists between what is prescribed and what people want and the shift from "doing to" to "being with". In particular, it fails to accommodate the proliferating market place in health care and is unable to do justice to the increasing heterogeneity of caring relationships arising out of the user movement and informal care initiatives (Fox, 1998).

Bracken and Thomas (2001: 727) argue for a new postpsychiatry in which "crucially . . . the voices of service users and survivors should now be centre stage". There is a strong tradition of self-help within addiction programmes and a growing interest in consumer involvement in service provision in mental health (Fisk et al, 2000). Service users seek to challenge the spoiled identities forced upon them by society and the professionals who participate in the construction of their disability. They look to exchange a dependent clinical relationship for one that focuses on empowerment and personal control. One way of resisting traditional models of caring is to behave otherwise than expected. Notions of people with substance misuse and psychosis as weak or irrational can be undermined by the very action of helping others. The delivery of services by people who have recovered from substance misuse and psychosis may be inherently less stigmatizing. They may be more effective in negotiating issues of responsibility and engaging people in the recovery process. Their presence as role models may also tangibly promote positive self-concepts and generate the hope which is crucial to recovery (Fisk et al, 2000).

Threats to a realignment of the therapeutic relationship and the development of a new partnership between clinicians and service users come from several sources. Although user involvement in restructuring the social support networks of people with substance misuse and psychosis may be as beneficial as the provision of individually focused cognitive therapies (Drake et al, 1993), professionals may yet claim an ascendant expertise that is inaccessible to service users. Incipient opportunities to involve users in offering care to others risk all too quickly eliding into therapeutic relationships based on a negative dependency. It is unclear whether service users can work in existing psychiatric organizations or alongside mental health professionals and still be uniquely effective. Furthermore, it cannot be ignored that medical codes generate meaning in illness and may render patients better able to cope, or indeed that clinicians still occupy a significant place in the lives of patients. As Bury (1982: 179) points out:

> The deep involvement of medicine in reorganising the disruptive experiences of chronic illness, in re-ordering its arbitrary and threatening characteristics inevitably involves issues of social control. That medical sociology should seek to explore this is important but to suggest, as some writers do, that the experience of pain, illness and even death can be faced without recourse to such codes is patently false.

In Western society, social problems are increasingly set within a psychological framework (Rose, 1996). Long before they come into contact with services, this may create an imprint on people's experiences which both mental health staff and service users may find difficult to resist. The presence of severe mental illness will continue to challenge a person's competency and demand the involvement of caring agencies. Moreover, where affected persons pose a threat to others, regardless of their capacity to make decisions for themselves, paternalistic institutions may be expected to intervene in order to safeguard the public. The impact of these countervailing forces (Light, 1997) on the relationship between service users and providers is likely to be especially sharply felt within the field of combined substance misuse and psychosis, and it can be expected to have an enduring impact on the evolution of service models and interventions.

REFERENCES

Anspach, R.R. (1979) From stigma to identity politics: political activism among the physically disabled and former mental patients. *Social Science and Medicine*, **13A**: 765–773.
Bracken, P. and Thomas, P. (2001) Postpsychiatry: a new direction for mental health. *British Medical Journal*, **322**: 724–727.
Brown, P. (1987) Diagnostic conflict and contradiction in psychiatry. *Journal of Health and Social Behaviour*, **28**: 37–50.
Brown, P. (1989) Psychiatric dirty work revisited. Conflicts in servicing nonpsychiatric agencies. *Journal of Contemporary Ethnography*, **18**: 182–201.
Brown, P. (1990) The name game: toward a sociology of diagnosis. *Journal of Mind and Behaviour*, **11**: 385–406.
Buchanan, A. (1998) Treatment compliance in schizophrenia. *Advances in Psychiatric Treatment*, **4**: 227–234.
Bury, M. (1982) Chronic illness as biographical disruption. *Sociology of Health and Illness*, **4**: 167–182.
Commander, M.J., Odell, S. and Sashidharan, S.P. (1997) Birmingham community mental health team for the homeless: one year of referrals. *Psychiatric Bulletin*, **21**: 74–76.
Conrad, P. and Schneider, J.W. (1982) *Deviance and Medicalisation: From Badness to Sickness*. St Louis, CV Mosby.
Department of Health (1998) *Modernising Health and Social Services: National Priorities Guidance. 1999/2000–2001/02*. London, Stationery Office.

Department of Health (1998) *Saving Lives: Our Healthier Nation*. London, Stationery Office.

Drake, R.E., Bebout, R.R. and Roach, J.P. (1993) A research evaluation of social network case management for homeless persons with dual disorders. In M. Harris and H.C. Bergman (Eds.), *Case Management for Mentally Ill Patients—Theory and Practice*. Langhorne, PA, Harwood Academic Publishers.

Drake, R.E., Yovetich, N.A., Bebout, R.R., Harris, M. and McHugo, G.J. (1997) Integrated treatment for dually diagnosed homeless adults. *Journal of Nervous and Mental Disease*, **185**: 298–305.

Fisher, D.B. (1994) Health care reform based on an empowerment model of recovery by people with psychiatric disabilities. *Hospital and Community Psychiatry*, **45**: 913–915.

Fisk, D., Rowe, M., Brooks, R. and Gildersleeve, D. (2000) Integrating consumer staff members into a homeless outreach project: critical issues and strategies. *Psychiatric Rehabilitation Journal*, **23**: 244–252.

Fox, N. (1998) The promise of postmodernism for the sociology of health and medicine. In G. Scambler, and P. Higgs (Eds.), *Modernity, Medicine and Health. Medical Sociology Towards 2000*, pp. 29–45. London, Routledge.

Graham, H.L., Copello, A., Birchwood, M., Orford, J., McGovern, D., Atkinson, E., Maslin, J., Mueser, K., Preece, M., Tobin, D. and Georgiou, G. (unpublished) *Cognitive–Behavioural Integrated Treatment (C-BIT). An Approach for Working with Your Clients Who Have Severe Mental Health Problems and Use Drugs/Alcohol Problematically*. Treatment Manual. Birmingham, Northern Birmingham Mental Health Trust.

Green, V.L. (1996) The resurrection and the life. *American Journal of Orthopsychiatry*, **66**: 12–16.

Ingleby, D. (1982) The social construction of mental illness. In P. Wright and A. Treacher (Eds.), *The Problem of Medical Knowledge: Examining the Social Construction of Medicine*, pp. 123–143. Edinburgh, Edinburgh University Press.

Jeffrey, R. (1979) Normal rubbish: deviant patients in casualty departments. *Sociology of Health and Illness*, **1**: 90–107.

Kelly, M.P. and May, D. (1982) Good and bad patients: a review of the literature and a theoretical critique. *Journal of Advanced Nursing*, **7**: 147–156.

Kelly, M.P. and Field, D. (1996) Medical sociology, chronic illness and the body. *Sociology of Health and Illness*, **18**: 241–257.

Lerpiniere, P. (1998) Drug diagnosis and social control. Scottish Council on Alcohol. *Alcohol Update*, **Oct**: 10.

Light, D. (1997) The rhetorics and realities of community health care: the limits of countervailing powers to meet the health care needs of the 21st century. *Journal of Health, Politics, Policy and Law*, **22**: 105–145.

Linder, R. (1965) Diagnosis: description or prescription? *Perceptual and Motor Skills*, **20**: 1081.

Lowenberg, J.S. and Davis, F. (1994) Beyond medicalisation-demedicalisation: the case of holistic health. *Sociology of Health and Illness*, **16**: 579–599.

McGrew, J.H., Wilson, R.G. and Bond, G.R. (1996) Client perspectives on helpful ingredients of assertive community treatment. *Psychiatric Rehabilitation Journal*, **19**: 13–21.

McHugh, P. (1970) A common-sense conception of deviance. In J.D. Douglas (Ed.), *Deviance and Respectability: The Social Construction of Moral Meanings*. New York, Basic Books.

McIntosh, J. and McKeganey, N. (2000) Addicts' narratives of recovery from drug use: constructing a non-addict identity. *Social Science and Medicine*, **50**: 1501–1510.

Mills, C.W. (1959) *The Sociological Imagination*. New York, Oxford University Press.

Muijen, M. (1996) Scare in the community: Britain in moral panic. In T. Heller, J., Reynolds, R., Gomm, R., Muston, and S. Pattison (Eds.), *Mental Health Matters. A Reader*. London, MacMillan.

O'Neill, M.M. (1993) Countertransference and attitudes in the context of clinical work with dually diagnosed patients. In J. Solomon, S. Zimberg and E. Shollar (Eds.), *Dual Diagnosis: Evaluation, Treatment, Training and Program Development*. New York, Plenum Press.

Parsons, T. (1951) *The Social System*. London, Routledge and Keegan Paul.

Perkins, R.E. and Repper, J.M. (1999) Compliance or informed choice. *Journal of Mental Health*, **8**: 117–129.

Pleace, N. (1998) Single homelessness as social exclusion: the unique and the extreme. *Housing Studies*, **13**: 46–59.

Quimby, E. (1995) Homeless clients' perspectives on recovery in the Washington, DC, dual diagnosis project. *Contemporary Drug Problems*, **Summer**: 265–289.

Rollnick, S. and Miller, W.R. (1995) What is motivational interviewing? *Behavioural and Cognitive Psychotherapy*, **23**: 325–334.

Rose, N. (1996) The discipline of mental health. In *The Power of Psychiatry*. Cambridge, Polity Press.

Smith, J. and Hucker, S. (1994) Schizophrenia and substance abuse. *British Journal of Psychiatry*, **165**: 13–21.

Strong, P.M. (1979) Sociological imperialism and the profession of medicine. A critical examination of the thesis of medical imperialism. *Social Science and Medicine*, **13A**: 199–215.

Szmukler, G. and Holloway, F. (2000) Reform of the Mental Health Act. Health or safety? *British Journal of Psychiatry*, **177**: 196–200.

Szmukler, G. (2001) A new mental health (and public protection) act. Risk wins in the balance between providing care and controlling risks. *British Medical Journal*, **322**: 2–3.

Taussig, M.T. (1980) Reification and the consciousness of the patient. *Social Science and Medicine*, **14B**: 3–13.

Taylor, P.J. and Gunn, J. (1999) Homicides by people with mental illness: myth and reality. *British Journal of Psychiatry*, **174**: 9–14.

Turner, B. (1995) *Medical Power and Social Knowledge*, London, Sage.

Young, S.L. and Ensing, D.S. (1999) Exploring recovery from the perspective of people with psychiatric disabilities. *Psychiatric Rehabilitation Journal*, **22**: 219–231.

Chapter 5

A COGNITIVE CONCEPTUALIZATION OF CONCURRENT PSYCHOSIS AND PROBLEM DRUG AND ALCOHOL USE

Hermine L. Graham

> Without a case formulation, the therapist is proceeding like a ship without a rudder, drifting aimlessly through the session.
>
> (Beck et al, 1993: 80)

INTRODUCTION

The importance in clinical practice of the interface between an understanding of the development, maintenance and treatment of a client's problems and theoretical models is often overlooked. "When one asks a novice cognitive therapist how they would handle a specific clinical problem . . . they usually can give a variety of techniques. . . . A few might suggest strategies . . . [but] rarely does the novice address the most important step—conceptualisation" (Beck et al, 1985: 181). A case conceptualization is a systematic way of making sense of the problems a client may present with; it answers questions such as how the problems developed and are maintained, and what is the most appropriate intervention (Beck et al, 1993; Persons, 1989; Liese and Franz, 1996). However, such an understanding of a case and treatment can be focused and effective only if based on evidence-based theoretical models (Persons, 1989; Bruch, 1998). Beck et al (1993)

Substance Misuse in Psychosis: Approaches to Treatment and Service Delivery.
Edited by Hermine L. Graham, Alex Copello, Max J. Birchwood and Kim T. Mueser.
© 2003 John Wiley & Sons, Ltd.

have suggested that case formulations/conceptualizations are essential to provide focus and direction to clinical interventions.

Cognitive based models and interventions have been developed separately for both problem substance use and psychosis. In addition, there has been an emergence in the literature of a range of cognitive-behavioural-based treatment approaches developed specifically for those with psychosis who use substances problematically (e.g., Kavanagh, 1995; Drake et al, 1998; Weiss et al, 1999; Mueser et al, 1998; Barrowclough et al, 2000; Drake and Mueser, 2000; Kavanagh et al, 1999) However, the lack of an identifiable cognitive conceptualization or model that has driven such approaches means that the specific targets and focus treatment remain unclear. Graham (1998) proposed a cognitive-developmental model based on a number of case conceptualizations that could be applied to this client group and serve as a guide to appropriate treatment. This chapter will seek to expand on that conceptualization and model in an attempt to help clinicians make sense of the problems their clients present with and the relationship between the experience of psychosis and problematic drug and alcohol use, within a cognitive framework. The purpose of the cognitive-developmental conceptualization and model of problem substance use and concurrent psychosis that will be expanded on here is not to explain the causal links between psychosis and substance use. The issue of aetiology is addressed in Chapter 2 of this book and has been thoroughly debated in the wider literature (e.g., Mueser et al, 1998). Nor is it intended to account for the experiences of all people with a psychosis who use substances problematically. Rather, this discussion attempts to offer an understanding of the relationship between the two for some people, and the higher incidence of problematic substance use among this population. The discussion will consider how problems may develop and the maintenance factors, and it will also serve as a guide to appropriate treatment.

Although, within the cognitive model, the focus is on cognitions, "environmental" factors are seen as influencing the development and maintenance of cognitions (Greenberger and Padesky, 1995). The cognitive-developmental model of substance use takes into account that drug and alcohol use and problem use occur within society and thus are greatly influenced by social, cultural and environmental factors, particularly in the development and maintenance of beliefs about use (Liese and Franz, 1996). The area of social and community perspectives on psychosis and problem substance use is clearly one of importance, and it is addressed in more detail in Chapters 3 and 4 of this book. Thus, this chapter will focus primarily at the level of an individual's cognition, but with an acute awareness that problematic substance use occurs within a wider social, community and cultural context (Orford, 2001).

DIAGNOSIS VERSUS CASE CONCEPTUALIZATION

It is possible that the effect of the terminology commonly applied to people with psychosis who use drugs or alcohol in problematic patterns—for example, "dual diagnosis"—has limited our understanding of this area. Such terminology evokes a tendency to use psychiatric classifications, which are useful nosological descriptions, but result in the development of standardized treatment approaches matched to a diagnosis, rather than individualized conceptualizations which meet the needs of individual clients (Bruch, 1998). Thus, a case conceptualization seeks to move beyond a diagnostic description, which can be in some instances static and limiting, to a more dynamic understanding or set of hypotheses about a client's problems, based on theoretical models, that can be tested (Bruch, 1998). This chapter will therefore seek to explore and conceptualize, within a cognitive framework, the dynamic and fluid interrelationship between the experience of psychosis and the use of drugs and alcohol for some of the people who experience such difficulties.

COGNITIVE UNDERSTANDING OF PSYCHOSIS

A number of cognitive models have been put forward in an attempt to understand psychosis. Some models have conceptualized components of the psychotic experience or symptoms (e.g., Chadwick and Birchwood, 1994; Chadwick and Lowe, 1994; Morrison et al, 1995; Fowler et al, 1998; Garety and Freeman, 1999). Others have sought to make sense of the development and maintenance of psychosis (e.g., Kingdon and Turkington, 1994; Fowler et al, 1995). One such model suggests that psychosis and the associated experiences can be viewed as a trauma which disturbs the equilibrium of a person's life (e.g., McGorry et al, 1991; Lundy, 1992; Shaw et al, 1997; Meyer et al, 1999). These researchers have sought to extend the diagnostic classification of post-traumatic stress disorder (PTSD) beyond an emphasis on the threat to physical integrity, to that on psychological integrity. They and others have found that there is a high incidence of symptoms of acute stress reactions in patients recovering from psychotic illnesses. Shaw et al (1997) found evidence of symptoms such as avoidance, and intrusive and distressing recollections of the experience of psychosis and hospitalization. McGorry et al (1991) have suggested that the postpsychotic period is characterized by PTSD-type reactions. Not only the psychotic symptoms but also the related hospitalization and subsequent treatment are said to be perceived as a stressor that triggers PTSD reactions, (Shaw et al, 1997; Meyer et al, 1999). Psychosis has been linked with intense anger, helplessness, sense of disintegration of self, and disconnectedness with others. Shaw et al (1997) suggest that, although there are few experiential accounts of psychosis documented, the "available accounts poignantly reveal the anguish and terror associated with psychosis along with the intense anger and ambivalence many patients feel toward treatment and mental health professionals". Birchwood et al (2000) found that about a third of people with schizophrenia in their study developed postpsychotic depression. Those who experienced postpsychotic depression were more likely to have a greater sense of loss, humiliation and entrapment related to their psychosis, and to have lower self-esteem and engage in self-criticism. They suggest that the meaning or appraisal of the psychotic experience and its implications for the self increases vulnerability to depression.

COGNITIVE UNDERSTANDING OF PROBLEM SUBSTANCE USE

A significant contribution to the field of psychological models of addictions has been the cognitive-developmental model of substance abuse. The extension of the core cognitive therapy model of emotional disorders (Beck, 1976) to specific disorders and problem areas, including problem substance use (Salkovskis, 1996), was an important development within cognitive therapy. This model, unlike other cognitive-based models, such as the model of the relapse process (Marlatt and Gordon, 1985), not only provided a conceptualization of the relapse process but also gave some ideas of the developmental and maintenance processes. The cognitive-developmental model of substance abuse (Beck et al, 1993; Liese and Franz, 1996) not only provides a range of techniques for intervention but also is based on a cognitive conceptualization of problem drug and alcohol use and identifies a clear target for treatment: cognitions. Cognitions at a number of levels are seen as pivotal in the development and maintenance of problem drug and alcohol use. Some of these cognitions are general core beliefs (e.g., "I am inadequate") and dysfunctional assumptions/conditional beliefs (e.g., "If I try to please people they will think well of me"). Other beliefs and automatic thoughts said to be specific to substance use are termed substance-related beliefs (e.g., "If I have a drink, it will take away my depression") (Beck et al, 1993; Liese and Franz, 1996).

Substance-related beliefs are said to develop through environmental and cultural exposure to drug and alcohol use. These beliefs can become conditional in nature if the use of the substance starts to be perceived as a way of coping with underlying/core beliefs (e.g., "If I have a drink, I will fit in and people will like me"). The cognitive-developmental model of substance abuse suggests that with continued substance use and positive experiences of using, such beliefs become more rigid, absolute in nature and automatically activated in relevant situations. For example, "The only way to cope with meeting other people is to have a drink". When such beliefs prevent goal attainment and affect the person's well-being, they can be dysfunctional and substance use is likely to become problematic (Beck et al, 1993; Liese and Franz, 1996). With continued use of the substance, a network of idiosyncratic, substance-related beliefs is developed and is activated by particular situations or internal states ("activating stimuli"/"high-risk situations"). Once activated, these beliefs serve to intensify cravings and urges to use the substance and provide permission to use (e.g., "I'll just have one rock"). Problematic patterns of use are thus maintained by a number of cognitive distortions in these beliefs. These distortions minimize the negative consequences of such patterns of use by keeping the person focused on the positive benefits or outcomes of continued use (e.g., "Crack isn't the problem—the problem is that I don't have enough money. When I use I feel good"). In addition, such cognitive distortions provide justification for continued use (e.g., "The only way I can cope with this is to have a drink").

For example, Gavin is a 27-year-old single man. He is employed on a casual basis as a market trader, after losing his job as a photographic printer. He is the eldest of two children. His father, who used drugs problematically, left when Gavin was quite young. His mother has experienced mental health difficulties, and attributes them to the aggressive behaviour of her sons, and often withdraws. Gavin experiences strong feelings of anger and hatred toward his family, particularly his brother, who behaves in an aggressive and threatening manner, on a regular basis, toward Gavin and members of the public. Gavin is often in fights with his brother and is occasionally verbally aggressive to people on the street. Gavin uses cannabis on a regular basis (previously 1 g per day; currently one-eighth ounce per day) and cocaine powder/crack-cocaine occasionally. Gavin began using drugs, initially on a social-recreational basis, when aged 14/15 years. His use became more habitual at the age of 18 years. In the past, he has used alcohol on the weekends. Illustrated diagrammatically in Figure 5.1. is a cognitive conceptualization of Gavin's problematic substance use based on the cognitive-developmental model of substance abuse (Beck et al, 1993; Liese and Franz, 1996).

Within the cognitive developmental model, early life experiences and core beliefs/dysfunctional assumptions are viewed as increasing the individual's vulnerability to the development of substance use problems, particularly if the person is exposed to substance-using environments, and beliefs about substance use become more accessible and salient (Liese and Franz, 1996).

It has been suggested, as described in this chapter, that a similar process to that outlined in the cognitive-developmental model of substance abuse is

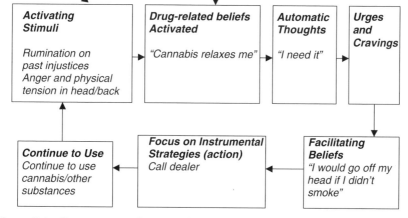

Figure 5.1   Case conceptualization of Gavin's problem substance use

operating in the development and maintenance of problematic substance use among those with psychosis (Graham, 1998).

For example, Irene has a long history of heavy drinking, and she experiences schizoaffective disorder. She drinks in a binge pattern and has had a number of periods of abstinence lasting up to about 8 months. Following a recent binge, she says she cannot understand why she started drinking again. When Irene is drinking heavily, her life becomes chaotic and she stops taking her medication. Often the result is that she becomes quite paranoid and disinhibited; on some occasions, this had led to her going into hospital. Illustrated diagrammatically in Figure 5.2 are the cognitive processes maintaining Irene's alcohol use problems and the relationship with her mood states/mental health, based on the cognitive model of substance abuse.

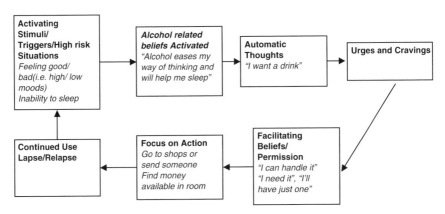

Figure 5.2   The cognitive processes maintaining Irene's alcohol-using cycle and the relationship with her mental health

COGNITIVE CONCEPTUALIZATION OF PSYCHOSIS AND PROBLEM SUBSTANCE USE

> The feeling that there is no escape from this internal chaos creates a sense of extreme helplessness and threat.
>
> (Shaw et al, 1997: 434)

Critical incident(s) or event(s) are viewed from a cognitive perspective as experiences that activate underlying schemas, core beliefs and dysfunctional assumptions. Beliefs are then generated about the critical incident(s) or event(s); that is, an appraisal is made of the event and/or meaning attached (Iqbal et al, 2000). From the classical cognitive therapy perspective

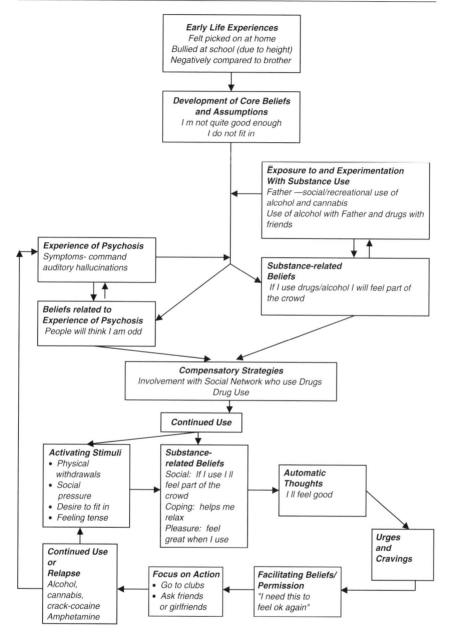

Figure 5.3 Jake's case conceptualization based on the cognitive-developmental model of concurrent psychosis and problem substance use

these beliefs are said to be closely related in content to the underlying beliefs. The meaning attached to an event or events or the appraisal of an event is said to influence the beliefs generated about the experience and the emotional reaction. It is the meaning attached and the related beliefs that cause emotional distress and drive attempts to cope. Hence, the same event can invoke different emotional and coping responses in different people (Salkovskis, 1996). Thus, the beliefs held about a psychotic illness and the treatment experiences or meaning attached to the psychosis/psychotic "event" affect the psychological sequlae (Birchwood et al, 2000; Iqbal et al, 2000).

In the proposed cognitive conceptualization (Figure 5.3), it is suggested that the meaning attached by people to the experience of psychosis and the related experiences or appraisal made of it influence their psychological adjustment. Environmental factors, early experiences, core beliefs and the dysfunctional assumptions held influence appraisals and psychological responses. "It is possible that certain basic assumptions may influence the process of coming to terms with trauma, either by preventing the emotional expression necessary to engage in processing . . . or by preventing the completion of the process" (Moorey, 1996: 460). Predisposing cognitive styles have been found to be important factors in determining responses to trauma. Secker et al (1999) found that young people's understanding or conceptualization of disturbances in mental health or behaviour was based on their own experiences or what they had been exposed to (i.e., salient others/media images). Any behaviour beyond their range of experience was inexplicable to them and classified as "abnormal" or mental illness. If general underlying beliefs are indeed activated by the experience of psychosis, substance-related beliefs will also be activated. Substance-related beliefs (e.g., "I feel less self-conscious and have a laugh with all my mates after a drink") are more likely to be activated if they have previously been associated with particular internal/external stimuli (e.g., feeling nervous, being with friends). Such associations are the product of earlier experiences through either exposure to (e.g., family members who drink alcohol) or experimentation with (e.g., drinking with friends as a teenager) substance-using behaviours.

The substance-related beliefs a person holds may, over time, become linked with the beliefs generated about the psychotic illness and/or the treatment experience (e.g., "I feel flat on my medication—cocaine makes me feel live, kicking and buzzing"). Thus, the experiences associated with psychosis (e.g., symptoms, social exclusion, loss issues, medication side-effects) activate substance-related beliefs that help people feel that they can self-manage or regulate the experience. Thus, drugs and alcohol may become a coping strategy, a means of increasing feelings of pleasure and an aid to socialization. Such reasons for use and the positive expectations

of use are often reinforced by continued use, despite the negative consequences of use (e.g., debt, increased feelings of paranoia, low mood and
anxiety). Cognitive distortions inherent in dysfunctional substance-related
beliefs (e.g., "Alcohol stops me feeling tense and helps me sleep so I can
shut things out"), such as dichotomous reasoning, overgeneralizations,
and magnification/minimization, maintain problematic patterns of drug
and alcohol use. The distortions in logical reasoning minimize the negative consequences of use and focus attention on its positive benefits. It has
been found, through psychological theories of health behaviour decision
making, that young people make active appraisal of personal benefits (coping, socialization, aid to pleasure enhancement) and costs to be gained from
alcohol and drug use (Boys et al, 1999). It has been suggested that people
often titrate the use of alcohol or drugs to achieve the most advantageous
cost-to-benefit ratio (Kavanagh, 1995). The three types of substance-related
beliefs and their relationship with the experience of psychosis will be
explored in more detail.

COPING-FOCUSED SUBSTANCE-RELATED BELIEFS

If the experience of psychosis is conceptualized as trauma, people will
search for understanding or meaning of the experience and ways to cope.
Birchwood et al (1993) see a person with a psychotic illness "as an active
agent searching for meaning and control over their illness and experiences". That is, such people are attempting to restore the equilibrium of
their life. It can be hypothesized that experiencing traumatic events often
stretches pre-existing coping repertoires to the limit. As such, it is unsur-
prising that higher rates of problematic substance use among those with
PTSD than in the general population have been well documented (Najavits
et al, 1996). Coping is one of the common motives or reasons cited for
substance use among those who use substances with (Warner et al, 1994;
Mueser et al, 1995; Drake et al, 1998) or without a psychosis (e.g., Cooper
et al, 1992). Thus, some people may already have pre-existing coping-
focused substance-related beliefs (e.g., "If I have a drink I will be able to
face the day") prior to the onset of psychosis. However, for others, beliefs
about the effectiveness of alcohol/drugs as a coping strategy may quickly
develop if drugs or alcohol are used in an attempt to alleviate distressing
symptoms or experiences (e.g., "When I smoke crack I feel good, and my
depression goes"). The result is that the immediate psychoactive effects of
drugs or alcohol, mediated by positive drug-related beliefs or expectancies,
quickly serve to reinforce and maintain use as an "immediate and effective" coping strategy, thus increasing the likelihood of substance use in
future under similar circumstances (Carpenter and Hasin, 1998), and even
in the light of conflicting evidence. Boys et al (1999) found that the negative

effects of using drugs or alcohol did not determine current patterns of use in people. Instead, the beliefs held about the function of drug and alcohol use and the extent of peer use was a more likely predictor of future use.

According to the trauma reaction model of psychosis, there is potentially a wide range of issues that a person experiencing a psychotic illness seeks to cope with. These include loss issues, such as loss of control due to treatment regimens and perceived inability to control one's own mind and thoughts (Shaw et al, 1997), and loss of social role and status (Iqbal et al, 2000). According to subjective reports, those with psychosis use alcohol or drugs to cope with a number of experiences. These have been found to range from psychotic symptoms (e.g., hallucinations, delusions, loss of energy and motivation), to depression and anxiety, to medication side effects, to boredom, to loss of self-esteem (Warner et al, 1994; Mueser et al, 1995; Wolf et al, 1986).

For example, Ray has a long history of poly-substance use and a diagnosis of schizophrenia. During the early stages of his drug-using career, Ray used LSD and enjoyed the hallucinogenic properties. He also liked some of the hallucinations he experienced when he first began having psychotic symptoms, but he has found that his depot medication has rid him of them. Over the years, Ray has been exposed to different drugs due to his drug-using network, and was initially introduced to crack-cocaine by a dealer/friend, as the availability of LSD was low. Ray feels left out by his brothers and believes that his family misattribute any changes in his behaviour to mental health problems. He is also anxious about going out socially as he fears meeting people who saw him when he was acutely psychotic. To some extent, the coping-focused beliefs Ray holds about drugs existed pre-morbidly, but are now more likely to be activated to cope with the experiences associated with his mental health (e.g., social exclusion, boredom, loneliness, stigma). This is illustrated diagrammatically in Figure 5.4.

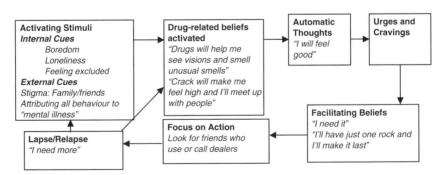

Figure 5.4   Ray's drug-using cycle—illustrating the role of coping-focused beliefs

SOCIALIZATION/PLEASURE ENHANCEMENT FOCUSED SUBSTANCE-RELATED BELIEFS

The perception and experience of loss following the onset of a psychotic illness has been found to result in significant levels of depression, demoralization and suicide among males who have a psychosis (e.g., Birchwood et al, 1993). Not only do the affected people lose a social role and social network but also, it can be suggested, are often bereft of or "excluded" from their original or "normative" routes of getting pleasure and social contact. Socialization and pleasure enhancement have been identified, in addition to coping, as two other self-identified reasons or motives for substance use among those who use substances with (Warner et al, 1994; Mueser et al, 1995; Drake et al, 1998) or without a psychosis (Cooper et al, 1992). Drug and alcohol use can give access to social groups and social contact (Drake et al, 1993; Drake et al, 1998; Orford, 2001). For some, substance-related beliefs about substance use as a way of increasing social contact and pleasure may have existed prior to the onset of psychosis. However, for others, it can be suggested that these beliefs may develop over time as a response to feelings of social isolation and exposure to substance-using networks. Often clients with psychosis and substance use problems describe their social networks as consisting almost exclusively of drinking and drug-using peers (Drake et al, 1993). It can thus be suggested that such a social group becomes one in which a more favoured identity and social acceptance can more readily be found in contrast to the difficulties that may be experienced in conventional society, where societal norms are less tolerant of apparently odd or bizarre behaviour. As substance use increases in severity, individuals' energy, source of pleasure, activities, social networks and relationships can be seen increasingly to revolve around their drug and/or alcohol use.

For example, Andrew had no history of drug use before the onset of his mental health difficulties in his early forties and his involvement with the mental health services. Andrew has a diagnosis of paranoid schizophrenia. Prior to the onset of his mental health symptoms, Andrew was self-employed and married with four children, and used alcohol on a social-recreational basis. He is currently separated from his wife although still in contact. Andrew is generally mentally quite well and visits regularly or is visited by old friends who smoke cannabis, as he is no longer working. He describes starting to use cannabis as a result of his contact with his friends and believes that "it is nice and relaxing to have a smoke and a drink with one's friends". However, after his flat was broken into, he began to drink four cans of strong lager and smoke cannabis every night whether or not he was with friends. He subsequently believes, in addition, that "cannabis and alcohol relax me", and this maintains his use when he is alone.

The morning after a substance-using session, he experiences persecutory voices and describes feeling "shaky, nervous and paranoid about leaving his flat". This subsequently increases the likelihood of his using alcohol and drugs, to cope with such difficulties, thus establishing a vicious cycle of problem use and mental health problems. Andrew's initial substance-related beliefs (socialization-focused) maintained his substance use in social settings and normalized substance use for him. However, the additional belief that emerged promotes use as a daily coping strategy.

CONCLUSIONS

The cognitive-developmental conceptualization of concurrent psychosis and problem substance use seeks to shed some light on the relationship between the experience of psychosis and problematic drug and alcohol use (see Figure 5.3). It also aims to help clinicians make sense of the dynamic and interrelated problems their clients present with, within a cognitive framework. It has been suggested that people with psychosis may or may not have pre-existing use or problematic use of drugs or alcohol. However, it is hypothesized that psychosis and the related social and treatment experiences result in a perceived loss of control and can be experienced as a stressor. Meaning is attached to these events and the beliefs generated about them. The response to such an experience, which threatens the integrity of the self, is an activation of underlying core beliefs and dysfunctional assumptions and substance-related beliefs, some of the results of which can be PTSD symptoms such as avoidance, and intrusive and distressing recollections; postpsychotic depression; and perceived loss of social role/status. Affected persons act to regain some equilibrium in their life, and this is restored, by some, through the use of alcohol and drugs, particularly if pre-existing substance-related beliefs are activated. It has been suggested that the use of alcohol and drugs is mediated by positive substance-related beliefs which can be classified into coping, socialization and pleasure enhancement. Such beliefs, it is suggested, become linked to the experience of psychosis, and the beliefs held about psychosis. Thus, a person attempting to regain control over distressing symptoms, treatment experiences, social exclusion/stigma, or lack of pleasure/boredom may find more immediate and "effective" results, albeit short-lived, through the use of drugs or alcohol. Problematic substance use is said to occur when substance-related beliefs become dysfunctional, that is, more rigidly held, are based on overgeneralizations, and are all-or-nothing in nature. Typically, such cognitive styles lead to patterns of use and associated problems that interfere with a person's self-identified goals and impair well-being (spiritual, social, physical, psychological/mental health and occupational).

IMPLICATIONS FOR TREATMENT TARGETS: COGNITIONS

Understanding the dynamic relationship between the use of substances and psychosis is essential in preventing or managing potential relapses to acute psychosis and relapses to problematic drug or alcohol use. The fact that both problems and the relationship between the two are, to some extent, mediated by cognitions means that clear targets and focus for treatment exist. Once a conceptualization of a case exists, it can be used on a set of hypotheses that can be tested, act as a guide for treatment interventions, and provide indicators of what may or may not be effective. The key benefit of a cognitive conceptualization is that it provides a framework for clients to begin to understand the vulnerability factors that influenced the development and maintenance of their problems. The person can become aware of and then learn how to self-manage the interaction between mental health and substance use problems that may precipitate relapses not only to problematic substance use but also to acute mental health problems. The focus for the self-regulation of the use of substances is to have in place more realistic beliefs about the efficacy of drug or alcohol use and a recognition of the role the perceived experience of psychosis and its treatment will play in the cycle of use. Therefore, when generating relapse signatures/plans, one must focus with clients not only on the monitoring of early earning signs of psychosis (Birchwood et al, 2000) but also on the perceived role of drugs/alcohol and medication in that process (Graham, 1998). Indeed, unless dysfunctional substance-related beliefs are tackled, engagement with treatment services and medication adherence will be hindered and a greater risk of relapse to problematic drug/alcohol use and acute psychosis will exist. An intervention based on the cognitive-developmental model of concurrent psychosis and substance use is described more fully in Chapter 11 in this book.

REFERENCES

Barrowclough, C., Haddock, G., Tarrier, N., Moring, J. and Lewis, S. (2000) Cognitive behavioural intervention for severely mentally ill clients who have a substance use problem. *Psychiatric Rehabilitation Skills, 4*: 216–233.

Beck, A.T. and Emergy, G. (with Greenberg, R.L.) (1985) *Anxiety Disroders and Phobias: A Cognitive Perspective*. New York, Basic Books.

Beck, A.T., Wright, F.D., Newman, C.F. and Liese, B.S. (1993) *Cognitive Therapy of Substance Abuse*. New York, Guilford Press.

Beck, A.T. (1976) *Cognitive Therapy and the Emotional Disorders*. New York, International Universities Press.

Birchwood, M., Mason, R., MacMillan, F. and Healy, J. (1993) Depression, demoralization and control over psychotic illness: a comparison of depressed and non-depressed patients with a chronic psychosis. *Psychological Medicine, 23*: 387–395.

Birchwood, M., Spencer, E. and McGovern, D. (2000) Schizophrenia: early warning signs. Early Advances in Psychiatric Treatment, Vol 6, 93–101.

Birchwood, M., Iqbal, Z., Chadwick, P. and Trower, P. (2000) Cognitive Approach to depression and suicidal thinking in psychosis—ontogeny of post-psychotic depression. *British Journal of Psychiatry*, **177**: 316–321.

Boys, A., Masden, J., Griffiths, P., Fountain, J., Stillwell, G. and Strang, J. (1999) Substance use among young people: the relationship between perceived functions and intentions. *Addiction,* **94**: 1043–1050.

Bruch, M. (1998) The development of case formulation approaches. In M. Brunch and F. W. Bond (Eds), *Beyond Diagnosis: Case Formulation Approaches in CBT*. Chichester, Wiley.

Carpenter, K.M. and Hasin, D.S. (1998) A prospective evaluation of the relationship between reasons for drinking and DSM-IV alcohol use disorders. *Addictive Behaviours*, **23**: 41–46.

Chadwick, P.D.J. and Birchwood, M. (1994) The omnipotence of voices—a cognitive approach to auditory hallucinations. *British Journal of Psychiatry*, **164**: 190–201.

Chadwick, P.D.J. and Lowe, C.F. (1994) A cognitive approach to measuring and modifying delusions. *Behaviour Research and Therapy,* **32**: 355–367.

Cooper, M.L., Russell, M., Skinner, J.B. and Windle, M. (1992) Development and validation of a three-dimensional measure of drinking motives. *Psychological Assessment*, **4**: 123–132.

Drake, R.E., Brunette, M.F., and Mueser, K.T. (1998) Substance use disorders and social functioning in schizophrenia. In K.T. Mueser, and N. Tarrier (Eds.), *Handbook of Social Functioning in Schizophrenia*. Boston, Allyn and Bacon.

Drake, R.E., Bebout, R.R., and Roach, J.P. (1993) A research evaluation of social network case management for homeless persons with dual disorders. In M. Harris and H. C. Bergman, *Case Management for Mentally Ill Patients: Theory and Practice*. Pennsylvania, Harwood Academic Publishers.

Drake, R.E. and Mueser, K.T. (2000) Psychosocial approaches to dual diagnosis. *Schizophrenia Bulletin*, **26**: 105–118.

Fowler, D., Garety, P. and Kuipers, E. (1995) *Cognitive Behaviour Therapy for Psychosis: Theory and Practice*. Chichester, Wiley.

Fowler, D., Garety, P. and Kuipers, E. (1998) Understanding the inexplicable: an individually formulated cognitive approach to delusional beliefs. In C. Perris and P.D. McGorry (Eds), *Cognitive Psychotherapy of Psychotic and Personality Disorders: Handbook of Theory and Practice*. Chichester, Wiley.

Garety, P.A. and Freeman, D. (1999) Cognitive approaches to delusions: a critical review of theories and evidence. *British Journal of Clinical Psychology*, **38**: 113–154.

Graham, H.L. (1998) The role of dysfunctional beliefs in individuals who experience psychosis and use substances: implications for cognitive therapy and medication adherence. *Behavioural and Cognitive Psychotherapy*, **26**: 193–208.

Greenberger, D.S. and Padesky, C.A. (1995) *Mind Over Mood: A Cognitive Therapy Treatment Manual for Clients*. New York, Guilford Press.

Iqbal, Z., Birchwood, M., Chadwick, P. and Trower, P. (2000) Cognitive approach to depression and suicidal thinking in psychosis—testing the validity of a social ranking model. *British Journal of Psychiatry*, **177**: 522–528.

Kavanagh, D.J. (1995) An intervention for substance abuse in schizophrenia. *Behaviour Change*, **12**: 20–30.

Kavanagh, D.J., Young, R., Boyce, L., Clair, A., Sitharthan, T., Clark, D. and Thompson, K. (1998) Substance treatment options in psychosis (STOP): a new intervention for dual diagnosis. *Journal of Mental Health,* **7**: 135–143.

Kingdon, D.G. and Turkington, D. (1994) *Cognitive Behavioural Therapy of Schizophrenia*. Hove, Psychology Press.

Liese, B.S. and Frantz, R.A. (1996) Treating substance use disorders with cognitive therapy: lessons learned and implications for the future. In P. Salkovskis (Ed.), *Frontiers of Cognitive Therapy*. New York, Guilford Press.

Lundy, S.M. (July 1992) Psychosis-induced post traumatic stress disorder. *American Journal of Psychotherapy*, **46**: 485–490.

Marlatt, G.A. and Gordon, J.R. (Eds.) (1985) *Relapse Prevention: Maintenance in the Treatment of Addictive Behaviour*. New York, Guilford Press.

Meyer, H., Taiminen, T. Vuori, T., Aijala, A. and Helenius, H. (1999) Post traumatic stress disorder symptoms related to psychosis and acute involuntary hospitalization in schizophrenic and delusional patients. *Journal of Nervous and Mental Disease*, 187, 343–353.

McGorry, P.D., Chanen, A., McCarthy, E., Van Riel, R., McKenzie, D. and Singh, B.S. (1991) Post traumatic stress disorder following recent onset psychosis: an unrecognized postpsychotic syndrome. *Journal of Nervous and Mental Disease*, **179**: 253–258.

Moorey, S. (1996) When bad things happen to Rational People: cognitive therapy in adverse life circumstances. In P. Salkovskis (Ed.), *Frontiers of Cognitive Therapy*. New York: Guilford Press.

Morrison, A.P., Haddock, G. and Tarrier, N. (1995) Intrusive thoughts and auditory hallucinations: a cognitive approach. *Behavioural and Cognitive Psychotherapy*, **23**: 265–280.

Mueser, K.T., Nishith, P., Tracy, J.I., De Girolamo, J. and Molinaro, M. (1995) Expectations and motives for substance use in schizophrenia. *Schizophrenia Bulletin*, **21**: 367–378.

Mueser, K.T., Drake, R.E., and Wallach, M.A. (1998) Dual diagnosis: a review of etiological theories. *Addictive Behaviors*, **23**: 717–734.

Najavits, L.M., Weiss, R.D. and Liese, B.S. (1996) Group cognitive-behavoural therapy for women with PTSD and substance use disorder. *Journal of Substance Abuse Treatment*, **13**: 13–22.

Orford, J.O. (2001) *Excessive Appetites: A Psychological View of Addiction*, 2nd edn. Chicester, Wiley.

Persons, J.B. (1989) *Cognitive Therapy in Practice: A Case Formulation Approach*. New York, Norton.

Salkovskis, P. (1996) Preface, In P. Salkovskis (Ed.), *Frontiers of Cognitive Therapy*. New York, Guilford Press.

Salkovskis, P. (1996) The cognitive approach to anxiety: threat beliefs, safety seeking behaviour, and the special case of health anxiety and obsessions, In P. Salkovskis (Ed.), *Frontiers of Cognitive Therapy*. New York, Guilford Press.

Secker, J., Armstrong, C. and Hill, M. (1999) Young people's understanding of mental illness. *Health Education Research*, **14**: 729–739.

Shaw, K., McFarland, A. and Bookless, C. (1997) The phenomenology of traumatic reactions to psychotic illness. *Journal of Nervous and Mental Disease*, **185**: 434–441.

Warner, R., Taylor, D., Wright, J., Sloat, A., Springett, G., Arnold, S. and Weinberg, H. (1994) Substance use among the mentally ill: prevalence, reasons for use, and effects on illness. *American Journal of Orthopsychiatry*, **64**: 30–39.

Weiss, R.D., Najavits, L.M. and Greenfield, S.F. (1999) A relapse prevention group for patients with bipolar and substance use disorders. *Journal of Substance Abuse Treatment*, **16**: 47–54.

Wolf, B., Ruther, E., Brenner, P.M., Poser, W. and Schmidt, L.G. (1986) Abuse of and dependence on stimulants and anorexigenic drugs in psychiatric inpatients. *Pharmacopsychiatry*, **19**: 296–297.

Part II

INTEGRATED SERVICE DELIVERY MODELS

INTRODUCTION

Kim T. Mueser

In the mid-1980s, integrated service delivery models for the treatment of substance misuse in patients with severe mental health problems ("dual disorders") began to be developed, with research over the following decade demonstrating their superiority over traditional separate services for the two disorders. With the initial successes of integrated treatment programmes, the number of treatment models has proliferated, and specialized integrated programmes have been developed. This section introduces several integrated service delivery models, including both community-based and inpatient-based programmes. Two of the chapters reflect variations in community-based integrated service delivery models that have been implemented at an organizational level in the USA and in parts of Europe, namely, England (Chapter 6 by Mueser and Drake and Chapter 7 by Graham et al). Chapter 8 (by Addington) illustrates the advantages of developing specialized treatment programmes to address the unique needs of specific subgroups of patients, those with a recent onset of their psychosis. In Chapter 9, Rosenthal describes a different specialized integrated treatment programme, an inpatient programme for those with substance misuse and psychosis. These chapters show the breadth of integrated treatment programs that have evolved in recent years, and discribe the policy, social and contextual factors that have shaped these models in their respective settings.

Chapter 6

INTEGRATED DUAL DISORDER TREATMENT IN NEW HAMPSHIRE (USA)

Kim T. Mueser and Robert E. Drake

The impetus to develop more effective services for persons with severe mental illness and comorbid substance use disorders (dual disorders) began in New Hampshire (USA) in the 1980s, as state mental health authorities and local mental health providers became increasingly concerned about the high use of costly treatment services in this group. Through a public academic liaison, coordinated efforts were undertaken by the state of New Hampshire and the New Hampshire-Dartmouth Psychiatric Research Center to begin to understand the scope of dual disorders and to develop more effective treatments. Over the subsequent years, a general model of integrated dual disorder treatment evolved and was implemented at the community mental health centres throughout the state. This model of integrated dual disorder treatment has continued to evolve to the present day.

In this chapter, we describe this model of integrated dual disorder treatment. While the mental health systems in New Hampshire differ in the specific components of treatment they offer, they share the core components of treatment, as guided by the integrated model. Furthermore, the centres share a focus on the importance of serving clients with the most severe and persistent of mental illnesses, including those with schizophrenia, schizoaffective disorder, bipolar disorder, and major depression. We begin this chapter with a brief description of New Hampshire and its mental health system, followed by an explication of the integrated dual disorder treatment model that guides the provision of services for these clients.

Substance Misuse in Psychosis: Approaches to Treatment and Service Delivery.
Edited by Hermine L. Graham, Alex Copello, Max J. Birchwood and Kim T. Mueser.
© 2003 John Wiley & Sons, Ltd.

NEW HAMPSHIRE'S MENTAL HEALTH SYSTEM

New Hampshire is a relatively small state, populated chiefly by persons of European ancestry, and with a relatively small minority population of about 5%. Approximately 1.2 million persons live in New Hampshire, with most of the population in the southeastern part of the state. Most of the state is rural, with several small cities located in the south of the state. Alcohol and cannabis abuse are fairly common throughout the state, with cocaine abuse mainly limited to the urban areas (Mueser et al, 2000; 2001)

Publicly funded mental health services are provided in New Hampshire by private, non-profit agencies that contract with the state to provide psychiatric services. Ten different mental health centres serve the population of New Hampshire, each centre covering a moderately large geographical area. The primary mission of mental health centres is to serve individuals designated by the state as having severe persistent mental illness, defined as a DSM-IV Axis I diagnosis (or Axis II diagnosis of borderline personality disorder) and substantial impairment in independent functioning, ability to work, or ability to maintain social relationships. Within each mental health centre, a range of services is provided, such as psychopharmacology, case management, and rehabilitation.

INTEGRATED DUAL DISORDER TREATMENT

The integrated treatment model developed in New Hampshire (Drake et al, 1991; Mueser et al, 1998) shares many characteristics with other models developed over the past decade (Carey, 1996b; Minkoff, 1991; Ziedonis and Fisher, 1996). *"Integrated care"* is defined as provision of mental health and substance abuse treatment services by the same team of clinicians at the same time, and in which the team assumes the responsibility for integrating the treatment of the two disorders. Integrated treatment is in contrast with traditional treatment approaches that predominated before the 1990s, in which separate services were provided in either a parallel or a sequential fashion (Polcin, 1992; Ridgely et al, 1990). The advantages of integrated treatment over parallel or sequential treatment approaches are that clinicians can ensure that both disorders are treated, the interactions between mental health and substance abuse problems can be directly addressed, and treatment team members are forced to arrive at a consensus on how to treat the two disorders, thereby avoiding conflicts and inconsistencies between different treatment providers.

While integration of mental health and substance abuse treatment services can occur at either the level of the clinical team or of the treatment systems themselves, integration of services at the treatment level is critical in order for integration to translate into clinical benefits for clients (Mercer-McFadden et al, 1998). In New Hampshire, the primary approach to integrating treatment has been for the community mental health centre treatment teams to assume responsibility for treating both disorders (Drake et al, 1991), while maintaining separate mental health and substance abuse treatment systems. Development of expertise in the treatment of substance abuse in persons with severe mental illness has occurred through a combination of methods, including the hiring of substance abuse professionals to work on mental health treatment teams and obtaining specialized training through the New Hampshire-Dartmouth Psychiatric Research Center.

In addition to integration, dual disorder services are characterized by six core features, including comprehensiveness, assertiveness, motivation-based intervention, reduction of negative consequences, multiple psychotherapeutic modalities, and a long-term perspective. The rationale for each of these features and examples of each are briefly described below.

COMPREHENSIVENESS

Clients with dual disorders have multiple needs, and an effective integrated treatment programme must be capable not only of addressing substance abuse, but also meeting the range of other important needs. Thus, integrated treatment programmes must be *comprehensive* in order to meet the needs of clients. In addition to services directly targeting substance abuse, common interventions to address areas of need include housing assistance to address housing instability and homelessness (Osher and Dixon, 1996); medical care for problems such as hepatitis C and other infectious diseases (Rosenberg et al, 2001); psychopharmacology to reduce symptoms and risk of relapse (Rush et al, 1999); vocational rehabilitation (Bond et al, 2001a); family psychoeducation (Dixon et al, 2001); social rehabilitation methods, such as social skill training (Heinssen et al, 2000); and opportunities for peer support and self-help to address self-esteem, provide clients with positive role models, and encourage individuals to becoming engaged in formulating and pursuing their own personal recovery goals (Anthony, 2000). Comprehensive services are critical to the recovery process because they help clients learn how to live a satisfying life without alcohol and drugs, rather than just avoiding substances.

ASSERTIVENESS

Assertiveness refers to the provision of services to clients in their natural environments, including their homes, the homes of family members, and community settings, such as restaurants, parks, and coffee shops. The ability to provide assertive outreach is a critical feature of integrated dual disorder treatment programmes because many such clients fall out of the treatment system and cannot be engaged in treatment conducted only at the mental health centre. In the absence of assertive outreach, many clients with dual disorders are never engaged in treatment (Mercer-McFadden and Drake, 1995).

In addition to the role of assertiveness in engaging clients in treatment, meeting and working with clients in their own natural settings provides valuable opportunities for assessing the conditions in which they live, and for making contacts with, and potentially engaging in treatment, members of the clients' social networks. Assertive outreach can also facilitate the teaching of new skills that are relevant and that do not require transfer from the clinic to the community. Finally, assertive treatment is helpful in monitoring the course of the dual disorder; by meeting with clients in their homes, clinicians are privy to information concerning the clients' use of substances they might otherwise not be aware of. Thus, assertiveness is an important component of treatment because it is more effective at engaging clients and significant others in treatment than clinic-based services, teaching the skills is often easier, and it often provides additional valuable information about the client's problems.

The importance of assertive outreach for engaging clients with severe mental illness in treatment and monitoring the course of illness has been amply documented in numerous controlled studies of the assertive community treatment model (Bond et al, 2001b). In recognition of the importance of assertiveness, during the early years of integrated dual disorder treatment, the state of New Hampshire developed a specific funding category for assertive outreach. After creation of a financial incentive for mental health centres to provide community-based services, outreach became common practice in the treatment of all clients with severe mental illness; consequently, the overall population of clients with severe mental illness has low rates of hospitalization, and there are relatively few long-term psychiatric beds in the state.

MOTIVATION-BASED INTERVENTION

Treatment for dual disorders must take into account clients' motivation for addressing their substance abuse problems, and avoid assuming that clients want to change self-destructive behaviour patterns in the absence of clear evidence of such desire. *Motivation-based* interventions in New Hampshire are guided by the application of the stages-of-change theory (Prochaska et al, 1992; 1994) to individuals with severe mental illness to achieve remission of a substance use disorder during the course of treatment. Four *stages of treatment* have been identified (Osher and Kofoed, 1989), with each stage characterized by a different motivational state of the client, and different goals that guide the selection of interventions (Mueser et al, 1998). The four stages of treatment include engagement, persuasion, active treatment and relapse prevention. Through assessing clients' stage of treatment, and identifying treatment goals and interventions appropriate for that stage, clients can be engaged and retained in treatment; as a result, outcomes can be optimized. We describe each stage below, including client behaviours that can be reliably rated by clinicians to facilitate team-based decision-making (McHugo et al, 1995).

The first stage of dual disorder treatment is the *engagement stage*. Before any effective treatment can be provided, clients need to be engaged, and a therapeutic relationship must be established. Therefore, the goal of the engagement stage is to establish a working alliance with the client that will serve as the basis for collaborative work. Successful engagement is defined as having regular meetings between the client and clinician for a significant period of time (e.g., 2 months). Examples of engagement strategies include assertive outreach, resolving a crisis or pressing issue (such as loss of housing), and social network support.

The second stage of treatment is the *persuasion stage*. Efforts to change behaviour cannot succeed unless the client views such change as desirable. Therefore, the goal of the persuasion stage is to help clients discover for themselves that the use of substances is problematic, and that decreasing substance use or attaining abstinence is in their best interest. Successful persuasion is defined as when clients begin to reduce their substance use, or show clear evidence of making concerted efforts to decrease the use of substances. Examples of persuasion strategies include psychiatric stabilization to address persistent symptoms, persuasion groups designed to create opportunities for clients to explore the effects of substance abuse on their lives in a supportive and non-confrontational setting, rehabilitation-based strategies designed to help clients learn more effective strategies for getting their needs met, psychoeducation about the interactions between mental illness and substance abuse, and motivational interviewing to help clients see how using substances interferes with their personal goals.

The third stage of treatment is the *active treatment stage*. When clients are sufficiently motivated to reduce their substance use, the goal of treatment shifts to reducing substance use. The goal of active treatment is to help the client further reduce substance use (preferably achieving abstinence) to the point where the individual no longer experiences substance abuse problems. Examples of active treatment strategies include self-monitoring urges to use substances and actual use of substances; cognitive-behavioural substance abuse counselling to address cravings to use in high-risk situations for use; self-help groups (e.g., Alcoholics Anonymous) to support abstinence; and rehabilitation-based interventions to address persistent symptoms, socialization needs, and recreation needs related to substance use.

The final stage of substance abuse treatment is the *relapse prevention stage*. Clients have progressed from active treatment to relapse prevention when they have not met criteria for substance use disorder for more than 6 months. The goals of the relapse prevention stage are to maintain awareness of the possibility of substance abuse relapse and to expand the client's recovery to other areas of functioning, including health (e.g., diet, exercise, smoking); social relationships; independent living; and work, school, or parenting. Examples of relapse prevention strategies include participation in self-help groups, supported employment to address work-related goals, and cognitive behavioural strategies to address social and independent living skills.

REDUCTION OF NEGATIVE CONSEQUENCES

Reducing the negative consequences of substance abuse, such as homelessness, infectious diseases, and exposure to violence, is an important goal of integrated dual disorder treatment (Carey, 1996a). Examples of harm-reduction strategies include providing clients with clean hypodermic needles to avoid the spread of diseases through contaminated needles, teaching safe sex practices to persons who exchange sex for drugs, encouraging clients to substitute a less destructive substance for a more destructive one, and securing safe housing to avoid victimization related to substance abuse on the street (Denning, 2001; Marlatt, 1998).

Minimizing the harmful effects of substance abuse in clients with dual disorders is often helpful in engaging clients in treatment; as clients experience the benefits of working with a caring professional, a therapeutic relationship evolves, and with this relationship, motivation to address destructive substance abuse habits grows. Many clients with dual disorders succeed in overcoming their substance abuse problems through the process of gradually reducing their substance use, rather than immediately endorsing abstinence as a goal. Focusing initially on collaborating with clients to reduce the negative effects of substances on their lives helps to gradually build motivation for reducing substance use, while avoiding unnecessary and potentially destructive confrontation over the issue of abstinence.

MULTIPLE PSYCHOTHERAPEUTIC MODALITIES

Integrated dual disorder treatment programmes benefit from having a variety of different psychotherapeutic modalities available. Individual, group, and family treatment modalities all have unique advantages, and being able to provide all three modalities in a system of care results in maximal flexibility for meeting clients' needs. Clients may benefit from participating in any one of the different treatment modalities, or a combination of modalities.

Individual treatment approaches, including cognitive-behavioural substance abuse counselling (Marlatt and Gordan, 1985) and motivational interviewing (Miller and Rollnick, 1991), have the advantage of focusing solely on the client's needs in the context of a therapeutic relationship. The attainment of specific skills or motivation is facilitated by the narrow focus on just one client in an individual treatment format. Early motivational work with clients is especially convenient to do in an individual format.

Group treatment approaches may be more economical, and provide unique opportunities for support from other clients and role models of clients in later stages of treatment. Several group treatment modalities have been developed in New Hampshire, including stage-wise treatment groups and social skills training groups (Mueser and Noordsy, 1996). Stage-wise treatment groups are aimed at addressing the needs of clients primarily in the persuasion stage of treatment, or the active treatment or relapse prevention stages. In *persuasion groups* (when clients are not yet motivated to work on their substance abuse problems), a non-confrontational approach is taken to developing a group milieu in which clients are encouraged to talk about their substance use, their mental illness, and their lives in a supportive environment that is conducive to exploring both positive and negative aspects of substance abuse. In *active treatment groups* (when clients want to achieve sobriety, and have made progress in reducing substance use or attaining abstinence), clients focus on supporting each other's sobriety goals, with cognitive-behavioural strategies often used to deal with cravings, high-risk situations, and partial or full relapses. Social skills training groups help clients to develop more effective interpersonal skills for getting their social needs met and dealing with substance abuse situations.

Family intervention is a critical treatment modality because of the high level of contact between clients with dual disorders and their relatives (Clark, 1996), increased family conflict caused by the presence of substance abuse in clients with severe mental illness (Dixon et al, 1995; Salyers and Mueser, 2001), and the problem of loss of family support leading to homelessness in this population (Caton, 1995). Family treatment is aimed at developing a collaborative relationship with the family, providing education and dual disorders, and using problem-solving training to reduce substance abuse and its negative effects on the family (Mueser and Fox, 2002). Family work is most successful when it strives to improve the functioning of all family members, and is not focused solely on the client.

LONG-TERM PERSPECTIVE

Integrated treatment services take a long-term perspective on intervention for persons with dual disorders. Artificial constraints on the length of dual disorder programmes are avoided because they fail to take the needs of individual clients into account, and they ignore the reality that both mental illness and substance abuse are often chronic and relapsing disorders that persist over significant periods of time. Long-term studies of integrated treatment programmes provide encouragement that many clients experience sustained remissions of their substance abuse over extended periods of time (Drake et al, 1998b). As severe mental illness typically requires long-term pharmacological and psychosocial treatment (Bellack and Mueser, 1993), it is no great surprise that dual disorders do as well.

STATEWIDE TRAINING IN INTEGRATED TREATMENT OF DUAL DISORDERS

Throughout the development of integrated treatment services in New Hampshire, the feasibility and effectiveness of several different approaches to training clinicians were explored. First, a clinician-researcher with expertise in the treatment of dual disorders was assigned to consult with each of the 10 mental health centres to help them develop appropriate services and to train clinicians. This approach proved unsuccessful, as the clinician-researcher's time was spread too thinly across the different mental health centres and not enough time was allowed to establish trust, leading to burnout of the clinician-researcher.

The second approach was a "train-the-trainers" method in which at least one expert ("trainer") at each mental health centre was designated to participate in a series of trainings in dual disorder treatment by the clinician-researcher expert, with the expectation that those newly trained trainers would conduct regular, ongoing trainings and supervision of clinicians at each centre. The approach also proved unsuccessful; while most trainers conducted initial trainings in dual disorder treatment at their mental health centres, there was poor follow-through on providing regular supervision to clinicians, resulting in minimal sustained change in treatment practices.

The third approach involved conducting central trainings and supervisory meetings at the New Hampshire-Dartmouth Psychiatric Research Center, in which clinicians and supervisors from each mental health centre were invited to participate on a monthly basis. At first, these trainings focused on didactic presentations about the core principles of dual disorder treatment, but they rapidly shifted to an interactive forum in which clinicians could share their treatment experiences and receive peer supervision from one another. These meetings also included occasional didactic presentations on special topics, invited speakers, and case consultations involving live interviews. In addition, clients were invited to attend and participate in some of these meetings, to share their experiences in receiving dual disorder treatment, to describe their personal experiences of recovery, to give tips to clinicians, and to answer questions. Teams of clinicians who participated in these trainings were successful in grasping the basic concepts and clinical skills of integrated treatment, and honing their skills over time through the process of ongoing feedback, sharing with other clinicians and continued training experiences.

RESEARCH ON DUAL DISORDERS

As part of the public academic liaison that first stimulated interest in the treatment of dual disorders in New Hampshire, mental health centres throughout the state have served as minilaboratories for the development and evaluation of promising interventions for dual disorders. The principles of Assertive Community Treatment were first adapted to address the problem of integrated treatment for dual disorders in New Hampshire, with a small pilot study showing excellent rates of substance abuse remission over 4 years (Drake et al, 1993). This study was followed up by a large multicentre controlled study comparing the Assertive Community Treatment model with standard case management for the delivery of integrated dual disorder treatment. The findings indicated modest advantages for the Assertive Community Treatment approach in achieving better outcomes for alcohol use disorders, and good substance abuse outcomes across both programmes, probably due to treatment diffusion (Drake et al, 1998a). Of particular importance, higher fidelity to the Assertive Community Treatment programme across the different mental health centres was associated with better outcomes (McHugo et al, 1999).

Several other pilot studies in the area of dual disorder treatment have also shown positive results. One naturalistic follow-up study of clients conditionally discharged from the state mental hospital and monitored closely as outpatients (a legal procedure similar to outpatient commitment) found significant decreases over 2 years in substance abuse problems (O'Keefe et al, 1997). Second, a study examined the effects of clozapine on substance abuse in clients with schizophrenia or schizoaffective disorder (Drake et al, 2000). Among 151 clients with dual disorders, the 36 clients who received clozapine demonstrated significantly better alcoholism outcomes than the other clients who did not receive clozapine (79% versus 34% remission for 6 months or more). Third, a study evaluated the outcomes of 33 clients with severe mental illness and alcohol use disorders who were prescribed disulfiram for their alcoholism. The results indicated that disulfiram was associated with significant remissions in alcohol abuse over the subsequent 3 years (64% of clients achieved a remission of their alcohol use disorder for 1 year or more) and that, contrary to expectations, few side effects or episodes of drinking while on disulfiram were observed (Mueser et al, in press). A fourth study involved the development of a family intervention programme for dual disorders, with a pilot test indicating that the programme was associated with high rates of substance abuse remission in clients with dual disorders over 2 years of treatment (Mueser and Fox, 2002). A fifth study employed a quasi-experimental design to compare the effects of a short-term residential programme (3–4 months) for dual disorders with a long-term programme, the Gemini House programme (2 years). In addition to its longer-term nature, Gemini House also provided a gradual transition for all clients from the residence back into the community. The results indicated that more clients in the long-term programme were successfully engaged in treatment, and they had better substance abuse outcomes, than clients in the short-term programme, whereas clients in the two programmes did not differ in symptom and hospitalization outcomes (Brunette et al, 2001).

The success of developing dual disorder programmes in New Hampshire has been followed by controlled research conducted outside New Hampshire in urban areas with higher proportions of minority clients. Several controlled studies have been conducted or are under way in cities throughout the USA, including Washington, DC; Hartford and Bridgeport, CT; Boston, MA; Los Angeles, CA; St Louis, MO; and Austin, TX. In addition, programmes in New Hampshire and related programmes in urban settings have been frequently visited over the past decade by clinicians and mental health authorities from other states and countries. Thus, while the state and population base of New Hampshire is small, by developing and studying new interventions in real world settings, and exploring their applicability in different settings with different client populations, new and effective dual disorder services have been developed and continue to be refined in an on-going, evolutionary process.

CONCLUSIONS

The public academic liaison established between the New Hampshire Division of Behavioral Health and the New Hampshire-Dartmouth Psychiatric Research Center has led to the development of guiding principles for integrated dual disorder treatment. While the principles of treatment remain much the same as they have over the past 15 years, the actual practices have evolved as clinicians and researchers working together have developed interventions to address specific problems in populations of dual disorder clients. The combination of research and clinical practice in typical mental health centre settings has been fruitful for the clients in the state, the mental health administrators, and the field at large. The New Hampshire experience supports the common observation that applied research in clinical settings often improves the overall standard of care for clients in those settings, as well as for other clients who are the beneficiaries of research as clinical practice improves, based on an understanding of what works.

REFERENCES

Anthony, W.A. (2000) A recovery-oriented service system: setting some system level standards. *Journal of Psychiatric Rehabilitation*, **24**: 159–168.
Bellack, A.S. and Mueser, K.T. (1993) Psychosocial treatment for schizophrenia. *Schizophrenia Bulletin*, **19**: 317–336.
Bond, G.R., Becker, D.R., Drake, R.E., Rapp, C.A., Meisler, N., Lehman, A.F., Bell, M.D. and Blyler, C.R. (2001a) Implementing supported employment as an evidence-based practice. *Psychiatric Services*, **52**: 313–322.
Bond, G.R., Drake, R.E., Mueser, K.T. and Latimer, E. (2001b) Assertive community treatment for people with severe mental illness: critical ingredients and impact on clients. *Disease Management and Health Outcomes*, **9**: 141–159.
Brunette, M.F., Drake, R.E., Woods, M., and Hartnett, T. (2001) A comparison of long-term and short-term residential treatment programs for dual diagnosis patients. *Psychiatric Services*, **52**: 526–528.
Carey, K.B. (1996a) Substance use reduction in the context of outpatient psychiatric treatment: a collaborative, motivational, harm reduction approach. *Community Mental Health Journal*, **32**: 291–306.
Carey, K.B. (1996b) Treatment of co-occurring substance abuse and major mental illness. In R.E. Drake and K.T. Mueser (Eds.), *Dual Diagnosis of Major Mental Illness and Substance Abuse: Volume 2: Recent Research and Clinical Implications* (Vol. 70, pp. 19–31). San Francisco, CA, Jossey-Bass.
Caton, C.L.M. (1995) Mental Health service use among homeless and never-homeless men with schizophrenia. *Psychiatric Services*, **46**: 1139–1143.
Clark, R.E. (1996) Family support for persons with dual disorders. In R.E. Drake and K.T. Mueser (Eds.), *Dual Diagnosis of Major Mental Illness and Substance Abuse Disorder II: Recent Research and Clinical Implications. New Directions for Mental Health Services* (Vol. 70, pp. 65–77). San Francisco, CA, Jossey-Bass.
Denning, P. (2001) *Practicing Harm Reduction Psychotherapy: An Alternative Approach to Addictions*. New York, Guilford.
Dixon, L., McFarlane, W., Lefley, H., Lucksted, A., Cohen, C., Falloon, I., Mueser, K.T., Miklowitz, D., Solomon, P. and Sondheimer, D. (2001) Evidence-based practices for services to family members of people with psychiatric disabilities. *Psychiatric Services*, **52**: 903–910.
Dixon, L., McNary, S., and Lehman, A. (1995) Substance abuse and family relationships of persons with severe mental illness. *American Journal of Psychiatry*, **152**: 456–458.
Drake, R.E., Antosca, L.M., Noordsy, D.L., Bartels, S.J. and Osher, F.C. (1991) New Hampshire's specialized services for the dually diagnosed. In K. Minkoff and R.E. Drake (Eds.), *New Directions for Mental Health Services* (Vol. 50, pp. 57–67). San Francisco, CA, Jossey-Bass.

Drake, R.E., McHugo, G., and Noordsy, D.L. (1993) Treatment of alcoholism among schizophrenic outpatients: four-year outcomes. *American Journal of Psychiatry*, **150**: 328–329.

Drake, R.E., McHugo, G.J., Clark, R.E., Teague, G.B., Xie, H., Miles, K. and Ackerson, T.H. (1998a) Assertive community treatment for patients with co-occurring severe mental illness and substance use disorder: a clinical trial. *American Journal of Orthopsychiatry*, **68**: 201–215.

Drake, R.E., Mercer-McFadden, C., Mueser, K.T., McHugo, G.J. and Bond, G.R. (1998b) Review of integrated mental health and substance abuse treatment for patients with dual disorders. *Schizophrenia Bulletin*, **24**: 589–608.

Drake, R.E., Xie, H., McHugo, G.J. and Green, A.I. (2000) The effects of clozapine on alcohol and drug use disorders among schizophrenic patients. *Schizophrenia Bulletin*, **26**: 441–449.

Heinssen, R.K., Liberman, R.P. and Kopelowicz, A. (2000) Psychosocial skills training for schizophrenia: lessons from the laboratory. *Schizophrenia Bulletin*, **26**: 21–46.

Marlatt, G.A. (Ed.). (1998) *Harm Reduction: Pragmatic Strategies for Managing High-Risk Behaviors*. New York, Guilford.

Marlatt, G.A. and Gordan, G.R. (1985) *Relapse Prevention: Maintenance Strategies in the Treatment of Addictive Behaviors*. New York, Guilford.

McHugo, G.J., Drake, R.E., Burton, H.L. and Ackerson, T.H. (1995) A scale for assessing the stage of substance abuse treatment in persons with severe mental illness. *Journal of Nervous and Mental Disease*, **183**: 762–767.

McHugo, G.J., Drake, R.E., Teague, G.B. and Xie, H. (1999) Fidelity to assertive community treatment and client outcomes in the New Hampshire dual disorders study. *Psychiatric Services*, **50**: 818–824.

Mercer-McFadden, C. and Drake, R.E. (1995) *Review and Summaries: National Demonstration of Services for Young Adults with Severe Mental Illness and Substance Abuse*. Rockville, MD, Center for Mental Health Services, Substance Abuse and Mental Health Services Administration.

Mercer-McFadden, C., Drake, R.E., Clark, R.E., Verven, N., Noordsy, D.L. and Fox, T.S. (1998) *Substance Abuse Treatment for People with Severe Mental Disorders: A Program Manager's Guide*. Concord, NH, New Hampshire-Dartmouth Psychiatric Research Center.

Miller, W.R. and Rollnick, S. (1991) *Motivational Interviewing: Preparing People to Change Addictive Behavior*. New York, Guilford.

Minkoff, K. (1991) Program components of a comprehensive integrated care system for seriously mentally ill patients with substance disorders. In K. Minkoff and R.E. Drake (Eds.), *Dual Diagnosis of Major Mental Illness and Substance Disorders. New Directions for Mental Health Services* (Vol. 50, pp. 13–27). San Francisco, CA, Jossey-Bass.

Mueser, K.T., Drake, R.E. and Noordsy, D.L. (1998) Integrated mental health and substance abuse treatment for severe psychiatric disorders. *Practical Psychiatry and Behavioral Health*, **4**: 129–139.

Mueser, K.T., Essock, S.M., Drake, R.E., Wolfe, R.S. and Frisman, L. (2001) Rural and urban differences in dually diagnosed patients: implications for service needs. *Schizophrenia Research*, **48**: 93–107.

Mueser, K.T. and Fox, L. (2002) A family intervention program for dual disorders. *Community Mental Health Journal*, **38**: 253–270.

Mueser, K.T. and Noordsy, D.L. (1996) Group treatment for dually diagnosed clients. In R.E. Drake and K.T. Mueser (Eds.), *Dual Diagnosis of Major Mental Illness and Substance Abuse Disorder II: Recent Research and Clinical Implications*.

New Directions for Mental Health Services (Vol. 70, pp. 33–51). San Francisco, CA, Jossey-Bass.

Mueser, K.T., Noordsy, D.L., Fox, L. and Wolfe, R. (2002, in press) Disulfiram treatment for alcoholism in severe mental illness. *American Journal on the Addictions.*

Mueser, K.T., Yarnold, P.R., Rosenberg, S.D., Swett, C., Miles, K.M. and Hill, D. (2000) Substance use disorder in hospitalized severely mentally ill psychiatric patients: prevalence, correlates, and subgroups. *Schizophrenia Bulletin,* **26**: 179–192.

O'Keefe, C., Potenza, D.P. and Mueser, K.T. (1997) Treatment outcomes for severely mentally ill patients on conditional discharge to community-based treatment. *Journal of Nervous and Mental Disease,* **185**: 109–111.

Osher, F.C. and Dixon, L.B. (1996) Housing for persons with co-occurring mental and addictive disorders. In R.E. Drake and K.T. Mueser (Eds.), *Dual Diagnosis of Major Mental Illness and Substance Abuse Disorder II: Recent Research and Clinical Implications. New Directions for Mental Health Services* (Vol. 70, pp. 53–64). San Francisco, CA, Jossey-Bass.

Osher, F.C. and Kofoed, L.L. (1989) Treatment of patients with psychiatric and psychoactive substance use disorders. *Hospital and Community Psychiatry,* **40**: 1025–1030.

Polcin, D.L. (1992) Issues in the treatment of dual diagnosis clients who have chronic mental illness. *Professional Psychology: Research and Practice,* **23**: 30–37.

Prochaska, J.O., DiClemente, C.C. and Norcross, J.C. (1992) In search of how people change: applications to addictive behaviors. *American Psychologist,* **47**: 1102–1114.

Prochaska, J.O., Norcross, J.C. and DiClemente, C.C. (1994). *Changing for Good.* New York, Avon Books.

Ridgely, M.S., Goldman, H.H. and Willenbring, M. (1990) Barriers to the care of persons with dual diagnoses: organizational and financing issues. *Schizophrenia Bulletin,* **16**: 123–132.

Rosenberg, S.D., Goodman, L.A., Osher, F.C., Swartz, M., Essock, S.M., Butterfield, M.I., Constantine, N.T., Wolford, G.L. and Salyers, M.P. (2001) Prevalence of HIV, hepatitis B and hepatitis C in people with severe mental illness. *American Journal of Public Health,* **91**: 31–37.

Rush, A.J., Rago, W.V., Crismon, M.L., Toprac, M.G., Shon, S.P., Suppes, T., Miller, A.L., Trivedi, M.H., Swann, A.C., Biggs, M.M., Shores-Wilson, K., Kashner, T.M., Pigott, T., Chiles, J.A., Gilbert, D.A. and Altshuler, K.Z. (1999) Medication treatment for the severely and persistently mentally ill: the Texas Medication Algorithm Project. *Journal of Clinical Psychiatry,* **60**: 284–291.

Salyers, M.P. and Mueser, K.T. (2001) Social functioning, psychopathology, and medication side effects in relation to substance use and abuse in schizophrenia. *Schizophrenia Research,* **48**: 109–123.

Ziedonis, D. and Fisher, W. (1996) Motivation-based assessment and treatment of substance abuse in patients with schizophrenia. *Directions in Psychiatry,* **16**: 1–7.

Chapter 7

THE COMBINED PSYCHOSIS AND SUBSTANCE USE (COMPASS) PROGRAMME: AN INTEGRATED SHARED-CARE APPROACH

Hermine L. Graham, Alex Copello, Max J. Birchwood, Jenny Maslin, Dermot McGovern, Jim Orford and George Georgiou

This chapter will outline the development and evaluation of a community-based intervention for clients with severe mental health problems who use drugs and/or alcohol problematically. The intervention was a strategic response to an identified need within a statutory provider of mental health and substance misuse services, in an inner-city area of Birmingham, UK. In addition, we will seek to describe the context in which these service developments occurred and the factors that influenced the development of this integrated shared-care approach.

THE SERVICE CONTEXT: NORTHERN BIRMINGHAM MENTAL HEALTH SERVICES

As part of the shift within the UK to deliver community-based treatment services for people who experience severe mental health problems (National Service Framework, Department of Health [DOH], 1999), the Northern Birmingham Mental Health NHS Trust (NBMHT) has evolved into a provider of well-developed, functionalized community mental health teams. These teams have been derived from community-based

Substance Misuse in Psychosis: Approaches to Treatment and Service Delivery.
Edited by Hermine L. Graham, Alex Copello, Max J. Birchwood and Kim T. Mueser.
© 2003 John Wiley & Sons, Ltd.

treatment models developed specifically to improve the treatment and re-covery of people who experience the range of mental health problems, and underpin the structure of mental health services, as outlined in the National Health Service (NHS) Plan (2000). Specialized in function and tailored to the needs and profile of particular client groups with mental health difficul-ties, these teams include Primary Care Liaison Mental Health Teams, Home Treatment Teams, Rehabilitation and Recovery Teams, and Assertive Out-reach Teams. The Primary Care Liaison Teams are the first point of contact with mental health services, working closely with general practitioners to assess the level of input needed, and referring on if appropriate. The Home Treatment Teams are based on the psychiatric emergency teams model originally developed by Hoult and Reynolds (1984) and Dean and Gadd (1990). These teams aim to provide an alternative to inpatient admission and respond with intensive input during a crisis. The Rehabilitation and Recovery Teams provide long-term support and mental health treatment to facilitate the "recovery" of people with severe mental health problems. The Assertive Outreach Teams are based on the assertive community treatment model (Stein and Test, 1980; McGrew and Bond, 1995; Drake and Burns, 1995). They provide intensive case management to those with severe men-tal health problems who have a history of poor engagement with treat-ment services, high relapse and rehospitalization rates, and a forensic/risk history. The catchment area of the NBMHT is broken down into six geo-graphically based localities. In each locality, there are four functionalized community mental health teams. The NBMHT also has specialist mental health services that cover the complete catchment area. These include an early intervention service for those experiencing their first episode of psy-chosis (Birchwood et al, 2001) and an assertive outreach team focused on people who are homeless. Some inpatient and respite facilities continue to be available for those people who are unable to be treated in the community.

The NBMHT is also a provider of community-based treatment services for those who use drugs and alcohol problematically. These services de-liver care in parallel to the functionalized mental health services. Although some level of liaison existed historically, this has been strengthened since the development of the COMPASS Programme, as described later. The Substance Misuse Services comprise four geographically-based commu-nity drug teams and one community alcohol team. Specialist services that cover the complete catchment area include a community drug team focused on the needs of those who use crack-cocaine problematically. The Substance Misuse Services are based on a social learning model approach to substance use (McMurran, 1997), and a harm reduction philosophy (Marlatt, 1998). Thus, they are not focused on complete abstinence but offer a range of interventions to reduce the overall harm associated with drug/alcohol use (Wilks, 1989). These services can be accessed either directly or via a referral from a professional. A trust-wide specialist tertiary service (the Addictive Behaviour Centre) is also available for those with substance use problems who also have psychiatric or other complex or specialist needs (i.e., mother and baby services). The Addictive Behaviour Centre also includes a 12-bed inpatient facility.

The NBMHT provides mental health and substance misuse services to a catchment population of approximately 570 000 in an urban area of the UK. The area is inner city and has been classified as one of high social deprivation, ranking fifth in the country (Department of the Environment, Transport and the Regions, 1998). Currently, unemployment rates among different localities in the region are in the range of 5–28%. The area is also a blend of cultural/racial groups, and "minority populations" (Asian, from the Indian subcontinent, and Black, typically African-Caribbean) comprise 3–69% in the different localities of the region (1991 Census).

CONTEXTUAL FACTORS INFLUENCING THE COMPASS PROGRAMME'S MODEL OF SERVICE DELIVERY

A general increase in the availability and use of drugs and alcohol (Parker et al, 1998) has inevitably meant that people with severe mental health problems are increasingly exposed to drugs and alcohol and are more at risk of becoming involved in problematic drug use (Smith and Hucker, 1993; Marshall, 1998; Johnson, 1997). The move towards community-based treatment for those with severe mental health problems has contributed to a heightened awareness of problematic drug and alcohol use among this group and its negative impact on treatment and recovery (Blowers, 1998). In addition, the use of alcohol and drugs has also been highlighted as a risk factor in a number of highly publicized homicides carried out by those with severe mental health problems in the UK (Ward and Applin, 1998). Such factors have contributed to an acute awareness among clinicians and service providers of the need to address problematic drug and alcohol use among those with severe mental health problems.

In common with the situation elsewhere, it became apparent that the needs of those with severe mental health problems who use drugs/alcohol problematically were not being met by the existing separate service provision (Drake et al, 2001). Four main factors were identified as contributing to this. First, within the NBMHT, as previously outlined, services for the treatment of substance misuse were provided in parallel to mental health treatment. Thus, substance misuse and mental health services, although provided by the same organization, were structurally and geographically separate. As this client group did not fit neatly into these well-defined services, they often fell somewhere between the two. In addition, liaison between the two types of services was variable, depending on who dealt with the enquiry or referral.

The second factor was that the treatment and engagement philosophies of the two types of services differed significantly. Mental health services tended to adopt a more assertive approach to engaging clients in treatment, whether clients felt they had mental health problems or not. In contrast, substance misuse services in the UK have typically required clients to be motivated for change as a prerequisite for treatment services to be offered. A common pattern would have been for persons with severe mental health diagnoses who did not perceive themselves as having a mental health problem or regard their drug use as problematic to be assertively engaged in mental health treatment by a mental health team. However, they would be reluctant to accept treatment and generally would engage poorly. In addition, they would be referred to substance misuse services to tackle their "drug problem". Typically, they would be poorly engaged with the mental health team and hence be unlikely to attend a community drug team. Consequently, the drug team would respond by highlighting their difficulty in offering treatment to people who are "unmotivated" or "pre-contemplative", fuelling frustration on both sides. It is important to add that there has also been a tendency for mental health services to disown some drug users, putting problems down to a "drug psychosis", based on an either or conceptualization of the cause of psychosis.

The third factor was that the focus of the two types of services, in terms of assessment and treatment, was on either mental health or substance use. Finally, the fourth factor was that a major disparity existed between the availability of skilled staff and the needs of people with both substance use and mental health problem. Each service tended to focus on its area of expertise, and staff generally lacked the confidence, skills and basic awareness of the other area. (Maslin et al, 2001).

The major unmet need for substance misuse treatment for people with severe mental health problems was the backdrop for a fundamental shift in service provision. The NBMHT's plan to address this shortfall of services was to develop a new initiative, spearheaded by the COMPASS Programme, aimed at integrating current service provision for this client group. Extra resources were made available through an application for centrally allocated resources. A multiagency steering group and a number of groups within the NBMHT were put in place to direct and facilitate the development of this initiative.

A number of issues emerged from a review of the literature and a visit to seven services in the USA, providing a range of treatment approaches for those with severe mental health and substance use problems that guided the model of service delivery forming the basis of the COMPASS Programme. These included the paucity of UK prevalence and treatment evaluation studies and the contextual differences between service provisions in the UK and the USA. The lack of studies in the UK meant that there was insufficient information on national and, in particular, local prevalence rates of problem substance use among those with severe mental health problems to guide local service developments. On visiting services in the USA, it became clear that a lot could be learned from these services and treatment approaches. However, these models could not be wholly imported and implemented in the UK due to significant differences in the contextual factors that guide service provision in the two countries. For example, in the USA, treatment is funded by medical insurance, a fact which means that treatment typically has to be well defined, in some residential programmes is time-limited, and is provided by an independently operating treatment provider to maximize funding and minimize costs. In contrast, treatment services in the UK are provided as part of the National Health Service, funding is not time-limited, and the services are to some extent centrally controlled.

In the USA, the integrated models that have been developed for the treatment of problem substance use among those with severe mental health problems have been based on improving the skills of clinicians in mental health teams to tackle drug/alcohol problems to the exclusion of specialist substance misuse services. The rationale behind this can be attributed to the confrontational, abstinence, disease model that has historically been adopted in the USA by substance misuse treatment services (Edwards, 1992; Smith and Hucker, 1993). Thus, integrated "dual diagnosis" services in the USA have sought to facilitate the use of more harm-minimization, motivational-based approaches, as the client group often found the approaches of their substance use treatment services, typically based on the disease model, too confrontational (Mueser et al, 1998; Ziedonis and Trudeau, 1997; Carey, 1996). However, in the UK, the harm-minimization approach is predominant and has traditionally been adopted by substance misuse services. In addition, these services are often provided by statutory agencies. Thus, in the NBMHT, it was not necessary to develop services for this client group wholly separate from existing substance misuse services on the grounds of either finance or treatment philosophy. The principles of "integrated treatment" (Mueser et al, 1998; Drake et al, 2001) were, to some extent, easy to integrate with the philosophy of our substance misuse services.

A further factor in the USA influencing the delivery of services that differs significantly from the UK is the common use of legislation in relation to state benefits. Such laws enable health professionals/treatment agencies to gain legal control over a client's state benefits. Payeeships are often used by clinicians, who act as a representative payee, to manage clients' money and hook them into treatment (Shaner et al, 1997; Ries and Dyck, 1997; Satel, 1998). Some services visited in the USA were inpatient/residential treatment programmes with day facilities (e.g., Greenfield et al, 1995); others were outpatient oriented. Those based on the New Hampshire model are community-based similar to that used in the UK, as described in Chapter 6.

The contextual differences between the USA and the UK highlighted the need for UK-relevant solutions.

DEFINING THE PROBLEM

The strategic plan incorporated a first stage of mapping local need, which included assessments of prevalence and associated clinical correlates, staff training, and support needs. The results of these assessments revealed a 1-year prevalence rate of combined problems of 24% (324/1369) across the NBMHT's community-based mental health and substance misuse services (Graham et al, 2001). The largest proportion of those with severe mental health problems who used drugs/alcohol in an impaired/dependent pattern (abuse/dependence as classified by DSM-IV) were located within the Assertive Outreach Teams (up to 41% of the teams' caseloads). This was not surprising, as problematic use of substances is one of the criteria for assertive outreach teams. These clients were typically white males, in their mid-thirties. The two most commonly used substances were alcohol and cannabis, with a significant proportion using crack-cocaine. Polysubstance use was common with this client group, who were often using 2–7 substances simultaneously.

The results of an assessment of the training and support needs of 136 community-based clinicians supporting these clients revealed that they often came into contact with this client group, were interested in working with these clients and saw it as part of their role. However, they felt they needed more information and training to improve their knowledge and skills to enable them to work confidently with this client group. Typically, substance use problems were not addressed in mental health services/teams (Maslin et al, 2001).

THE COMPASS PROGRAMME: AN INTEGRATED "SHARED-CARE" TREATMENT APPROACH

An "integrated shared care" model was developed that sought to "meet the unmet needs of this client group" and complement the existing service provision within the NBMHT. The model aims to achieve integration of

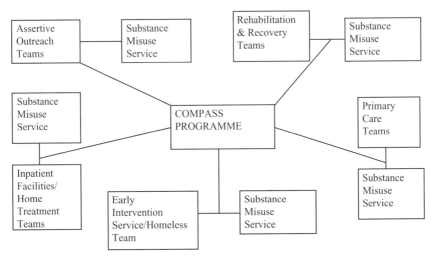

Figure 7.1   COMPASS Programme: NBMHT Integrated shared care model

treatment at the level of both the clinician and the service. The key principle underlying this integration is that both the mental health and substance use problems and the relationship between the two are addressed simultaneously. The main thrust of this model is that this work with a client out is carried by one clinician. However, if, in some cases, it may be necessary that more specialist input is required, this can be achieved via shared care between mental health and addiction services, as illustrated in Figure 7.1. Sharing care between service levels means that there needs to be in place agreed protocols for closer and/or joint working between mental health and substance misuse services.

Overall, the focus of the COMPASS Programme is on training and coworking, with staff in the teams supporting those with severe mental health problems. In addition, it aims to build bridges between substance misuse and mental health services. The COMPASS Programme developed a "hub and spoke" model of service delivery (see Figure 7.1), as opposed to creating an additional specialist third service that took on a caseload. Thus, the COMPASS Programme evolved as a specialist multidisciplinary team that aims to train and support existing mental health and substance misuse services to provide integrated treatment, where appropriate to their client group. As such, we are working toward a situation where clients with mental health problems remain engaged and are case-managed within mental health, and, if necessary, the client's care is shared with substance misuse services. This has been achieved to a greater extent in the Assertive Outreach Teams. In the other teams/services, the focus is on facilitating closer working between services.

STAFF: THE COMPASS PROGRAMME TEAM

The COMPASS Programme's multidisciplinary team consists of six clinicial staff; one consultant clinical psychologist/head of programme, one research psychologist, three senior graded community psychiatric nurses, and one senior occupational therapist, with sessional support from a consultant psychiatrist working with the substance misuse services.

INTERVENTIONS

Outlined below are the two main services that have been developed and are being evaluated by the COMPASS Programme, namely, intensive intervention in the Assertive Outreach Teams and a consultation-liaison service.

WORKING WITH THE ASSERTIVE OUTREACH TEAMS

Two key issues led to the deployment of the bulk of the resources to conduct more intensive work within the Assertive Outreach Teams in the NBMHT. First, there was the higher prevalence of more complex and severe problems within these teams (Graham et al, 2001). Second, there was the need for service users with severe and enduring mental health problems to remain engaged and be case-managed within the Assertive Outreach Teams. These teams are being trained intensively to provide integrated treatment for problematic substance use alongside other needs that are routinely met. In order to achieve the required level of competence in delivering this integrated treatment, members of the COMPASS Programme team are allocated to work alongside and to train members of the Assertive Outreach Teams and in some instances work jointly on specific cases.

Intervention model

The intervention cognitive-behavioural integrated treatment (C-BIT) is an approach specifically designed to help clinicians to engage and work with clients who have severe mental health problems and use drugs/alcohol problematically, particularly those clients who do not initially perceive substance use as problematic. It is in essence an approach that helps clinicians to put substance use on the agenda. It encourages clients to begin to think about the negative impact of problematic use on areas of their life including mental health, and physical and social well-being (Graham et al, unpublished). This treatment approach is described in more detail in Chapter 11.

The aim of this intervention is to reduce the harm associated with problematic drug/alcohol use in this client group and promote self-management of psychosis/substance use and recovery.

Training

All Assertive Outreach Team members are trained to use this manualized treatment approach over an intensive 7-day period. This is followed by clinicians from the COMPASS Programme team being placed in each of the Assertive Outreach Teams to work alongside the team members for 2 days of the week on a long-term basis. The role of these clinicians is to provide on-going training (through modelling the skills embodied in the C-BIT approach) and wider support to the Assertive Outreach Team. The COMPASS Programme team member works jointly with each case manager as coworker within the Assertive Outreach Team to develop individualized treatment plans to address problematic substance use in conjunction with mental health, social problems and other difficulties for those clients identified as having severe mental health and substance use problems. This is incorporated within the client's overall "Care Plan" (i.e., a coordinated case-management plan designed to address the individual needs of clients).

The COMPASS Programme team members also aim to facilitate, within their allocated teams monthly case discussions to highlight any difficulties encountered in attempting to engage clients in addressing their drug/alcohol use; review how they have utilized the C-BIT approach and for the Assertive Outreach Team to identify the best way forward; and encourage fidelity to the C-BIT approach and team approach. Where appropriate, the COMPASS Programme team member may also liase with substance misuse services if more specialist input is required (i.e., substitute prescribing, detoxification, and residential rehabilitation). This is achieved through the COMPASS Programme consultant psychiatrist or designated liaison clinicians in the community drug/alcohol teams.

Evaluation

This model is being evaluated over a 2-year period, details of the evaluation of which are presented in Chapter 11.

CONSULTATION-LIAISON

The results of the assessment of prevalence in the NBMHT indicated that, although mental health teams (teams other than Assertive Outreach) and substance misuse services did not have the highest proportion of those with severe mental health and substance use problems, a number of clients with such combined problems were still present in these services (Graham et al, 2001). It was clear from consultations with these teams and services that they did not all require the intensive input of the Assertive Outreach Teams. However, they often experienced difficulties in accessing services and felt they lacked particular skills and knowledge to carry out specialist assessment of this client group and offer brief motivational-based interventions (Maslin et al, 2001). The initial consultation-liaison service offered by the COMPASS Programme was based on an adaptation of a model developed by Greenfield et al (1995). This service is offered to inpatient facilities as well as non-assertive outreach community mental health teams and substance misuse services within the NBMHT. Clinicians within these services can make specific requests for input from the COMPASS Programme, either an assessment and brief intervention or training and support.

Brief Intervention

Based on the initial pilot of the consultation-liaison service, it was felt necessary to improve the structure and focus of the assessments and brief interventions, offered as part of this service, and to make them time limited. From the developments in the area of brief interventions developed for substance use treatment (Miller et al, 1995; Franey and Thom, 1995; Richmond et al, 1995) and substance use in psychosis (Saunders et al, unpublished), a number of principles were incorporated into this service. The aim of the modified brief intervention is to engage clients in discussing their drug and/or alcohol use and mobilize their motivation, so that they are then able to makes changes appropriate to their stage of change. "Significant others" (if possible and appropriate) and key workers are included in the process. Key workers are involved in the intervention from the outset to ensure that there is joint ownership and that they feel able to continue the work once the COMPASS Programme is no longer involved. The inclusion of significant others is to promote social support, through the client's social network, for change.

The brief intervention is carried out over a 12-week period and comprises two sessions of a motivational enhancement intervention and two follow-up sessions. The treatment sessions are preceded by an in-depth assessment, carried out over two sessions, that includes the C-BIT assessment phase and a battery of assessment tools for the client and key worker. The results of the assessment are fed back to the client. The two motivational enhancement sessions include identifying negative consequences associated with use, reviewing the advantages and disadvantages of continued use, re-evaluation and modification of substance-related beliefs

(Beck et al, 1993), and reviewing the pros and cons of behaviour change and obstacles to behaviour change (Miller and Rollnick, 1991). The aims of these motivational sessions are to get a decision for change and build commitment to change. The two follow-up sessions focus on monitoring and encouraging progress.

Evaluation

A basic method of before and after series design (with multiple follow-up data points) is being utilized to evaluate the effectiveness of the pilot consultation-liaison service. When a request for assessment/treatment is made as part of the consultation-liaison service, a range of brief assessment tools are utilized as a way of establishing a baseline. They are then repeated at 3 and 6 months to evaluate outcome. The staff member who made the request is asked to complete the Clinicians' Rating Scale for Alcohol Use (CAUS) and Drug Use (CDUS) (Drake et al, 1996). This scale is based on DSM-IV diagnostic criteria for substance-related disorders and has been reliably used to classify the severity of substance use among people with severe mental health problems (Mueser et al, 1995). The staff member also completes the Substance Abuse Treatment Scale (SATS). This scale seeks to assess the extent to which clients are engaged in discussing their substance use or receiving substance abuse treatment (Drake et al, 1996).

Over the period of 1 year, 71 requests were made for the consultation-liaison service. The majority of these requests were for assessment and the brief intervention (61%). The main sources of requests were inpatient facilities, primary care mental health teams and community drug teams. The clients were mainly male (82%), with a mean age of 31 years. The two most commonly used substances by the clients in a problematic pattern were alcohol and cannabis. The majority were poly-drug users, and were using 2–6 drugs at the same time.

Training

As part of the consultation-liaison service, a two-staged training package was offered to the inpatient facilities and primary care mental health teams, the aim of which was to encourage integration of treatment at a basic level and to improve understanding and links with substance misuse services. The first stage of training involved an awareness raising session offered to all clinicians in the mental health inpatient facilities/community-based teams. This training included raising staff awareness of drugs and alcohol, and the use and problematic use of these substances. Raising awareness of the reasons for problematic substance use among those with severe mental health problems and its impact on mental health and functioning was also incorporated within this training. The second stage of training involved team/inpatient managers identifying two members of staff who would take a specialist interest/lead in this area and serve as a designated liaison person for other services, especially substance misuse services. These identified staff received the second stage of specialist training to support their inpatient facility/team. The focus of this skills-based training was to help the staff learn how to engage clients in talking about problematic substance use, build motivation to change, and screen and assess for problematic substance use and its relationship with mental health. This training was based on a brief version of the C-BIT approach encompassing components from Treatment Phase 1 and the Assessment Phase (for details, see Chapter 11). The aim was twofold. First, it was intended that these designated staff would eventually pass on their skills to other members of staff in the inpatient facilities/teams, supported by a designated COMPASS Programme team member to attend ward rounds/primary mental health team meetings on a regular basis. Second, it was intended that the designated staff members would act as formalized points of contact for substance misuse services/teams.

Similarly, mental health awareness-raising sessions were offered to substance misuse services. Community drug teams have identified staff members who have been designated as a liaison person/point of contact for the mental health teams/services. The aim of having designated liaison people in both mental health and substance misuse services is to have a point of contact within each service and a formalized link. This seeks to improve access to services, and movement between services, where appropriate, for this client group.

FUTURE DIRECTIONS

A number of developments have taken place within the COMPASS Programme since its inception. The programme is still in its early days, but a number of important lessons have been learned. Internationally, a number of "integrated" service models exist, some of which are being or have already been evaluated. However, there is a need for the development of service models in the UK that fit within the National Service Framework (DOH, 1999) and the NHS Plan (2000), are evaluated for effectiveness, and are tailored to local need. It is essential that developments within this area, particularly within the UK, lead to improvements in the pathways of care for people who experience severe mental health problems and use substances problematically, and the integration of treatment and continuity of care between substance misuse and mental health services.

ACKNOWLEDGEMENTS

We thank Professor Kim Mueser, Dartmouth, New Hampshire, USA, who has served as an external consultant in the development of this service model; Emma Atkinson, Mike Preece and Derek Tobin for their role in these developments, as part of the COMPASS Programme Team; and the Staff and service users in NBMHT for their continued support during the developmental process.

REFERENCES

Beck, A.T., Wright, F.D., Newman, C.F. and Liese, B. (1993) *Cognitive Therapy of Substance Use*. New York, Guilford.

Birchwood, M., Spencer, E. and McGovern, D. (2001) Schizophrenia: early warning signs. *Advances in Psychiatric Treatment*, **6**: 93–101.

Blowers, A.J. (1998) Drugs and mental health. *Mental Health Review*, **3**: 3–5.

Carey, K.B. (1996) Substance use reduction in the context of outpatient psychiatric treatment: a collaborative, motivational, harm reduction approach. *Community Mental Health Journal*, **32**: 291–306.

Dean, C. and Gadd, E.M. (1990) Home treatment for acute psychiatric illness. *British Medical Journal*, **301**: 1021–1023.

Department of the Environment, Transport and the Regions (1998) *Index of Local Deprivation*, UK.

DOH (1999) *National Service Framework for Mental Health: Modern Standards and Service Models*. Department of Health.

Drake, R., McHugo, G., Clark, R., Teague, G., Xie, H., Miles, K. and Ackerson, T. (1998) Assertive community treatment for patients with co-occuring severe mental illness and substance use disorder: a clinical trial. *American Orthopsychiatric Association*, **68**: 201–215.

Drake, R.E. and Burns, B.J. (1995) Special section on assertive community treatment: an introduction. *Psychiatric Services*, **46**: 667–668.

Drake, R.E., Essock, S.M., Shaner, A., Carey, K.B., Minkoff, K., Kola, L., Lynde, D., Osher, F.C., Clark, R.E. and Rickards, L. (2001) Implementing dual diagnosis services for clients with severe mental illness. *Psychiatric Services*, **52**: 469–476.

Drake, R.E., Mueser, K.T. and McHugo, G.J. (1996) Clinician rating scales: Alcohol Use Scale (AUS), Drug Use Scale (DUS) and Substance Abuse Treatment Scale (SATS). In L.I. Sederer and B. Dickey (Eds.), *Outcomes Assessment in Clinical Practice*. Baltimore, Williams & Wilkins.

Edwards, G. (1992) Problems and dependence: the history of the two dimensions. In M. Lader, G. Edwards and D.C. Drummond (Eds), *The Nature of Alcohol and Drug Related Problems*. Oxford, Medical Publications.

Franey, C. and Thom, B. (1995) The effectiveness of alcohol interventions. Centre for Research on Drugs and Health Behaviour, *Executive Summary, 38*.

Graham, H.L., Copello, C., Birchwood, Orford, J.M., McGovern, D. Atkinson, E., Maslin, J., Mueser, K., Preece, M., Tobin, D. and Georgiou, G. (Unpublished) Cognitive-behavioural integrated treatment: an approach for working with your clients who have severe mental health problems and use drugs/alcohol problematically. *Treatment Manual: COMPASS Programme*, Northern Birmingham Mental Health (NHS) Trust.

Graham, H.L., Maslin, J., Copello, C., Birchwood, M., Mueser, K., McGovern, D. and Georgiou, G. (2001) Drug and alcohol problems amongst individuals with severe mental health problems in an inner city area of the UK. *Journal of Social Psychiatry and Psychiatric Epidemiology*, **36**: 448–455.

Greenfield, S., Weiss, R., and Tohen, M. (1995) Substance abuse and the chronically mentally ill: a description of dual diagnosis treatment services in a psychiatric hospital. *Community Mental Health Journal*, **31**: 265–277.

Hoult, J. and Reynolds, I. (1984) Schizophrenia: a comparative trial of community oriented and hospital oriented psychiatric care. *Acta Psychiatrica Scandinavica*, **69**: 359–372.

Johnson, S. (1997) Dual diagnosis of severe mental illness and substance misuse: a case for specialist services? *British Journal of Psychiatry*, **171**: 205–208.

Marlatt, G.A. (1998) Basic principles and strategies of harm reduction. In G.A. Marlatt (Ed.), *Harm Reduction: Pragmatic Strategies for Managing High-Risk Behaviours*. New York, Guilford.

Marlatt, G.A. (1998) Harm reduction around the world: a brief history. In G.A. Marlatt (Ed.), *Harm Reduction: Pragmatic Strategies for Managing High-Risk Behaviours*. New York, Guilford.

Marshall, J. (1998) Dual diagnosis: co-morbidity of severe mental illness and substance misuse. *Journal of Forensic Psychiatry*, **9**: 9–15.

Maslin, J., Graham, H., Cawley, M., Copello, A., Birchwood, M., Georgiou, G., McGovern, D., Mueser, K. and Orford, J. (2001) Combined severe mental health and substance use problems: what are the training and support needs of staff working with this client group? *Journal of Mental Health*, **10**: 131–140.

McGrew, J.H. and Bond, G.R. (1995) Critical ingredients of assertive community treatment: judgement of the experts. *Assertive Community Treatment*, **22**: 113–125.

McMurran, M. (1997) *The Psychology of Addiction*. London, Taylor & Francis Ltd.

Miller W.R., Zweben, A., DiClemente, C.C. and Rychtarik, R.G. (1995) *Motivational Enhancement Therapy Manual: A Clinical Research Guide for Therapists Treating Individuals with Alcohol Dependence*. NIAAA, Project Match Monograph Series, 2.

Miller, W.R. and Rollnick, S. (1991) *Motivational Interviewing: Preparing People To Change Addictive Behaviour*. London, Guilford.

Mueser, K.T., Drake, R.E. and Noordsy, D.L. (1998) Integrated mental health and substance abuse treatment for severe psychiatric disorders. *Journal of Practical Psychiatry and Behavioural Health*, **May**: 129–139.

Mueser, K.T., Drake, R.E., Clark, R.E., McHugo, G.J., Mercer-McFadden C. and Ackerson, T.H. (1995) *Toolkit for Evaluating Substance Abuse in Persons with Severe Mental Ilness*. Unpublished.

NHS Plan (2000) *A Plan for Investment, A Plan for Reform*. Department of Health.

The 1991 Census and the Health of Birmingham. (2000) Report of the Healthy Birmingham 2000 Information Group.

Parker, H., Aldridge, J. and Measham, F. (1998) *Illegal Leisure: The Normalisation of Adolescent Recreational Drug Use*. London, Routledge.

Richmond, R., Heather, N., Wodak, A., Kehoe, L. and Webster, I. (1995) Controlled evaluation of a general practice-based brief intervention for excessive drinking. *Addiction*, **90**: 119–132.

Ries, R.K. and Dyck, D.G. (1997) Representative payee practices of community mental health centers in Washington state. *Psychiatric Services*, **48**: 811–813.

Satel, S. (1998). When disability benefits make patients sicker. In R. Drake, C. Mercer-McFadden, G. McHugo, K. Mueser, S. Rosenberg, R. Clark and M. Brunette (Eds.), *Readings in Dual Diagnosis*. Columbia, MD, IAPRS.

Saunders, J., Kavanagh, D.J., Young, R., Jenner, L. and Clair, A. (Unpublished) *Start Over and Survive (SOS) Treatment Manual: Evaluation of a Brief Intervention for Substance Abuse in Early Psychosis*. Department of Psychiatry, University of Queensland.

Shaner, A., Roberts, L., Eckman, T., Tucker, D., Tsuang, J., Wilkins, J. and Mintz, J. (1997) Monetary reinforcement of abstinence from cocaine among mentally ill patients with cocaine dependence. *Hospital and Community Psychiatry*, **48**: 807–810.

Smith, J. and Hucker, S. (1993) Dual diagnosis patients: substance abuse by the severely mentally ill. *British Journal of Hospital Medicine*, **50**: 650–654.

Stein, L.I. and Test, M.A. (1980) Alternative to mental hospital treatment. *Archives of General Psychiatry*, **37**: 392–397.

Ward, M. and Applin, C. (1998) *The Unlearned Lesson: The Role of Alcohol and Drug Misuse in Homicides Perpetrated by People with Mental Health Problems*. London, Wyne Howard Books.

Wilks, J. (1989) Drug treatment and prescribing practice: what can be learned from the past? In G. Bennett (Ed.), *Treating Drug Abusers*. London, Routledge.

Ziedonis, D.M. and Trudeau, K. (1997) Motivation to quit using substances among individuals with schizophrenia: implications for a motivation based treatment model. *Schizophrenia Bulletin*, **23**: 229–238.

Chapter 8

AN INTEGRATED TREATMENT APPROACH TO SUBSTANCE USE IN AN EARLY PSYCHOSIS PROGRAMME

Jean Addington

INTRODUCTION

The prevalence of drug and alcohol use and misuse is high among individuals newly diagnosed with a psychotic disorder (Hambrecht and Häfner, 1996). This has a major impact on efforts to improve early detection and intervention. Substance use may precede the onset of the illness and thus be considered a precipitant. For example, certain drugs, such as stimulants, can precipitate onset at an earlier age in biologically vulnerable people (Tsuang et al, 1982). Cannabis abuse has been associated with earlier psychotic relapses in young people experiencing a first episode of psychosis (Linszen et al, 1994). In this study, these authors suggested that cannabis use 1 year prior to the illness was an independent risk factor. Secondly, substance abuse may follow the onset of the illness and may possibly be an attempt to alleviate certain symptoms (Dixon et al, 1991; Addington and Duchak, 1997). A recent study has attempted to clarify the position (Hambrecht and Häfner, 1996) by retrospectively assessing the onset and course of schizophrenia and substance abuse in 232 first-episode schizophrenic patients. In this study, one-third of first-episode patients with a high rate of comorbid substance abuse began using substances prior to the first signs of psychosis, whereas the remainder began use around or after the start of the illness. In a study comparing current abusers, past abusers and

Substance Misuse in Psychosis: Approaches to Treatment and Service Delivery.
Edited by Hermine L. Graham, Alex Copello, Max J. Birchwood and Kim T. Mueser.
© 2003 John Wiley & Sons, Ltd.

non-abusers, the most notable difference among the groups was that the past substance abusers had a significantly younger age of onset than the non-abusers (Addington and Addington, 1998). This has been shown by other studies. It is possible that for the "past abusing group" the first psychotic episode was exacerbated by the use of substances. Alternatively, early-onset symptoms may be a risk factor for using substances.

Clearly, substance use interferes with the lives of these young people, and there is no doubt about the havoc that serious abuse and dependence can cause. However, what is equally important is what Drake et al (1990) have termed "use without impairment" as a marker for potential problems. Recent work has implied that substance use may have more profound effects on the course of psychotic illnesses than perhaps was previously thought. McGlashan and Fenton (1993) have suggested that the processes that make schizophrenia a long-term disorder may be most active and do the most damage early in the course of the disorder. Several studies of first-episode psychosis have examined the average time between onset of psychotic symptoms and the first effective treatment, (i.e., the duration of untreated psychosis). This has been estimated to be between 1 and 2 years (Larson et al, 1996; Loebel et al, 1992). It has been hypothesized that initially untreated psychosis may reflect an active, morbid process that is associated with increasingly poor long-term outcome unless ameliorated by antipsychotic drugs (Waddington et al, 1997).

This hypothesis has been extended by Lieberman et al (1997) into a theoretical model of the pathophysiology of schizophrenia. To summarize, this model hypothesizes three stages of schizophrenia. The first stage arises in the gestational and perinatal periods. This consists of the cytoarchitectural abnormalities in the cerebral cortex that may have resulted from a failure of normal neural development and synaptogenesis. Thus, a deficiency matrix for the subsequent neuromaturational events is established. This is what is known as the vulnerability to the illness. It is then hypothesized that the second stage arises in adolescence or early adulthood. This occurs during the prodrome, psychosis onset, and early course of the illness, and involves the development of neurochemical sensitization in response to environmental stimulation or stress. Stress can include life events or, what is important for this current discussion, drug abuse. Finally, Lieberman et al (1997) hypothesized that the third stage is the development of a limited neurotoxicity, which occurs as a consequence of progressive sensitization and underlies the deterioration and residual phases of the illness. In terms of support for these three stages, there is extensive support for the first stage, there is substantial evidence for the second stage, but the third stage is more speculative.

This hypothetical model has important implications for treatment. It is necessary to minimize the potential for neurochemical sensitization. Thus, one goal is to reduce the amount of time an individual is experiencing psychosis. This can be accomplished by attempting to reduce the duration of untreated psychosis. Secondly, we can attempt to reduce the stressors that exacerbate or maintain psychotic symptoms. One such stressor is the misuse of substances. Thus, the implication for substance misuse from Lieberman's theoretical model (Lieberman et al, 1997) is that substance misuse through the process of neurochemical sensitization can have an effect on maintaining psychotic symptoms, a result which in turn may have a neurotoxic effect on the brain that could lead to irreversible change. Thus, it is extremely important to consider potential problems of substance use when an individual first presents with a psychotic illness.

This chapter will discuss how the problem of substance use is addressed in a comprehensive early psychosis programme. The Calgary Early Psychosis Program (EPP) is situated in Calgary, Alberta, in Western Canada. It serves a population of 930 000 through a publicly funded health-care system. This is a comprehensive outpatient programme for individuals experiencing a first episode of psychosis. The EPP offers psychiatric management, case management, family intervention, and individual and group therapy. There is also a small clinic within the EPP to address the needs of individuals who may be experiencing prodromal symptoms of psychosis or who are deemed to be at high risk of psychosis. This chapter will describe how substance use is addressed through all aspects of the programme, and how several intervention strategies for substance use are integrated within the range of available psychosocial treatments.

THE CALGARY EARLY PSYCHOSIS TREATMENT AND PREVENTION PROGRAM

The Early Psychosis Treatment and Prevention Program is an established programme which began in October 1996. The programme is provided without charge to the patients and their families. It is available to anyone in the city of Calgary, and funding is provided through a provincially administered Medicare Program, governed by a Canada Health Act. This offers a 3-year treatment programme to individuals diagnosed with a first episode of psychosis and their families.

Overview of the programme

The goals of the programme are early identification of the psychotic illness, reduction in the delays in initial treatment, treatment of the primary symptoms of psychosis, reduction of secondary morbidity, reduction of

Table 8.1 DSM-IV diagnoses of current substance abuse for the 46% of initial referrals who have a diagnosis of substance abuse

Substances used	Numbers	Percentage
Cannabis and alcohol	28	26%
Cannabis and hallucinogens	1	1%
Cannabis	30	28%
Alcohol	27	26%
Hallucinogens	1	1%
Combinations of two or more of alcohol, cannabis, hallucinogens, cocaine	19	18%
Total	106	100%

the frequency and severity of relapse, promotion of normal psychosocial development, and reduction of stress for families and caregivers.

In the Early Psychosis Program, we offer five areas of treatment: case management, psychiatric management, and medication strategies; cognitive behaviour therapy; group therapy; and family interventions. We conduct comprehensive assessments initially on entering the programme; at 3, 6, 9, 12, 15, 18, 21, and 24 months; and at discharge. Assessments focus on positive, negative, and depressive symptoms. Medication side effects are continually monitored. Social and cognitive functioning are assessed to help determine prognosis and future planning. Substance abuse is routinely monitored.

After 4 years of operating, we have admitted over 300 individuals to the programme. The majority of the referred patients are between 16 and 25 years of age. Initial DSM-IV diagnoses include schizophrenia (43%), schizophreniform disorder (39%), psychosis NOS (13%), and other psychotic disorders (5%). Forty-six per cent of new admissions also met DSM-IV criteria for a current diagnosis of substance abuse or dependence. The majority abuse cannabis. These percentages are presented in Table 8.1. Very few have severe and none have extremely severe levels of use. Thus, it may be that individuals with severe addiction problems and experiencing a first episode of psychosis are not being referred or are not willing to attend our programme. It is also possible that the severity typically worsens gradually over time. However, our programme does serve the entire population, and there are no barriers to access to the programme.

Focus on substance use in the Early Psychosis Program

Philosophy

The stress vulnerability model underlies the philosophy of our programme. This fits with the pathophysiological model of Lieberman et al (1997) previously described. In our education and discussions with patients and families, we actually use a simpler version of the model, which is well described by Mueser and Glynn (1995). We teach that certain individuals have a vulnerability to schizophrenia or other psychotic disorders. This may be a result of genetics, neurodevelopment, trauma in utero or at birth, or any combination of these factors. This vulnerable person has what we term "a sensitive brain". The brain is sensitive to stress; that is, the vulnerable individual may not be as resilient to certain kinds of stress as other people might be. Thus, we advocate avoiding stress, developing better coping mechanisms for stress, and avoiding or eliminating the use of substances.

In our teaching about substance use, we add that since a psychotic illness is a brain disease, substances are clearly detrimental to this condition. They may increase or exacerbate positive symptoms. They may have an impact on negative symptoms. This is over and above any sequelae of substance use on interpersonal, social, and economic functioning. When these theories of neurotoxicity are considered, a possible consequence of substance misuse is damage to an already compromised brain. Thus, the focus on avoiding substances does not have to be one of disapproval or morals. Rather it is an issue of working with a patient who has a specific disease and eliminating a behaviour that potentially compromises improvement or long-term outcome. This is an important stance to take when dealing with these young individuals.

First experiences

In developing the Early Psychosis Program, our decision was to address substance use throughout the programme. We first addressed the problem through several intervention strategies within the range of psychosocial treatments being offered. These will be discussed in more detail below. Since we had previously had some success in a more chronic population with a specialty group addressing substance use (Addington and el-Guebaly, 1998), we modified the manual for our first-episode patients to make it more relevant and appropriate for young individuals who were experiencing their first psychotic episode and who continued to use substances. Our plan was to offer a specialty group early in the programme.

Our clinical impressions were that those individuals who abused substances generally were not interested in receiving help for their substance problems. In fact, they often stated that they did not want to attend special groups and often did not believe that they had a problem. Those who did accept that they might have a substance-abuse problem usually thought they could address the problem themselves. In the first few years of the programme, we did not have enough people to run a substance group for first-episode patients. This was initially disappointing. Despite this, on examining our outcome data, we found that after 1 year in the programme there was a significant reduction in the level of use as rated by the Case Manager Rating Scale for Substance Use Disorder (Drake et al, 1989). This has been reported elsewhere (Addington and Addington, 1998). We found that for the first 90 patients in the programme who completed a 1-year assessment there was a significant decline overall in the use of hallucinogens and cannabis, but not in alcohol. This included the whole programme population, not just those who had a problem. For those who met DSM-IV criteria for alcohol, cannabis, or hallucingen abuse or dependence, there was a significant reduction overall on all three substances at the 1-year assessment with the Case Manager Rating Scale.

There are several possible reasons why this improvement occurred. It is possible that for many young people there comes a time when they stop using substances as a function of maturity, or life or developmental changes. Others may have stopped because of the education, information, encouragement, and suggested strategies offered in various aspects of the programme throughout the first year. Thus, we felt that there were components of the programme that had an impact on substance use prior to starting a specialty group. This encouraged us to develop further all components of our programme to address the problem of substance misuse.

However, there remains a concern about those who continue to use, especially after having been in the programme for 1 year. These are the individuals we are currently attempting to engage in our speciality group on substance use. Certainly, all individuals in the programme who are using substances are encouraged to come to the group at any time during their stay in the programme. However, for those who are not interested in coming and who perhaps do not feel they have a problem, we wait until after the 1-year assessment. Often they are more willing to consider this treatment when they are presented with data demonstrating that they have clearly been unable to stop using over the course of the past year, and that one consequence is that there has been no improvement in symptoms. Linszen and Lenoir (1999) reported that in their clinic in Amsterdam some young patients who abuse cannabis do stop once they see the impact of cannabis use on their symptoms.

ADDRESSING SUBSTANCE USE THROUGH THE DIFFERENT COMPONENTS OF THE EARLY PSYCHOSIS PROGRAM

Use of substances is assessed throughout all aspects of the programme. Secondly, the programme offers a specific treatment for those who continue to use. Immediately after admission of clients to the programme, case management, psychiatric management, and family interventions continue on a regular basis. Individual cognitive-behaviour therapy occurs once the individual is stabilized. The groups are phase specific and occur at various times throughout the 3 years of the programme. Since our programme is small, the three case managers, two family workers, and three group and individual therapists are able to meet together with the psychiatrists on a weekly basis. Thus, there is excellent communication between all team members in terms of continuity of care of any one patient.

Assessment

Substance abuse is assessed routinely as part of the ongoing evaluation. A DSM-IV diagnosis using the SCID (Spitzer et al, 1992) is completed at the initial assessment and again at the 1-year assessment. A diagnosis of substance abuse or dependence is considered at these times as well as diagnoses of schizophrenia spectrum disorders. The Case Manager Rating Scale (Drake et al, 1989) is routinely used at the initial assessment and then every 3 months for 2 years to assess the level of severity of substance use. This is a short checklist that is administered by the case manager and is used to determine the level of substance misuse for each substance used (Drake et al, 1990). Level of use is ranked as follows: none = 0, mild = 1, moderate = 2, severe = 3, or extremely severe = 4. A rating of 2 is similar to the criterion for abuse and ratings of 3 or 4 are similar to the criterion for dependence. Drug screens are used if use is suspected.

Case management

Case management involves participation in medication clinics with a psychiatrist as well as offering patients education and supportive therapy, and the coordination of programme, hospital, and community services. Patients have the same case managers for the duration of their time in the programme. Case managers are responsible for the ongoing assessment of substance abuse, and they offer support and counselling with respect to minimizing or quitting substance use. For those who do have a substance-abuse problem, the case manager continually addresses this. In individual sessions with the case manager, there is a focus on triggers and on strategies to minimize or stop use. All of our case managers have previous experience in working with individuals who have substance problems as well as psychotic illnesses. For those whom programme treatments are not helping and those whose addiction problems may be too severe to manage initially on an outpatient basis, the case manager also addresses readiness for treatments that may be offered outside the programme. These include attending a dual disorders programme or admission to a detoxification centre or residential treatment centre. When working with individuals who are experiencing a first episode, we do have patients whose recovery is good enough that they can cope with and gain from a residential treatment programme. This may not be the case for those who have an established schizophrenia illness.

Psychiatric management

Our overall medication strategy within the programme is that all clients are started on new low extrapyramidal side-effect (EPS) medications. This may help counteract some of the reasons that individuals with schizophrenia give for using substances (Addington and Duchak, 1997). We routinely assess akathisia and EPS, and thus attempt to find appropriate solutions for such problems if they arise to avoid any chance of self-medication for these side effects. In regular clinic meetings, the psychiatrist continues to ask about the amount of substance use. This allows another opportunity for education on how substances may be affecting thoughts, mood and effectiveness of medication.

Family intervention

The family intervention programme offers help for family members to understand the illness, and strategies for coping with the disorder. Families are seen individually and patients are welcome at and encouraged to attend the family sessions. Each family has their own family worker who is available to them for the duration of the programme. The family work focuses on education about the disorder and its management, problem solving and communication skills training. The vulnerability model is the basis for the family education. With all families, the issue of substance misuse is addressed in the initial sessions regardless of whether substance misuse is a specific problem. We usually find that if patients attend the family sessions, they will admit to some use, a fact which facilitates the discussion. Furthermore, this often allows for the extent of the use to become apparent to the family if they are not already aware of it.

After receiving education about the effects of substance use on the "sensitive brain", the majority of the families are then able to begin to work towards discouraging the patient from excessive use. With patients who continue to use, the family is offered help in setting limits both on the use and the resultant behaviours. The family is made aware of various options for substance use treatment either within the EPP or in the community. Help is sought in encouraging this from the family.

Cognitive behaviour therapy (CBT)

CBT is offered on an individual basis. Two different models are being used in our programme. Both include psychoeducation about the illness, treatment, and outcome. The first model is based on the work of Henry Jackson in Melbourne, Australia (Jackson et al, 2000). The second model of CBT that we offer is for the reduction of psychotic symptoms. This treatment is based on the British models of coping enhancement strategies (CSE) (Tarrier, 1992), and CBT for psychosis (Fowler et al, 1995).

The first model of Jackson et al (2000) is more relevant to addressing substance abuse. This model addresses depression, anxiety, demoralization, lowered self-esteem, and vulnerability to future episodes. In this approach, the first goal is adaptation to a psychotic illness. This can be accomplished through a search for meaning in the experience, helping the individual to promote a sense of mastery, protecting and enhancing self-esteem, and trying to enable the individual to have a positive attitude to the illness. The second goal is to avoid secondary morbidity, which is the result of a failure to adapt, and which includes depression, anxiety, and substance abuse. It may be that secondary morbidity has already occurred and will need to be addressed through this same model. Thus, through individual CBT, we are actively addressing the issues that may sustain substance misuse. As part of the work in the individual sessions, ways to cope with substance use can be addressed.

Group programme

Our group programme offers several short-term groups—psychosis education, personal support, and good health modules (nutrition, exercise, weight loss, and smoking cessation). Our four-session psychosis education group offers education about psychotic illness, symptoms, diagnoses, and medications. Explanatory models and theories of psychoses are explored. All patients in the programme are encouraged to attend this group, which is held 5–6 times per year. Most of a session focuses on substance use, which is discussed in the context of vulnerability, stress to a "sensitive" brain, and the problems of continued substance use. The emphasis here is for individuals to understand the impact of substance use as a stressor on the symptoms, management, and course of their illness. We want to emphasize the importance of stopping substances and the potential help available to them.

Group approach to stopping substance use

The Stopping Substances Group is a speciality group addressing substance use in psychosis. Patients can attend this group as soon as they are stable or at any other time during their 3 years in the programme. Previously, we used this group for individuals who were experiencing their first episode of schizophrenia and individuals who had experienced multi-episodes of schizophrenia (Addington and el-Guebaly, 1998). However, we have made modifications to it to make it more relevant to the individual experiencing a first episode of psychosis. A manual to guide therapists and a workbook for group participants is available on request from the author.

The goals of this group are as follows:

- to educate participants about current knowledge of the effects of drugs and alcohol and the interaction of these substances with psychosis
- to develop commitment to reduce or abstain from substance use
- to develop awareness of barriers to achieving these goals
- to learn and develop strategies to reduce or abstain from substance use.

The Stopping Substances Group has several components. These include engagement, support, interaction, and psychoeducation. It is important to engage with these young people to get them to come to the group so that they can get help for their difficulties with substances. The group is supportive and offers interaction. The group is psychoeducational and uses a problem-solving skills training approach to address some of the interpersonal issues that may arise because of the substance abuse. For example, we may try to bolster the ability of the members to resist peer pressure to abuse drugs and alcohol. We can teach them skills to avoid relapses by anticipating and avoiding risk situations or even altering the composition of their social network so that they can reduce their exposure to substance-abusing peers. Once they have stopped use, members can learn new skills to cope with daily living, particularly in areas where they may once have used substances.

We take advantage of motivational-interviewing techniques, which are well described by Miller and Rollnick (1992). Using these techniques, we explore the factors associated with members' use of substances with the goal of assessing and influencing motivation to change the substance-using behaviour. It is important that the interventions that are offered in the group fit with the stage of readiness to change of the group members. These stages are pre-contemplation, contemplation, preparation, action, and maintenance, as described by Prochaska et al (1992). Finally, we have to remember that individuals with schizophrenia and other psychotic illnesses may have impaired neurocognitive functioning. It is not unusual to find difficulties in areas such as sustained attention, processing information, memory, conceptual organization, or abstraction. Therefore, when we are planning for the teaching of the group, we have to take into account the possibility that members may be suffering from these deficits. These various components occur throughout the group and are an important part of most, if not all, sessions.

Before starting the group, there is opportunity for individual sessions. Usually, one or two sessions are provided, but more can be offered if necessary. In those sessions, potential group members are given an outline of the group, and boundaries are clarified. We emphasize that this is a special intervention with a particular focus on substance use. There is opportunity for other issues to be dealt with elsewhere in our programme. In these individual sessions, we review thoroughly the history of alcohol and drug abuse. We want to explore the individuals' knowledge of substance use and the explanatory model that they have adopted with regard to psychosis and substances. By doing this, we are validating their personal experience and acknowledging that their own viewpoint is important. This helps therapists gain information regarding the degree of pathology a person is experiencing. The therapists can also determine the discrepancy between the individual's explanatory model and what they as therapists might be proposing.

The group is for approximately 10 sessions. The first four sessions are specific and focus on assessment and feedback incorporated with a motivational-interviewing framework. Psychoeducation emphasizes the risk of continuing to use substances in the context of having experienced a psychotic episode or having a psychotic disorder. The first two sessions focus on education about alcohol, drugs, tolerance, dependence, and withdrawal. We review the interaction between psychosis and substance use and the effects of substances on psychosis and treatment. There is a discussion about the advantages and disadvantages of using and what the past, present, and future effects of substances are or will be. We review the vulnerability model and put great emphasis on the effect of drugs as a stressor within this model. Although these first two sessions have a major focus on education, we encourage a commitment to action, action being a change in the clients' substance-use behaviours.

The third session focuses on goal setting. Goals are set that are related to harm reduction and/or abstinence. Goals have to be stage appropriate, according to Prochaska et al (1992). In the fourth session, we address reasons why people are using, what their attitude is to quitting, and what they see as barriers to quitting or reducing their use. We identify such barriers in session 4 and they will again be addressed in later sessions. At the end of these initial sessions, the individuals will have learned about the interrelationship of the use of substances and psychosis and will have a good understanding about the impact of their substance use on both their general health and their psychotic illness. Hopefully, they will be ready to try to make some changes.

In the later sessions, the focus is on learning strategies and techniques to help change substance-use behaviour. We devote one session to teaching social problem-solving skills that can be used to overcome some of the barriers to change. Two sessions focus on exploring the reasons why individuals may relapse or increase their use. In these sessions, members are helped to identify the situation, and to learn and develop solutions and problem-solving strategies for such situations. Similarly, we provide an approach to learning about high-risk situations and warning signs of impending relapse. In the group, we develop contingency plans for high-risk situations.

At the end of these sessions, the group members are aware of the potential difficulties in achieving their goals. They possess a range of strategies to overcome the difficulties, and, most importantly, they have practised and utilized several different strategies to help reduce or stop their substance use. It is very important that strategies that are being taught are actually practised through role-play in the group. Group members can leave the group and try to practise these strategies in the real world and return to the group for feedback about how successful or unsuccessful they were with various strategies. Other issues, such as dealing with cravings, high-risk situations, relapse prevention, and unrealistic expectations, are also addressed.

Integration

The Early Psychosis Program focuses on offering optimal treatment to patients and their families for a psychotic illness. The majority of the young people in the EPP use substances, and for some it is a major problem. Rather than focus only on those who are abusing substances or have diagnosis of a substance problem, we consider substance use to be a stressor that has implications for psychosis and one with which we have the potential to intervene. Thus, avoiding the use of substances is part of all education in the clinics, in individual and group therapy, in family work, and in psychosis education for the patients. Substance use is routinely assessed so that the degree of the use can be identified. Thus, we address substance use for everyone in the programme and are aware that what may not be a problem at the initial assessment could become a problem as the illness progresses.

Having all staff in the programme, as well as the patient and all family members, give due attention to substance use is paramount. Only then can the various treatment modalities offer specific interventions for substance use. Interventions can take place on an individual basis with a CBT therapist, with the case manager, with the psychiatrist, or with all three. Additionally, intervention can take place in the context of the family work, and the family can be engaged to either help with the problem or be offered help themselves to manage the problem. Finally, intervention can occur within one of the groups or in the speciality group itself. All staff are familiar with the techniques and strategies used in the speciality group, so that they can reinforce these strategies and/or use them in their own work with the patient.

One of the most difficult issues is engaging these young people to attend the substance use group. They often attend some of the treatments offered in the programme but seem to be least likely to be willing to attend a specialized group for this. This is not an unusual problem. Our strategy is to have the whole team work together around this issue and also engage the help of the family so that we can make the best possible effort to engage the patients as much as possible. With the whole team working on substance misuse, there is the opportunity for some help even if they do not attend a speciality group. One of the therapists who conducts the Stopping Substance Group has scheduled time to approach potential group members, visit them at home, or meet with them in any way they are willing, in order to attempt to engage them in specific treatment for substance use.

CONCLUSIONS

Substance misuse clearly has serious implications for the treatment of recent-onset psychosis. First, there is the possibility of increasing or exacerbating positive symptoms. Second, there is the risk of further damage to an already compromised brain. Regardless of the extent of the misuse, substance use remains an area of concern in terms of maximum recovery from a psychotic illness. Thus, substance use needs to be addressed regardless of the degree of the use or misuse. In our Early Psychosis Program, we are focusing on maximizing the short-and long-term recovery from a psychotic illness, and, as such, addressing substance use is a priority in all interventions. Finally, the impact of the different interventions on substance needs to be assessed in a rigorous manner, and we are attempting to do that.

REFERENCES

Addington, J. and Addington, D. (1998) The effects of substance abuse in early psychosis. *British Journal of Psychiatry*, **172** (Suppl 33): 134–136.

Addington, J. and Duchak, V. (1997) Reasons for substance use in schizophrenia. *Acta Psychiatrica Scandinavica*, **96**: 329–333.

Addington, J. and el-Guebaly, N. (1998) Group treatment for substance abuse in schizophrenia. *Canadian Journal of Psychiatry*, **43**: 843–845.

Dixon, L., Haas, G., Weiden, P.J., Sweeney, J. and Frances, A.J. (1991) Drug abuse in schizophrenic patients: clinical correlates and reasons for use. *American Journal of Psychiatry*, **48**: 224–230.

Drake, R.E., Osher, F.C., Noordsy, D.L., Teague, G.B., Hurlbut, S.C. and Beaudett, M.S. (1990) Diagnosis of alcohol use disorders in schizophrenia. *Schizophrenia Bulletin*, **16**: 57–67.

Drake, R.E., Mercer-McFadden, C., Mueser, K., McHugo, G.J and Bond, G.R. (1998) Review of integrated mental health and substance abuse treatments for patients with dual disorders. *Schizophrenia Bulletin*, **24**: 589–608.

Drake, R.E., Osher, F.C. and Wallach, M.A. (1989) Alcohol use and abuse in schizophrenia. *Journal of Nervous and Mental Disease*, **177**: 408–414.

Fowler, D., Garrety, P. and Kuipers, E. (1995) *Cognitive Behavior Therapy for Psychosis*. Chichester, Wiley.

Hambrecht, M. and Häfner, H. (1996) Substance abuse and the onset of schizophrenia. *Biological Psychiatry*, **39**: 1–9.

Jackson, H., Hulbert, C. and Henry, L. (2000) The treatment of secondary morbidity in first episode psychosis. In M. Birchwood, D. Fowler and C. Jackson (Eds.), *Early Intervention in Psychosis: Guide to Concepts, Evidence and Intervention* (pp. 213–235). Chichester, Wiley.

Larsen, T.K., McGlashan, T.H., Johannessen, J.O. and Vibe-Hansen, L. (1996) First-episode schizophrenia. II. Premorbid patterns by gender. *Schizophrenia Bulletin*, **22**: 257–269.

Lieberman, J.A., Sheitman, B. and Kinon, B.J. (1997) Neurochemical sensitization in the pathophysiology of schizophrenia: deficits and dysfunction in neuronal regulation and plasticity. *Neuropsychopharmacology*, **17**: 205–229.

Linszen, D.H. and Lenior, M.E. (1999) Early psychosis and substance abuse. In P. McGorry and H.J. Jackson (Eds.), *The Recognition and Management of Early Psychosis* (pp. 363–375). Cambridge, Cambridge University Press.

Linszen, D.H., Dingemans, P., Loebel, A.D. and Lenior, M.E. (1994) Cannabis abuse and the course of recent onset schizophrenic disorders. *Archives of General Psychiatry*, **51**: 273–279.

Loebel, A.D., Lieberman, J.A., Alvir, J.M.J., Mayerhoff, D.I., Geisler, S.H. and Szymanski, S.R. (1992) Duration of psychosis and outcome in first episode schizophrenia. *American Journal of Psychiatry*, **149**: 1183–1188.

McGlashan, T.H. and Fenton, W.S. (1993) Subtype progression and pathophysiologic deterioration in early schizophrenia. *Schizophrenia Bulletin*, **19**: 71–84.

Miller, W.R. and Rollnick, S. (1992). *Motivational Interviewing: Preparing People for Change*. New York, Guilford.

Mueser, K.T., Bellack, A.S. and Blanchard, J.J. (1992) Comorbidity of schizophrenia and substance abuse: implications for treatment. *Journal of Clinical and Consulting Psychology*, **60**: 845–856.

Mueser, K.T. and Glynn, S. (1995) *Behavioral Family Therapy for Psychiatric Disorders*, Boston, MA, Allyn & Bacon.

Prochaska, J.O., DiClemente, C.C. and Norcross, J.C. (1992) In search of how people change. *American Psychologist*, **47**: 1102–1114.

Spitzer, R.L., Williams, J.B., Gibbon, M., First, M. (1992) The structured clinical interview for DSM-IV SCID. I. History, rationale, and description. *Archives of General Psychiatry*, **49**: 624–629.

Tarrier, N. (1992) Management and modification of residual psychotic symptoms. In M. Birchwood and N. Tarrier (Eds.), *Innovations in the Psychological Management of Schizophrenia*. Chichester, Wiley.

Tsuang, M.T., Simpson, J.C. and Kronfol, Z. (1982) Subtypes of drug abuse with psychosis: demographic characteristics clinical features and family history. *Archives of General Psychiatry*, **39**: 141–147.

Waddington, J., Scully, P. and Youssef, H. (1997) Developmental trajectory and disease progression in schizophrenia: the conundrum, and insights from a 12-year prospective study in the Monaghan 101. *Schizophrenia Research*, **23**: 107–118.

Chapter 9

AN INPATIENT-BASED
SERVICE MODEL

Richard N. Rosenthal

INTRODUCTION AND CONTEXTUAL INFORMATION
THAT HAS SHAPED THIS DEVELOPMENT/APPROACH

In 1979, Henry Pinsker, MD, was the Associate Director for Clinical Services
in the Department of Psychiatry at Beth Israel Medical Center (BIMC) in
New York City. The Morris J. Bernstein Institute housed some 130 detoxification beds in a medical setting that was run by the department of medicine,
and had a medical model of chemical dependence. Dr Pinsker was struck
by the degree of psychopathology in this addicted population. Patients
frequently became agitated or disorganized and were not easily han-
dled by the non-psychiatric staff, except through physical intervention or
administrative discharge from hospital. Much of the disruption on the units
was attributed to bad behaviour by antisocial addicts, and although this
was true to some degree, much acute psychiatric illness was overlooked
or undertreated, as typical in traditional addiction recovery settings where
psychiatric services are underutilized. At this time, part-time psychiatric
staff were consultants to the detoxification units. It became clear that a
unit with a more restricted focus upon those who needed psychiatric hospitalization, and who also suffered from addictive disorders might prove
clinically and administratively advantageous to care. The proposal was
approved by the hospital administration, and, in 1979, probably the first
substance abuse unit in the USA for patients with psychiatric disorders
was opened as a 36-bed unit in the Bernstein Institute (Pinsker, 1997). It
moved into a new building in 1984 as a 28-bed unit.

Substance Misuse in Psychosis: Approaches to Treatment and Service Delivery.
Edited by Hermine L. Graham, Alex Copello, Max J. Birchwood and Kim T. Mueser.
© 2003 John Wiley & Sons, Ltd.

Over the next several years, a literature began to develop describing the young, chronic mentally ill patient (Pepper and Ryglewicz, 1984; Richardson, 1985). These patients were described as highly resistant to treatment engagement, non-compliant with prescribed medication (Solomon et al, 1984), and vulnerable to a course of repeated emergency room visits and hospitalizations (Craig et al, 1985; Richardson, 1985). One other important aspect of this newly described population was its penchant for drug abuse and dependence comorbid with severe and persistent mental illness (Richard et al, 1985; Schneier and Siris, 1987; Treffert, 1978). Data from the Epidemiologic Catchment Area survey of the 1980s supported the notion that comorbidity of mental disorders with substance-use disorders (SUDs) was more common than clinicians supposed; that is, the relative risk of SUDs was increased in those with mental disorders, and vice versa (Regier et al, 1990). As such, a treatment delivery system with disparate mental health and addiction services began to be viewed as an obstacle to engagement of those with comorbid drug and mental disorders. However, it took the National Comorbidity Study (Kessler et al, 1994) to demonstrate how widespread was the problem confronting clinical services: among people with severe disorders (those with psychosis, mania, or needing hospitalization in a 12-month period), 89.5% had three or more lifetime alcohol, drug, or mental disorders (ADM) (14% of the sample). Of the 48% of the US population with lifetime ADM disorders, the majority (27%) have two or more lifetime disorders. These data clearly demonstrated the existence of a population that traditional inpatient psychiatric and chemical dependency services neither properly diagnosed nor specifically treated.

UNIT STRUCTURE

At a New York State Office of Mental Health licensed inpatient unit, patients can be admitted on voluntary or involuntary status. Licensed addiction inpatient treatment units in the USA are allowed to admit only on voluntary status. As such, this 28-bed unit has the distinct advantage of being able to admit for detoxification, medical stabilization, and early engagement into treatment for substance abuse patients who are acutely psychotic, suicidal, or otherwise behaviourally dyscontrolled, as compared with some other dual-diagnosis inpatient models (cf. Wilens et al, 1993). The unit has safe observation rooms equipped for restraint or seclusion and capacity for emergency admission 24 h a day, 7 days per week.

The staffing include a nursing care coordinator; registered nurses and licensed practical nurses; nursing aides; occupational therapists; a clinical psychologist; three second-year psychiatric residents, who rotate for 3–4 months; a senior psychiatric resident or an addiction psychiatry fellow;

and a half-time psychiatrist and a full-time unit chief, both of whom are board-certified addiction psychiatrists. All permanent staff are either knowledgeable or formally trained in addictions work. In addition, as part of the medical centre's academic mission, all disciplines have students on rotation at various times. There are daily rounds with interdisciplinary discussion of treatment and discharge planning and patient responses to current treatment interventions. Highly complex or difficult-to-manage cases are presented in weekly case conference or walking rounds.

THEORY/RESEARCH AND ITS CLINICAL IMPLICATIONS

In parallel with the focus upon developing integrated services to patients with comorbid SUD and mental disorders in the 1980s, a convergent line of clinical thinking on supportive psychotherapy was being developed at Beth Israel, also under the auspices of the then clinical director, Henry Pinsker, and the author (Pinsker and Rosenthal, 1988). The predominant mode of psychotherapy offered by the outpatient clinic at that time was psychodynamically oriented supportive psychotherapy, yet, as a teaching service, it was practised by staff and trainees with neither a formal conceptual basis nor supervision. This was remedied by the development of a supportive psychotherapy manual for use in research and training (Pinsker and Rosenthal, 1988). Supportive psychotherapy has demonstrated comparable efficacy to more expressive treatments in personality-disordered subjects, with reductions in self-rated symptoms and interpersonal problems and sustained change 6 months after termination of treatment (Hellerstein et al, 1998; Rosenthal et al, 1999).

This approach, because it was specifically focused upon reduction in anxiety (Kaufman and Reoux, 1988) and building self-esteem through modelling, skills building, and empowerment, seemed an appropriate foundation for psychotherapeutic interventions with mentally ill chemical abusers. It formed the basis for outpatient research with substance-abusing patients with schizophrenia (Hellerstein and Meehan, 1987) and formed the core of the manualized COPAD integrated group therapy approach for the same research population (Rosenthal et al, 1992a; Hellerstein et al, 1995; Rosenthal et al, 1996). Supportive substance-abuse group therapy, as the foundation of an integrated treatment, engages patients with schizophrenia and substance abuse in treatment more effectively than parallel approaches (Hellerstein et al, 1995). As such, supportive approaches are the basis for both individual and group interventions on the inpatient unit.

The overall inpatient treatment approach is similar to that described by Wallen and Weiner (1988). Inpatient interventions include detoxification

Table 9.1   Criteria for admission to outpatient COPAD programme

Subjects are psychotic inpatients admitted to the inpatient dual-diagnosis unit

Inclusion criteria
1. DSM-IV schizophrenia, schizo-affective, or schizophreniform disorder†
2. diagnosis of drug and/or alcohol abuse or dependence
3. age 18–55 years
4. willingness to take psychiatric medications as indicated
5. willingness to attend groups and evaluation sessions
6. an expressed interest in decreasing drug use

Exclusion criteria
1. need for chronic hospitalization for symptom control
2. DSM-IV Axis V global assessment of functioning past year score of 20 or less (indicating extremely poor chronic functioning)
3. presence of significant cognitive impairment or organic mental syndrome (mini-mental state score of $\leq$24)
4. presence of life-threatening medical illness

†Patients were excluded in the original research study if a clear diagnosis of a schizophrenia continuum disorder could not be made as distinct from the symptoms of drug intoxication or withdrawal states. This is not true for the clinical programme.

(where necessary); diagnostic assessment; acute management of psychiatric, medical, and substance-abuse problems; and psychopharmacological treatment. Inpatient psychosocial interventions include family assessment; individual and group supportive psychotherapy; occupational, recreational, and movement therapy; preliminary group substance-abuse counselling and education; and on-site self-help groups (Alcoholics Anonymous, Narcotics Anonymous, "Double-Trouble", etc.). Patients with schizophrenia are assessed for the COPAD outpatient programme during inpatient hospitalization (admission criteria are listed in Table 9.1), and attend several outpatient group sessions before discharge, in an attempt to increase engagement in outpatient treatment. There are 7–8 twice-weekly COPAD outpatient groups running at any time in the BIMC outpatient department.

ASSESSMENT

In the initial phase of hospitalization, there is medical and psychiatric evaluation of patients by resident psychiatrists supervised by the unit chief or attending staff. Residents administer diagnostic tests including the Hamilton Depression Rating Scale (Hamilton, 1960) when indicated for patients presenting with symptoms of depression, as this is useful, when administered serially, to assist in discriminating substance-induced mood disorders, which typically have a steep decline in symptom intensity as compared to major depression (Brown and Schuckit, 1988). Furthermore, residents evaluate the need for use of sedative or antipsychotic medication when indicated, as well as for pharmacological treatment of withdrawal symptoms. Psychiatric residents and other trainees who present the new patients defend their working diagnoses to the unit chief, based upon current symptoms and history. Provisional clinical diagnoses are made, addressing the substance-related and non-substance-related components of the illness, past history, the patient's strengths, and the psychosocial context. The social worker delineates and engages the support systems available to the patient, including contact with significant others, and hypothesizes an expected outcome so that appropriate discharge planning can be incorporated into the initial treatment plan. The case is discussed with the full staff in morning rounds, and a definitive coordinated treatment plan is devised.

In typical clinical programmes, procedures usually focus upon the one or two addictive disorders with the most obvious implications for treatment. Standardized assessment provides a more comprehensive assessment of multiple substance abuse than routine clinical procedures. In a 1985 study of 146 BIMC inpatients with DSM-III schizophrenia and substance abuse/dependence, 10.9% abused three or more substances. In 1989, 16.0% of the substance-abusing schizophrenia patients met DSM-III-R abuse or dependence criteria for three or more substances by consensus diagnosis. By contrast, fully 90% of the COPAD inpatients in 1990–1 met DSM-III-R criteria for three or more concurrent substances. The 1985 data were obtained retrospectively upon chart review and were methodologically undersensitive in diagnosing multiple SUDs. The 1989 data were derived from routine clinical diagnosis and treatment. (Rosenthal et al, 1992b). The COPAD data from 1990–1, however, were derived from structured clinical interviews using standardized research instruments, and clearly had higher sensitivity, reflected in the much higher rates of diagnosis of polysubstance abuse. In an attempt to compensate for standard clinical approaches, residents and nursing staff are trained to ask about all classes of abused substances, and to obtain information from collateral sources, if available. Since research evaluation by trained raters is impractical in the routine clinical situation, it is essential that toxicological screening be done at admission along with the history and physical examination (Goldfinger et al, 1996), and that all results be presented at rounds where expert consensus opinion can be brought to bear (Ananth et al, 1989).

DIFFERENTIAL DIAGNOSIS

When patients present with a history of substance abuse, they may have acute psychotic symptoms due to exacerbation of non-substance-related disorders such as bipolar disorder or schizophrenia (Weiss and Collins, 1992), to direct effects of substance abuse (Szuster et al, 1990; Brady et al, 1991), or to both (Rosenthal et al, 1994). In the acute emergency-room/inpatient setting, it is difficult to establish the time of onset of symptoms of either independent psychosis or SUD. Thus, it is difficult to diagnose reliably a substance-induced versus a non-substance-related disorder (Kane and Selzer, 1991; Rosenthal et al, 1992a; Shaner et al, 1993), a fact which can affect treatment planning. Using our inpatient data, we derived a statistical model that may prove a useful adjunct to screening for SUDs in psychotic inpatients: psychotic patients with SUDs are more likely to have schizophrenia when formal thought disorder and bizarre delusions are present, and less likely when there is current suicidal ideation, a history of intravenous cocaine use, inpatient drug detoxification, or methadone maintenance (Rosenthal and Miner, 1997).

BIMODAL DISTRIBUTION

Differential diagnosis has a systemic as well as a treatment implication. The majority of those who have a substance-induced mental disorder have a shorter length of stay in hospital. As such, the length of stay in hospital has a bimodal distribution, and affects treatment planning. Patients with the shorter duration of hospitalization (mean length of stay [LOS] $\sim$ 4 days) tend to have self-limited acute disorders where the treatment is primarily targeted at detoxification and engagement into longer-term treatment for the SUD, and discharge planning to support intermediate plans. Representative diagnoses among this group are substance induced-mood disorder; substance-induced delusional disorder; cocaine, opiate, or alcohol dependence, usually in multiple; and concomitant personality disorders such as antisocial and borderline. Patients with longer lengths of stay (mean LOS $\sim$ 17 days) typically are suffering from an exacerbation of more severe mental disorders such as schizophrenia, bipolar mania, and major depression. The treatment for these consists firstly of acute stabilization: maintenance of safety, pharmacotherapy, supportive therapy, and concurrent detoxification; and then, as the patient becomes less psychotic or acutely disabled, the treatment attempts to engage the patient initially not only in individual but also group activities, such as low-demand recreational task groups.

ACTIVE TREATMENT

Once the working diagnosis is established, the patient in acute withdrawal can begin a detoxification schedule as indicated, and the patient requiring psychotropic medications can begin these. The therapeutic activities staff evaluate the patient for placement in treatment groups and protocols. Integrated into this programme is basic group substance-abuse counselling and education by videotape and discussion modes. In addition, patients attend on-unit self-help groups such as Alcoholics Anonymous, Cocaine Anonymous, Narcotics Anonymous, and "Double Trouble".

PSYCHIATRIC ADDICTION DETOXIFICATION (PAD)

The early component of the programme is the PAD programme which begins detoxification in the absence of a definitive diagnosis of a non-substance-induced mental disorder. The safest early approach to psychosis in the context of substance abuse is to consider the symptoms substance-induced. This strategy reduces the potential harm of untreated withdrawal states (Brown et al, 1988a; Becker and Hale, 1993) or the unnecessary exposure of patients to neuroleptic treatment (Olivera et al, 1990; Ziedonis et al, 1992). After several days of medical detoxification, patients with persisting symptoms of an acute or exacerbated mental disorder who also need an inpatient level of care are "transferred" to the dual-diagnosis inpatient programme proper, on the same unit.

TREATMENT CONTRACTS

At any point that the staff determine that a patient is capable of reading and comprehending a treatment contract, when indicated by history or behaviour, the patient is asked to read and sign a contract which will set overt limits as to acceptable behaviour. Generally, this document prohibits direct aggression, threatening behaviour, and sexual behaviour and makes clear the consequences of such actions. In addition, the contract outlines the patient's expected level of participation in the treatment and the expected benefits that will be derived. The contract demonstrates that patients bear responsibility for their treatment to whatever degree they is capable (Selzer et al, 1987). The timing of the contracting process is a factor of diagnosis, recovery of autonomy, and treatment history, including prior use of behavioural contracts (see "floating line model" below).

For example, a 28-year-old woman with many prior hospitalizations for acute suicidal ideation and behavioural dyscontrol in the context of cocaine dependence, opiate dependence, and borderline personality disorder was again admitted to the inpatient service for detoxification and stabilization of mood and cocaine-induced psychosis. Well known to the staff for years as a difficult and non-compliant patient who regressed with extended time on the inpatient service, and who was characterized by emotional volatility, manipulativeness and threatening behaviour, the patient was more than reluctant even to read the behavioural contract. However, after extended support and negotiation, she had the contract explained to her, read it, and signed it. Although she lost certain benefits due to impulsive infractions of the contract, the staff worked with her on giving positive feedback for the gains she was able to make in her inpatient stay, and she related better to others than usual. During her next hospitalization, in spite of a paranoid state, she was, without as much negotiation, able to read and sign the contract on admission, and the staff were struck by the increase in organization and treatment compliance the patient demonstrated during this briefer than usual admission. At a much later date, the patient was again readmitted to the inpatient service. This time, she asked for the contract upon admission. Her stay was characterized by its brevity, and the patient's relatively rapid return to a euthymic state, and the staff were struck not only at their lack of animosity but also their feelings of warmth toward this historically difficult and provocative patient.

INTEGRATED TREATMENT

Integrated treatment aims to do the following:

1. create a sense of group identity and cohesion among patients who historically are poorly compliant with treatment
2. educate patients about schizophrenia and SUD
3. control psychosis, preferably with second-generation antipsychotic drugs that reduce negative symptoms
4. support the attainment of sobriety though group discussion, counselling, motivational enhancement, and skills training
5. encourage the use of self-help participation where it is appropriate to the patient's needs and capacities
6. improve patients' socialization and community adaptation skills.

Psychoeducation includes lectures and discussion about mental illness, the medications used to treat it, SUDs with a disease model view (Jellinek,1952), and drugs of abuse. Information is given about signs and symptoms of both mental illness and substance abuse. Patients are encouraged to share their experience of how drugs affect their mental state, positively as well as negatively. Psychoeducation can also be delivered ad hoc in the course of the group process. This gives factual as well as emotional content in generating peer support for group attendance and sobriety. Information is thus used to tip the decisional balance towards medication compliance and sobriety.

The essence of supportive group psychotherapy is to maintain, restore, or improve self-esteem, adaptive skills, and psychological (ego) functioning

(Pinsker et al, 1991). Self-esteem, deemed the critical factor in this model, can be modelled as the top pole of a triangle resting upon the two foundations of ego functioning and adaptive skills. As a result of the current circumstances in their lives, and in addition to the burdens of addiction and mental illness, most dually diagnosed inpatients are acutely demoralized (see below). If patients are demoralized, they do not bother to try new things to improve their quality of life, because they believe that they have no power to effect change (Pinsker et al, 1991). Because patients are only there for days to weeks, the initial focus in the inpatient group is to engage patients in treatment through development of the therapeutic alliance and through increased motivation, to support their re-experiencing a sense of opportunity, to get them to come back to the group, and to highlight the dual problems of substance abuse and mental illness.

The main techniques of supportive group psychotherapy are clarification (restating, acknowledging), expression of interest and empathy, supporting healthy defences, giving expert advice, and giving data-based praise and reassurance. Praise for something the patient does not feel praiseworthy belittles the patient. Confrontation is limited to active drug use or when the frame of therapy is threatened. The therapist repeatedly models appropriate supportive behaviour for the group members to begin to emulate over time. The therapist, although limit setting, is active in a conversational mode, not withholding or anxiety provoking. The art of working with these patients is to be able to confront the disease without punishing the patient, and to be able to support patients without fostering regression.

TECHNICAL CONSIDERATIONS: THE FLOATING LINE MODEL

Having made initial diagnostic assumptions, obtained the history, and searched for signs of organic or substance-induced pathology, one can address certain interpersonal aspects of the acute treatment context for the dual-diagnosis patient. This context can be conceptualized among several different axes, such as autonomy or proximity. One way to conceptualize the shifting give-and-take between staff and a patient along the autonomy axis is the floating-line model (Rosenthal, 1993). This model may be applied to the acutely ill, non-dually diagnosed psychiatric patient, and it is what is done generally, albeit implicitly.

We can look at the responsivity of patients to staff intervention by diagnosis, by time, and by the degree of disruption of characterologic function by interpersonal, functional, or toxic stressors. For example, the degree of autonomy demonstrated over time by patients on an acute-care inpatient unit will clearly vary with diagnosis (Figure 9.1).

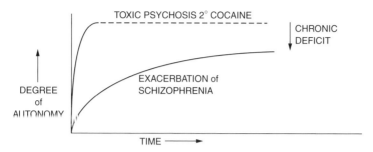

ACUTE RECOVERY OF AUTONOMY BY DIAGNOSIS

Figure 9.1   Diagnosis affects the rate of recovery of autonomy

A patient suffering a psychosis from the toxic effects of cocaine, but who has no other functional psychosis, will typically regain full autonomy in a short time, whereas patients with an acute exacerbation of a schizophrenic disorder will slowly recompensate to their baseline of psychosocial functioning, which usually shows chronic impairment. The acutely decompensated schizophrenia patient may be so regressed and overwhelmed as to need assistance with structuring the most basic functions such as eating, grooming, and dressing. The ability of patients to carry out basic functions will be contingent on their level of cognitive and emotional organization. Clearly, it would demonstrate little respect for autonomy and would also feel clinically inappropriate to treat the higher functioning patient as one would an acutely decompensated schizophrenia patient. As such, one uses clinical assessment and feedback, and diagnostic consideration, in order to assign most appropriately the level of personal responsibility that one can expect from the patient at any given time.

The extent to which the mentally ill patient needs time to regain autonomy can be related to the mood-altering or disorganizing effect of certain drugs. If one holds the functional diagnosis constant, it is not difficult to entertain a differential effect of drug type, route of administration, and use intensity upon the ability of the patient in the acute phase of inpatient treatment thus to understand and internalize external controls on behaviour, i.e., to make use of rules and restrictions. For example, the increase in the average peak dosage of smokable "crack" over that of intranasal cocaine correlates with increased risk of depressive symptoms in crack users versus cocaine snorters (Ringwalt and Palmer,1989). Indeed, one can demonstrate a differential effect of crack cocaine upon production of psychotic symptoms independent of the contribution of the schizophrenic disorder in patients with SUD and schizophrenia (Cleghorn et al, 1991; Rosenthal et al, 1992b). Understanding amounts and routes of administration of specific drugs can therefore have some predictive value in estimating the rate and trajectory of a patient's reorganization.

EFFECT OF CHARACTER UPON
INTERPERSONAL BALANCE

The degree of disruption of character functioning will also influence where one can set effective levels of restrictiveness upon behaviour. From the viewpoint of psychodynamic theory, the development of character is through a continuum of defensive structures, from the most primitive distortion, projection, and denial in young children, to mature defences such as suppression, humour, and altruism in healthy adults (Vaillant, 1971). The DSM-IV criteria propose that character traits in the personality disorders are chronic, pervasive, and maladaptive (American Psychiatric Association, 1994). As such, from a psychodynamic perspective, the primary attributes of personality disorders are the habitual use of ego defences that are typically immature, and individually and interpersonally maladaptive. Under functional or toxic stress, these characters can show increased intensity of the habitual defences or regress to the use of even more primitive ones. Clearly, people with certain personality disorders have an increased vulnerability to the development of affective instability and psychosis (Schuckit, 1985; Fyer et al, 1988).

Patients presenting with the acute and chronic effects of cocaine can be quite disorganized, showing irritability, dysphoria, agitation, hallucinations, and paranoid persecutory delusions (Szuster et al, 1990; Satel et al, 1991; Brady et al, 1991). At the extreme, they may need for a short time the kind of hands-on supportive care one generally provides to more regressed patients with functional psychosis. Two patients presenting with cocaine psychoses may look similar on first inspection, and be similarly lacking in organizational autonomy (Figure 9.2). However, patients with concurrent borderline personality disorder will only reorganize back to the level of their chronic maladaptive character defences. Thus, the clinician needs to follow the shifting line of increasing independence and reset the balance between permissiveness/support and responsibility/autonomy accordingly. This balance is therefore clinically derived by staff in an active fashion which is sensitive to positive and negative feedback, i.e., whether the patient is able to meet the expectations of staff to function at a particular level of autonomy.

As stated above, at one such arbitrary level, staff can ask the patient to read and agree to the behavioural contract which sets overt limits as to acceptable behaviour. If patients are still disorganized and agitated to the point that they are unable to understand or make use of the information, then they need more permissive support. An intervention which inaccurately assumes more autonomy on the part of the patient will frustrate the staff. In response to feelings of impotence, this frustration, if not identified (i.e., countertransference) may increase the likelihood of staff retaliatory

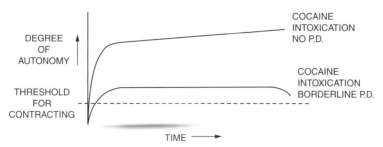

Figure 9.2 Character organization affects the recovery of autonomy after substance-induced psychosis

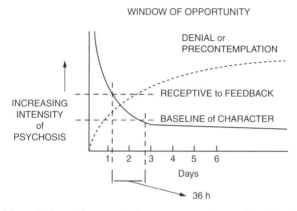

Figure 9.3 The window of opportunity may vary inversely with the rigidity of defences

behaviour. This will have the net effect of punishing the patient while wasting staff time and energy. Therefore, empathy and accurate clinical assessment make for better treatment.

It has been noted that a crisis can mobilize affects through previously held rigid defences. Indeed, some forms of brief psychotherapy make use of the relative plasticity of the ego defences in the crisis state in order to advance character change (Flegenheimer, 1982). There appears to be a "window of opportunity" for making certain acute interventions which appears to vary inversely with the strength of ego defensive functioning (Figure 9.3); that is, as the patient reorganizes from the psychotic episode or crisis, the more rigid the maladaptive structure, the less likely denial is to be affected by confrontation/education in the acute phase of treatment.

As patients becomes less psychotic, they reintegrate back to their specific baseline of character functioning. For someone with a personality disorder, this means that the patient will reintegrate using the defensive structures which are chronic, pervasive, and maladaptive. For example, in antisocial personality disorder, one can see a rapid return of typical utilitarian attitudes and behaviours after a crisis. If one tries to make an intervention while the patient's defences are grossly overwhelmed, the patient will not be able to make use of the information. Once patients have returned to their habitual mode of functioning, it is difficult in a short-term setting to address denial of illness. Between these two states is a varying interval within which to forge an alliance; unfortunately, this period often lasts only from a few hours to a few days.

PSYCHOTHERAPEUTIC IMPLICATIONS

The classical motivation for change in addiction recovery lore is "hitting bottom", or the patients' experience that their coping strategies have utterly failed. It may be that the artful clinician can "keep the window open" by supporting the continued sense of crisis in these patients, and present a healthier direction to move in, one that relieves demoralization. This pressure to "stay scared" may come in the form of clarifying the costs of the addiction to the patient, confronting minimization, supporting acceptance of the hopelessness of trying to maintain control, etc. Another way to look at the intervention is that it confronts maladaptive behaviour (denial of illness) while supporting better adaptive functioning (continuance of treatment). Without a clear direction for the patient to move towards, and in a less structured milieu, this type of confrontation is risky as it tends to increase anxiety in the patient that can trigger behavioural dyscontrol and increase drug use. Removing characterologic defences is more likely to be successful with higher functioning patients in later stages of rehabilitation and psychotherapy when the patient is stable in sobriety and has a firm working alliance with the therapist (Kaufman and Reoux,1988).

DEPRESSION VERSUS DEMORALIZATION

Depressed mood with or without suicidal ideation is among the most common presentations of dual-diagnosis patients. In addition to primary unipolar and bipolar depressions exacerbated by alcohol or substance abuse, primary alcoholism and substance dependence can cause depressive symptoms. Depressive symptoms in a dual-diagnosis patient often confuse the treatment team as to where and when to "draw the line" in responding with psychopharmacologic or psychotherapeutic interventions.

Patients are typically admitted to the dual-diagnosis inpatient service with suicidal ideation, depressed mood, decreased sleep and appetite, agitation, helplessness, and anhedonia. Most of these symptoms become less intense or clear completely in several days off the drug of abuse and do not require antidepressant medication; this is the typical course for a patient with a substance-induced mood disorder (Brown and Schuckit, 1988; Weiss et al, 1989). Some patients continue to appear depressed, and while some have major depression, many have a resolving DSM-IV substance-induced mood disorder. In addition to persisting substance-induced or withdrawal-related mood and anxiety symptoms, they may have what might be called a "demoralization syndrome". It becomes important then to distinguish the neurovegetative symptoms of depression, which, if persisting after several weeks of sobriety, respond to antidepressant treatment, from the dysphoria, anger, guilt, and sense of helplessness of demoralization. Since the critical feature of the demoralized state is subjective incompetence or helplessness (de Figueiredo, 1993), substance abusers, who typically demonstrate an external locus of control (Dohrenwend et al, 1980) or a dysfunctional attributional style (Peterson et al, 1982), may be at increased risk of demoralization.

The depressive-type symptoms which are related to demoralization may persist after those related to organic causes abate. However, there is no evidence that demoralization, as such, will respond to antidepressant medication. These patients often claim that their lives are miserable, and, generally, they are correct. One must take reality into consideration, and understand that patients having gained enough lucidity to recognize their current state of being may cause appropriate pain from which real motivation for change may come. Here is where the art of psychotherapeutic intervention is important. The patients must begin to realize that their prior course of action has directly contributed to their present state, and yet somehow feel hopeful of the possibility of change. The art comes in attacking the disease without attacking the patient. Here, the disease model of addiction may assist the clinician by giving the patients something they can ally with the clinician against, and by not blaming the patients for the addiction.

Another major characteristic of these patients is that they have particular difficulty in establishing an on-going therapeutic alliance, whether this be due to a lack of basic trust, paranoid ideation, help-rejecting complaints, or an exploitative stance as result of the shift in values seen in the addiction process. Clinicians must therefore take care not to increase the patient's sense of alienation and helplessness, in effect increasing demoralization. On the contrary, use of motivational-enhancement techniques (Rollnick and Miller, 1995) can build up patients' motivation for treatment by educating patients singly and in a group about the course of addictive illness; the effects of drugs on mood, thinking, and behaviour; and the real-life damage to psychosocial functioning. The intention is to offer enough information for the patient to experience an opportunity to change for the better. Perceived opportunity is an antidote to demoralization. Clearly within the supportive frame, active clinical interventions to engage dual-diagnosis patients into treatment are appropriate. The use of positive reinforcement, such as the offer of support for access to concrete services or entitlements, socialization, recreation, or vocational opportunities, and any other thing which is perceived by the patient as beneficial and is objectively not harmful or enabling can help foster alliance and motivation (Rosenthal, in press).

INTERPERSONAL DISTANCE

Another axis of interpersonal behaviour that can be usefully addressed in the dual-diagnosis inpatient is proximity, one pole of which is isolation/avoidance. One needs to assess real phobic anxiety in contrast to avoidant strategies, which are maladaptive and assist the patient in denial of illness. Patients with acute psychosis due to schizophrenia or depression may need to withdraw due to an inability to tolerate interpersonal contact, and, as with autonomy, will slowly regain the ability to participate in low-demand, one-to-one and then group activity. Patients with only substance-induced psychoses and mood disorders can be expected to shift more quickly from true contact intolerance back to habitual superficial interpersonal contact. This cursory style may be understood in the context of the shift in values that takes place in the development of addictions, where the nature of relationships changes from egalitarian to utilitarian. As at least some of this shift may be due to a learning process, the extent to which this is independent of character may be amenable to active limit-setting and exposure to traditional values by staff. Clearly, we do not expect character change on an acute basis. Rather, we attempt to direct and manage the character pathology of patients so as to maximize their ability to make use of current treatment. This treatment, in addition to resolving acute psychosis, mood disorders and withdrawal states, is aimed at educating patients about the illness they suffer from, offering substitutive behaviours for maladaptive ones, and forming enough of a therapeutic alliance to guide patients into longer-term treatment and rehabilitation.

AVOIDING "SPLITTING" WITH DUAL-DIAGNOSIS PATIENTS

Patients can use a specific "hook" to direct individual staff to depart from the treatment team's plan. These patients see others receive a certain treatment and therefore claim that for themselves not to receive this treatment is "not fair". This strategy attempts to coerce fair-minded clinicians to overextend their good judgement and limit-setting through induced feelings of guilt or inadequacy. Unfortunately, clinicians are susceptible because they are operating on the wrong model of treatment. "Everybody gets the same treatment here!" may sound egalitarian, but it is counter to the best principles of treatment. Clinical treatment is not democratic in the sense of participatory voting strength or "equal treatment". Patients have the right to respectful, reasonable, and fair treatment, but just because one patient receives insulin for diabetes does not mean that another patient with a broken arm should get the same treatment. Treatments are supposed to be specific. Indeed, the more specific treatments have become for psychiatric disorders over the past hundred years, the better the outcomes have been. Thus, with a patient suffering from a schizophrenic disorder, it may be appropriate to have more permissive treatment, but for a patient with antisocial personality disorder and cocaine dependence, even with some psychotic symptoms, more permissive treatment would be clinically less productive. This explanation is not to be considered solely professional/technical, and the reasoning may be made explicit to patients in confronting this form of interaction.

TRANSITIONAL PHASE

In the transitional phase, the patient's acute psychiatric symptoms have resolved with detoxification, medication, and milieu treatment, and the patient is involved in the unit programme. Decisions have been made about appropriate aftercare, and in this period, these plans are finalized. Interviews for outpatient programmes, therapeutic communities, etc., generally take place during this last phase, with the hope that linking patients directly may improve their ability to stay in treatment.

REFERENCES

American Psychiatric Association (1994) *Diagnostic and Statistical Manual of Mental Disorders* (4th edn), 629–673 Washington, DC, American Psychiatric Association.

Ananth, J., Vandeater, S., Kamal, M. and Brodsky, A. (1989) Missed diagnosis of substance abuse in psychiatric patients. *Hospital and Community Psychiatry*, **40**: 297–299.

Becker, H.C. and Hale, R.L. (1993) Repeated episodes of ethanol withdrawal potentiate the severity of subsequent withdrawal seizures: an animal model of alcohol withdrawal "kindling". *Alcoholism, Clinical and Experimental Research*, **17**: 94–98.

Brady, K.T., Lydiard, R.B., Malcolm, R. and Ballenger, J.C. (1991) Cocaine-induced psychosis. *Journal of Clinical Psychiatry*, **52**: 509–512.

Brown, M.E., Anton, R.F., Malcolm, R. and Ballenger, J.C. (1988a) Alcohol detoxification and withdrawal seizures: clinical support for a kindling hypothesis. *Biological Psychiatry*, **23**: 507–514.

Brown, S.A. and Schuckit, M.A. (1988) Changes in depression among abstinent alcoholics. *Journal of Studies on Alcohol*, **49**: 412–417.

Cleghorn, J.M., Kaplan, R.D., Szechtman, B., Szechtman, H., Brown, G.M., Franco, S. (1991) Substance abuse and schizophrenia: effect on symptoms but not on neurocognitive function. *Journal of Clinical Psychiatry*, **52**: 26–30.

Craig, T.J., Lin, S.P., El-Defrawi, M.H. and Goodman, A.B. (1985) Clinical correlates of readmission in a schizophrenic cohort. *Psychiatric Quarterly*, **57**: 5–10.

de Figueiredo, J.M. (1993) Depression and demoralization: phenomenological differences and research perspectives. *Comprehensive Psychiatry*, **34**: 308–311.

Dohrenwend, B.P., Shrout, P.E., Egri, G. and Mendelsohn, F.S. (1980) Non-specific psychological distress and other dimensions of psychopathology. *Archives of General Psychiatry*, **37**: 1229–1236.

Drake, R.E. and Sederer, L.I. (1986) Inpatient psychosocial treatment of chronic schizophrenia: negative effects and current guidelines. *Hospital and Community Psychiatry*, **37**: 897–90.

Dunner, D.L., Hensel, B.M. and Fieve, R.R. (1979) Bipolar illness: factors in drinking behavior. *American Journal of Psychiatry*, **136**: 583–585.

Flegenheimer, W.V. (1982) Techniques of brief psychotherapy. New York, Jason Aronson.

Fyer, M.R., Frances, A.J., Sullivan, T., Hurt, S.W. and Clarkin, J., (1988) Suicide attempts in patients with borderline personality disorder. *American Journal of Psychiatry*, **145**: 737–739.

Goldfinger, S.M., Schutt, R.K., Seidman, L.J., Turner, W.M., Penk, W.E. and Tolmiczenko, G.S. (1996) Self-report and observer measures of substance abuse among homeless mentally ill persons in the cross section and over time. *Journal of Nervous and Mental Disease*, **184**: 667–672.

Hamilton, M. (1960) A rating scale for depression. *Journal of Neurology, Neurosurgery and Psychiatry*, **23**: 56–60.

Hellerstein, D.J. and Meehan, B. (1987) Outpatient group therapy for schizophrenic substance abusers. *American Journal of Psychiatry*, **144**: 1337–1340.

Hellerstein, D.J., Pinsker, H., Rosenthal, R.N. and Klee, S. (1994) Supportive therapy as the treatment model of choice. *Journal of Psychotherapy Practice and Research*, **3**: 100–106.

Hellerstein, D.J., Rosenthal, R.N. and Miner, C.R. (1995) A prospective study of integrated outpatient treatment for substance-abusing schizophrenic patients. *American Journal on Addictions*, **4**: 33–42.

Hellerstein, D.J., Rosenthal, R.N., Pinsker, H., Wallner-Samstag, L., Muran, J.C. and Winston, A. (1998) A randomized prospective study comparing supportive and dynamic therapies: outcome and alliance. *Journal of Psychotherapy Practice and Research*, **7**: 261–271.

Jellinek, E.M. (1952) Phases of alcohol addiction. *Quarterly Journal of Studies on Alcohol*, **13**: 4.

Kane, J.M. and Selzer, J. (1991) Considerations on "organic" exclusion criteria for schizophrenia. *Schizophrenia Bulletin*, **17**: 69–73.

Kaufman, E. and Reoux, J. (1988) Guidelines for the successful psychotherapy of substance abusers. *American Journal of Drug and Alcohol Abuse*, **14**: 199–209.

Kessler, R.C., McGonagle, K.A., Zhao, S., Nelson, C.B., Hughes, M., Eshelman, S., Wittchen, H.U. and Kendler, K.S. (1994) Lifetime and 12-month prevalence of DSM-III-R psychiatric disorders in the United States: Results from the National Comorbidity Study. *Archives of General Psychiatry*, **51**: 8–19.

Khantzian, E.J. (1985) The self-medication hypothesis of addictive disorders: focus on heroin and cocaine dependence. *American Journal of Psychiatry*, **42**: 1259–1264.

LaPorte, D.J., McLellan, A.T., O'Brien, C.P. and Marshall, J.R. (1981) Treatment response in psychiatrically impaired drug abusers. *Comprehensive Psychiatry*, **22**: 411–419.

McLellan, A.T., Luborsky, L., Woody, G.E., O'Brien, C.P. and Druley, K.A. (1983) Predicting response to alcohol and drug abuse treatments—role of psychiatric severity. *Archives of General Psychiatry*, **40**: 620–625.

Olivera, A.A., Kiefer, M.W. and Manley, N.K. (1990) Tardive dyskinesia in psychiatric patients with substance abuse disorders. *American Journal of Drug and Alcohol Abuse*, **16**: 57–66.

Pepper, B. and Ryglewicz, H. (1984) The young adult chronic patient and substance abuse. *Tie Lines Bulletin*, **1**: 1–5.

Peterson, C., Semmel, A., von Baeyer, C., Abramson, L.Y., Metalsky, G.I. and Seligman, M.E.P. (1982) The attributional style questionnaire. *Cognitive Therapy and Research*, **6**: 287–299.

Pinsker, H. (1983) Addicted patients in hospital psychiatric units. *Psychiatric Annals*, **13**: 619–623.

Pinsker, H. and Rosenthal, R.N. (1988) *Beth Israel Medical Center Supportive Psychotherapy Manual*. Social and Behavioral Sciences Documents, vol., 18: no. 2.

Pinsker, H., Rosenthal, R.N. and McCullough, L. (1991) Supportive dynamic psychotherapy. In P. Crits-Christoph (ed.), *Handbook of Short-Term Dynamic Therapy*, pp. 220–247. Basic Books.

Pinsker, H. (1997) On co-occurring addictive and mental disorders [Letter]. *American Journal of Orthopsychiatry*, **67**: 158–159.

Rado, S. (1933) Psychoanalysis of pharmacothymia. *Psychoanalytic Quarterly*, **2**: 1–23.

Regier, D.A., Farmer, M.E., Rae, D.S., Locke, B.Z., Keith, S.J., Judd, L.L., Goodwin, F.K. (1990) Comorbidity of mental disorder with alcohol and other drug abuse. Results from the Epidemiologic Catchment Area (ECA) Study. *Journal of the American Medical Association*, **264**: 2511–2518.

Richard, M.L., Liskow, B.I. and Perry P.J. (1985) Recent psychostimulant use in hospitalized schizophrenics. *Journal of Clinical Psychiatry*, **46**: 79–83.

Richardson, M.A. (1985) Treatment patterns of young schizophrenic patients in the era of deinstitutionalization. *Psychiatric Quarterly*, **57**: 243–249.

Ringwalt, C.L. and Palmer, G.H. (1989) Cocaine and crack users compared. *Adolescence*, **24**: 851–859.

Rollnick, S. and Miller, W.R. (1995) What is motivational interviewing? *Behavioral and Cognitive Psychotherapy*, **23**: 325–334.

Rosenthal, M.S. (1984) Therapeutic Communities: a treatment alternative for many but not all. *Journal of Substance Abuse Treatment*, **1**: 55–58.

Rosenthal, R.N., Hellerstein, D.J. and Miner, C.R. (1992a) A model of integrated services for outpatient treatment of patients with comorbid schizophrenia and addictive disorders. *American Journal on Addictions*, **1**: 339–348.

Rosenthal, R.N., Hellerstein, D.J. and Miner, C.R. (1992b) Integrated services for treatment of schizophrenic substance abusers: demographics, symptoms and substance abuse patterns. *Psychiatric Quarterly*, **63**: 3–26.

Rosenthal, R.N. (1993) *Mental Illness/Chemical Addiction: A Guide to Emergency Services Assessment and Treatment.* Albany, New York State Office of Mental Health, Division of Clinical Support Systems.

Rosenthal, R.N., Hellerstein, D.J. and Miner, C.R. (1994) Positive and negative syndrome typology in schizophrenic patients with psychoactive substance use disorders. *Comprehensive Psychiatry,* **35**: 91–98.

Rosenthal, R.N., Pinsker, H. and Winston, A. (1996) Supportive group psychotherapy and counseling manual for patients with substance abuse and schizophrenia. The COPAD Program; Beth Israel Medical Center Psychotherapy Research Program. Unpublished Manuscript, 1993; Revised 1996.

Rosenthal, R.N. and Miner, C.R. (1997) Differential diagnosis of substance-induced psychosis and schizophrenia in patients with psychoactive substance use disorders. *Schizophrenia Bulletin,* **23**: 187–193.

Rosenthal, R.N., Muran, J.C., Hellerstein D.J., Pinsker H. and Winston, A. (1999) Interpersonal change in supportive psychotherapy. *Journal of Psychotherapy Practice and Research,* **8**: 55–63.

Rosenthal, R.N., Group treatments for schizophrenic substance abusers. (2002, in press) In D.W., Brook and H.I., Spitz (Eds), *The Group Psychotherapy of Substance Abuse,* New York, Haworth Press.

Satel, S.L., Southwick, S.M. and Gawin, F.H. (1991) Clinical features of cocaine-induced paranoia. *American Journal of Psychiatry,* **148**: 495–498.

Schneier, F.R. and Siris S.G. (1987) A review of psychoactive substance abuse and abuse in schizophrenia. *Journal of Nervous and Mental Disease,* **175**: 641–652.

Schuckit, M.A. (1983) Alcoholism and other psychiatric disorders. *Hospital and Community Psychiatry,* **34**: 1022–1027.

Schuckit, M.A. (1985) The clinical implications of primary diagnostic groups among alcoholics. *Archives of General Psychiatry,* **42**: 1043–1049.

Selzer, M.A., Koenigsberg, H.W. and Kernberg, O.F. (1987) The initial contract in the treatment of borderline patients. *American Journal of Psychiatry,* **144**: 927–930.

Shaner, A., Khalsa, M.E., Roberts, L., Wilkins, J., Anglin, D. and Hsieh, S.C. (1993) Unrecognized cocaine use among schizophrenic patients. *American Journal of Psychiatry,* **150**: 758–762.

Solomon, P., Davis, J., Gorson, B. (1984) Discharged state hospital patient's characteristics and use of aftercare—effect upon community tenure. *American Journal of Psychiatry,* **141**: 1566–1570.

Szuster, R.R., Schanbacher, B.L., McCann, S.C. and McConnell, A. (1990) Underdiagnosis of psychoactive-substance-induced organic mental disorders in emergency psychiatry. *American Journal of Drug and Alcohol Abuse,* **16**: 319–327.

Treffert, D.A. (1978) Marijuana use in schizophrenia: a clear hazard. *American Journal of Psychiatry,* **135**: 1213–1215.

Vaillant, G.E. (1971) Theoretical hierarchy of adaptive ego mechanisms. *Archives of General, Psychiatry,* **24**: 107–118.

Vaughn, C.E. and Leff, J.P. (1976) The influence of family and social factors on the course of psychiatric illness. *British Journal of Psychiatry,* **129**: 125–137.

Wallen, M. and Weiner, H. (1988) The dually diagnosed patient in an inpatient chemical dependency treatment program. *Alcoholism Treatment Quarterly,* **5**: 197–219.

Weiss, R.D., Griffin, M.L. and Mirin, S.M. (1989) Diagnosing major depression in cocaine abusers: the use of depression rating scales. *Psychiatry Research,* **28**: 335–343.

Weiss, R.D. and Collins, D.A. (1992) Substance abuse and psychiatric illness: the dually diagnosed patient. *American Journal of Addictions,* **1**: 93–99.

Wilens, T.E., O'Keefe, J., O'Connell, J.J., Springer, R. and Renner, J.A. (1993) A public dual diagnosis detoxification unit. I. Organization and structure. *American Journal of Addiction*, **2**: 91–98.

Ziedonis, D.M., Kosten, T.R. and Glazer, W.M. (1992) The impact of drug abuse on psychotic outpatients. American Psychiatric Association 145th Annual Meeting, New Research Program and Abstracts, p. 103, 2–7 May. Washington., DC.

Part III

TREATMENTS FOR SUBSTANCE MISUSE IN PSYCHOSIS

INTRODUCTION

Alex Copello

As Noordsy, McQuade and Mueser remind us in the first line of Chapter 10, "Individuals with psychosis and concurrent substance misuse represent a formidable challenge to their clinicians." Treatment providers are faced with the task of developing treatment approaches that can be effective in reducing the whole range of problems associated with this group.

The key first step in the treatment process is a good and thorough assessment of the problem. Noordsy, McQuade and Mueser deal with assessment issues in Chapter 10 and start by discussing a number of common impediments to assessment of this client group. They continue with a description of a four-step assessment process that include detection, classification, functional assessment and analysis, and treatment planning. A number of validated measures are also described, and the authors stress the need for continuous assessment throughout the treatment process.

In the next series of chapters, authors describe treatment approaches and provide an account of current attempts to evaluate their effectiveness.

Chapter 11 introduces us to a cognitive-behavioural approach delivered within the context of integrated services. The approach emphasizes the need to address dysfunctional, substance-related beliefs but also incorporates a range of strategies to work with clients from early engagement through to relapse prevention. A number of examples from cases are used throughout the chapter to illustrate the various treatment components.

In Chapter 12, Weiss, Greenfield and O'Leary discuss some of the particular problems presented by people with bipolar and substance use disorders. The authors describe a systematic relapse prevention group programme developed to work with this client group. A detailed description of the contents of the group sessions is followed by a case example illustrating both common issues faced by this group and treatment progress.

In contrast to the more individually based approaches described in other chapters, Christine Barrowclough takes a family perspective in Chapter 13, which describes in detail a family intervention for substance misuse in psychosis. The approach combines motivational interviewing, cognitive-behavioural therapy, and family and carer intervention into a coherent package delivered to people with psychosis and substance misuse. Details of the intervention as well as its evaluation are covered. Again, case examples are used to illustrate the way in which the intervention works.

In Chapter 14, Kavanagh and colleagues describe the development of a brief intervention ("Start Over and Survive") used for people with substance misuse problems in early psychosis. In their previous work, the authors became interested in the development of a relatively brief intervention that can be compatible with the demands faced by mental health workers. Drawing from motivational enhancement principles, the approach is delivered in over 3 hours of individual treatment. The approach is flexible and described and illustrated in the aforementioned chapter.

Finally, there are important considerations related to the pharmacological management of substance misuse in psychosis. In Chapter 15, Day, Georgiou and Crome discuss the pharmacological management of both psychosis and substance misuse by reviewing the available evidence. Practical strategies are also given, and a case example illustrates some of the challenges posed by this client group.

Chapter 10

ASSESSMENT CONSIDERATIONS

Douglas L. Noordsy, Debra V. McQuade
and Kim T. Mueser

INTRODUCTION

Individuals with psychosis and concurrent substance misuse present a formidable challenge to their clinicians. We know, from both research and clinical experience, that active substance use increases the likelihood of deleterious outcomes for patients with psychosis (Drake and Brunette, 1998). They experience increased risk of symptomatic relapse, hospitalization and suicide (Bartels et al, 1995; Linszen et al, 1996; Swofford et al, 1996). Disinhibition from substance use can increase violence, aggression and suicide risk, potentiating interpersonal conflicts and legal problems (Steadman et al, 1998; Swartz et al, 1998; Yesavage and Zarcone, 1983). Housing instability and homelessness increase in likelihood (Drake et al, 1989).

These prognostic complications make it important for treatment providers to recognize substance use in these clients. Unfortunately, despite a growing interest in substance misuse and psychosis (SMP), substance use remains underrecognized and undertreated (Ananth et al, 1989; Shaner et al, 1993). At the present time, assessment tools unique and appropriate for SMP are not widely implemented. This leaves mental health workers with little training or experience in identification of their clients with SMP (Carey and Correia, 1998).

The purpose of the current chapter is to present a model of assessment of substance misuse among people with severe mental illness. Also

Substance Misuse in Psychosis: Approaches to Treatment and Service Delivery.
Edited by Hermine L. Graham, Alex Copello, Max J. Birchwood and Kim T. Mueser.
© 2003 John Wiley & Sons, Ltd.

included in the chapter is a discussion of common impediments to proper assessment, as well as a presentation of useful evaluation and treatment tools. It is our intent to provide the reader with the knowledge and tools necessary for conducting comprehensive assessments and for planning treatment.

THE IMPORTANCE OF ASSESSMENT

Assessment is best viewed as ongoing and continuous throughout the course of all work with clients with SMP. It is the cornerstone of effective treatment; its impact is felt initially with identification of clients at risk. The treatment of clients with SMP cannot proceed until their clinicians identify the signs of substance abuse and subsequently determine whether diagnostic criteria for a substance-use disorder are met. Ideally, assessment involves the availability and implementation of appropriate evaluation tools, preferably those specific for use in this special population. These tools should clarify the nature of clients' substance use, including its temporal course; the context in which it occurs; and its functional significance to the clients' lifestyles and behaviours, as well as identification of the clients' personal interpretation of the role that substances play in their lives. Coherent, specific and realistic treatment plans are best designed with this information at hand.

Assessment continues after treatment plans are designed, as feedback regarding a plan's efficacy is used for its modification. The interactive nature of the relationship between assessment and treatment is particularly important for clients with SMP, as much literature implicates the importance of multiple modes and times of evaluation for diagnostic certainty (Ananth et al, 1989; Drake et al, 1990; Kranzler et al, 1994).

COMMON IMPEDIMENTS TO ASSESSMENT

The Epidemiologic Catchment Area Study (Regier et al, 1990) reports the lifetime prevalence of substance misuse among people with schizophrenia to be 47%; estimates obtained in smaller, more recent studies are similar (Fowler et al, 1998; Mueser et al, 2000; Ziedonis and Trudeau, 1997). Despite the estimated high frequency of SMP, it has been difficult, in practice, for clinicians to establish the presence of both severe mental illness and substance misuse in the same client. Numerous complicating factors contribute to this difficulty (Carey and Correia, 1998; Mueser et al, in press; Zeidonis and Stern, 2001).

The role of clinicians

Clinicians may fail to take a history adequate to recognize SMP. Numerous studies have demonstrated that clinicians are often unaware which of their clients abuse alcohol or drugs, and the most common reason for this lack of awareness is that they neglect to ask (Ananth et al, 1989; Barbee et al, 1989; Drake et al, 1990; Galletly et al, 1993; Shaner et al, 1993). However, stable outpatients have been shown to be quite accurate in their reporting of usage (Weiss et al, 1998). For initial evaluations, standardized self report questionnaires elicit more accurate responses than personal interviews (Pristach and Smith, 1990). Clinicians need to keep in mind that information about substance use is unlikely to be spontaneously offered, and they should be encouraged to ask in a manner designed to maximize reliable reporting (Shea, 1998).

The nature of the illnesses

Psychosis and substance misuse are frequently difficult to distinguish on the basis of their manifested symptoms. Both can produce dysregulation of cognition, mood, and behaviour, and altered patterns of thought, and both have a negative impact on the same areas of psychosocial functioning. Both syndromes unfold gradually in early stages, so even the most rigorous of initial assessments can fail to be accurate (Shaner et al, 1998). When substance misuse can be identified, it remains difficult to rule out underlying mental illness, as sufficient periods of abstinence are usually lacking. Where severe mental illness is documented, the frequently associated psychosocial dysfunction can make the negative impact of substance use less salient. The negative effects of the substance on mood or cognition may be misattributed to the original, or to a second, psychiatric condition (Schuckit, 1983). Given that diagnostic uncertainty is likely when the conditions present separately, this uncertainty becomes even more likely when the two illnesses present jointly (Lehman et al, 1994).

Traditional assessment approaches have attempted to designate either substance misuse or mental illness as being primary, indicating that one disorder preceded or caused the other (Mueser et al, 1998). However, scientific support for the utility of a primary/secondary distinction is virtually nonexistent. In a recent report by Shaner et al (1998), accurate diagnosis of mental illness and substance misuse was less than 20% at initial presentation and only 25% 18 months later. Given this imprecision, attempts to disentangle the causes and the effects of the different syndromes are likely to remain largely unsuccessful and may lead to errors in treatment approach. The alternative to the primary/secondary classification, which circumvents the practical and theoretical problems described above, is to assume that both syndromes are primary and to treat them simultaneously. This strategy has proven effective in treatment of clients with SMP (Drake et al, 1998).

Systemic problems

The simultaneous treatment of two individual and primary syndromes is not easy to achieve, given structural limitations on the current mental health-care delivery system. Currently, mental health clinicians who serve clients with psychosis tend not to treat those with substance misuse. Similarly, specialists in substance abuse tend not to treat individuals with severe mental illness. In many cases, the presence of one syndrome disqualifies individuals from treatment programmes for the other. In some countries, such as the USA, the provider reimbursement or public health system structure may support this fragmentation. Therefore, the burden of coordinating and following through on separate aspects of care falls on the clients, leaving them highly vulnerable to receiving inadequate care (Ziedonis and Stern, 2001).

Client characteristics

A final source of difficulty with the proper assessment of SMP involves client characteristics. Interference from negative and positive symptoms in schizophrenia may make it difficult for clients to engage fully in treatment. Cognitive limitations may make it difficult for them to assess adequately the impact that substance use has on them. Poor insight may impair their ability to identify cause-and-effect relationships between substance use and negative outcomes. Day-to-day variations in symptoms associated with their underlying mental illness may contribute to inconsistent reporting of substance use and/or its effects. However, the presence of symptoms and cognitive deficits alone does not mean that a client's self-reports are not valid. To enhance the validity of information, clinicians should gather information from various sources. Collateral information from family members and other caregivers, and periodic behavioural observations of the client can be helpful.

Additionally, individuals with psychosis frequently experience significant negative consequences with modest quantities of substance use (Cohen and Klein, 1970; Crowley et al, 1974; Lehman et al, 1994). Because of their moderate use, they are less likely to develop physical dependence (Corse et al, 1995; Drake et al, 1990; Test et al, 1989). Similarly, clients with SMP are less likely to use injectable drugs. To avoid underrecognition, clinicians need to be aware that persons with psychosis are prone to experiencing negative consequences from even low levels of alcohol or drug use.

Many clients with SMP are not motivated to address their substance-use problems, making them difficult to involve in the assessment process. Recognizing that most clients early in treatment are in a pre-motivational state, clinicians can focus their assessment attempts at understanding how clients perceive their own problems and goals. The acceptance and understanding of clients as they are, without prejudice or pre-conceived agendas for anticipated change, may facilitate their increasing participation. Additionally, clients' concerns regarding possible legal sanctions, such as restriction of access to their disability income, can also deter them from talking openly about substance use with their clinicians. Clinicians need to be aware of these disincentives in order to create a therapeutic relationship with the client that minimizes concerns over legal or financial sanctions associated with their substance use behaviours.

STEPS TO ASSESSMENT

Assessment of substance misuse among people with psychosis can be broken down into four steps: 1. detection, 2. classification, 3. functional assessment and analysis, and 4. formation of the treatment plan. Each of the initial three steps feeds directly into, and receives feedback from, the treatment-planning step. Thus, this is not a simple forward-flowing, sequential model, but rather one in which information gleaned in later stages of assessment has impact and bearing on earlier steps. Assessment is an ongoing process, with provisions for change based upon evaluation of treatment plan viability.

Step 1: detection

The goal of detection is to identify clients who may be at risk of experiencing problems with substance use. This step is undertaken with the assumption that it is preferable to "cast a wide net" in identification of these clients. Misidentifying clients who are later determined not to have substance misuse is considered more appropriate than failing to identify clients who do. To this end, it is useful for clinicians to have a high index of suspicion regarding any individual client's use of substances.

Many demographic, historical and clinical factors have been shown to be correlated with substance misuse (Mueser et al, in press), and clinicians should be aware of these. Young, unmarried males with little education are particularly likely to be abusers. There is frequently a family history of substance-use disorders (Noordsy et al, 1994). The individual may have had a conduct disorder evident in childhood; there may be a positive history of trauma and post-traumatic stress disorder (PTSD). Clinically, there is a high correlation between substance abuse and depression, suicidality, violent and/or disruptive behaviour, and antisocial personality disorder. Other behavioural correlates are involvement with the legal system, homelessness and non-compliance with treatment.

Astute clinicians will be wary of these signals, but will not limit their consideration of clients who fail to match these correlates when available information is suggestive of substance use. Other important indicators are the following common consequences of substance use in persons with psychosis: relapse and rehospitalization; financial problems; family conflict; housing instability; violence; victimization; suicidality; legal problems such as incarceration; trading sex, drugs, or money; health problems; and health risk behaviours for infectious diseases (such as exchanging needles and unprotected sex).

There are several tools appropriate for gathering information in the detection step. Personal interview is probably the most frequently used, as clinicians have many opportunities for contact with their clients, and discussions about substance use can occur in many of these. In order to lower clients' defence regarding discussions of their substance use, we recommend starting with discussions about their use in the past. Once clients are comfortable with discussions about past use, clinicians' gradual introduction of questions about current substance use may facilitate disclosure.

As previously described, structured self-report screening instruments are superior to the personal interview in attaining valid responses from substance users in some contexts. Numerous screening instruments have been developed for the detection of alcohol and drug use disorders in the general population; however, most lack sensitivity and specificity among individuals with psychosis (Drake et al, 1990). An alternative is the Dartmouth Assessment of Lifestyle Instrument (DALI) (Rosenberg et al, 1998), an instrument specifically tailored for use with this special population. The DALI is a brief, 18-item instrument that can be administered in a variety of formats (interview, self-report questionnaire, or computer), and which requires less than 5 min to administer and score. It has high sensitivity and specificity for the detection of recent use of alcohol, cannabis, and cocaine as well as other substance misuse. A positive score on the DALI indicates a high probability (80–90%) that the client meets DSM criteria for a recent substance-use disorder.

Finally, laboratory tests, such as breath, saliva, urine, blood or hair analysis, can aid in the detection of clients using various substances. These are reserved for clients who are already engaged in treatment. We recommend that laboratory tests for drug and alcohol use be performed during all hospital admissions and emergency room visits, and that they be considered at times of concern about substance use and at times when other routine laboratory testing is being performed.

Step 2: classification

The goal of classification is to determine whether the clients identified in the previous step meet specific diagnostic criteria for substance-use disorders. Such classification aids in communicating the nature and severity of the disorder between clinicians. It is also useful for monitoring the effects of treatment over time.

The DSM-IV (American Psychiatric Association, 1994) distinguishes between substance abuse and substance dependence. *"Substance abuse"* refers to a pattern of substance use which results in significant problems in one or more areas of functioning, such as work, school, family, personal care, or legal status, or the use of substances in hazardous situations, such as driving. *"Substance dependence"* refers to the use of substances in a manner meeting criteria for abuse, but also meeting criteria for either psychological or physical dependence. *Psychological dependence* is a syndrome of using more substances than intended, repeated unsuccessful attempts to cut down on substance use, giving up important activities to use substances, and/or spending excessive amounts of time obtaining substances. *Physical dependence* is a syndrome in which persistent substance use results in the development of physical tolerance to the effects of the substance and withdrawal symptoms following cessation of substance use.

It is relatively common for clients with SMP to develop psychological dependence on drugs or alcohol, despite relatively moderate amounts of use (Mueser et al, in press). Limited social outlets and recreational activities may be a contributing factor; substance use may fill a social/recreational void. In contrast, physical dependence is less common, probably due to the high sensitivity these clients have to the negative physical and psychosocial impact of psychoactive substance use.

We recommend the use of the Clinician Rating Scales for alcohol and drugs (Drake et al, 1990; Mueser et al, 1995) in order to classify substance misuse among people with psychosis. The Clinician Rating Scales are 5-point, behaviourally-anchored scales that correspond to the client's use and/or abuse of substances over the previous 6 months. A separate scale is provided for alcohol and drugs. In each, the clinician evaluates the extent to which substance use has had an impact on the areas of functioning identified by the DSM as contributing to either substance abuse or dependence. Evaluation focuses on the client's *worst* period of substance use over the 6-month period in question. A final rating of from 1 to 5 is determined, given this input. For each scale, a score of "1" corresponds to no use (abstinence) for that substance over the past 6 months. A rating of "2" corresponds to substance use over the past 6 months without evidence for substance abuse or dependence. A rating of "3" corresponds to meeting criteria for substance abuse, but not substance dependence. A rating of "4" means that the client meets DSM criteria for substance dependence, with either psychological or physical dependence evident. Finally, a rating of "5" means that, in addition to meeting criteria for substance dependence, the client's substance misuse has been so severe over the past 6 months that it has resulted in significant institutionalization, such as repeated hospitalizations, emergency room visits or time spent incarcerated.

The completion of the Clinician Rating Scales is best accomplished with input from a client's entire treatment team, as opposed to the primary clinician alone. This ensures that it reflects an opinion of consensus, rather than being one-sided. It has the further advantage of fostering team communication, leading to the accessibility of multiple avenues of information regarding an individual client's behaviour, increasing the likelihood that substance misuse will be identified, where appropriate. It further promotes a mutual agreement between team members with respect to treatment issues, minimizing potential conflicts in treatment.

Occasionally, a clinician will become aware of a client's substance use, but the impact of this use will be unclear. Two considerations are worth noting in this context: first, clinicians need to be reminded that evaluation of substance use should be based on all available sources of information, including client self-reports, direct observations of the client's various treatment providers, reports by significant others such as family members, medical records and laboratory tests. Comprehensive assessment is not accomplished without consideration of all of these.

Secondly, clinicians should not assume that their client is experiencing negative consequences from substance use when there is no supporting evidence. When all available information is gathered, and negative consequences do not become apparent, the client should not be classified as meeting criteria for substance misuse on the Clinical Rating Scales.

We recommend that the Clinician Rating Scales be completed on each client every 6 months. This enables clinicians to track improvement of substance use, as well as to identify emergent cases of substance abuse, in a timely manner. Similarly, clients who have met criteria for a substance misuse in the previous 6 months, but who are demonstrating improvement, remain at high risk of relapse. Classification of their substance use on the basis of the worst prior period ensures that this high risk of relapse is considered in treatment planning. Finally, biannual reviews cue clinicians to the importance of considering SMP in their service planning for all their clients.

Step 3. Functional assessment and analysis

The goal of the functional analysis is to identify the factors which maintain (or reinforce) a client's use of substances, or, in a state of remission, to identify the factors which contribute to risk of relapse. A thorough functional analysis provides a compelling description of the role that substances play in a client's life. Furthermore, it provides important clues for treatment planning in terms of controlling substance use.

Data for the functional analysis are acquired in the functional assessment. This is the most information intensive step in the overall assessment process, as information is sought from many areas of the client's current and past life domains. It includes information directly related to substance use as well as information only indirectly related. This is necessary since integrated treatment requires an understanding of the interactions between mental illness, substance use, and general social, emotional, and physical functioning.

Collection and coordination of information obtained from a wide range of relevant sources is organized with the use of the functional analysis interview (FAI) (Mueser et al, in press). The FAI is organized into six different topics: 1. background information, 2. psychiatric illness, 3. physical health, 4. psychosocial adjustment, 5. substance use and 6. functional analysis. It is best conducted as a series of meetings with a client, with additional information being collected independently from family and friends, other treatment providers, and medical records. Meetings with the client may be held formally or informally, with the discussion paced and intermingled with case management according to the client's comfort and need.

Background information

This includes demographic descriptors, as well as information on family relationships, living circumstances, performance of activities of daily living, and educational experiences. One area of potential importance in this section concerns clients who have children, especially women. Many parents with SMP experience difficulties in managing their relationships and responsibilities with their spouses and children. As a consequence, these clients often lose custody of their children. Issues of lost mother-hood are critical to these clients (Fox, 1999). Helping clients improve their relationships with their children, and potentially regain their parenting roles, are important goals that can contribute to their motivation to work on their substance-abuse problems (Schwab et al, 1991).

Psychiatric illness

Information about the client's psychiatric illness is obtained, including the diagnosis, the characteristic symptoms, use of medications and the client's understanding of the illness and its treatment. Rather than being a comprehensive psychiatric assessment, this part of the FAI is intended to be a summary of the information most relevant to developing an inte-grated treatment plan. The FAI identifies common psychiatric symptoms including mood problems, sleep disturbances, cognitive impairments, and apathy and anhedonia, as well as hallucinations and delusions. Medical records, client interview, or a meeting with a team member more experi-enced in the evaluation of psychiatric symptoms, such as a psychiatrist, may be useful.

Medication issues are not limited to an accurate list of current prescriptions, but include important information regarding clients' perceptions about particular medications and medication use in general. Patients may have concerns about side effects which influence compliance. They may have delusions regarding the use of medications which increase or decrease use patterns. They may have ideas about the interactions of their medications with substances which affect treatment compliance. Any of these issues can have bearing on the functional analysis to follow.

Some caveats regarding client interview are warranted. When enquiring about the client's understanding of a psychiatric illness, it is important not to attempt to persuade the clients about their diagnosis. Many clients will deny having a specific psychiatric disorder, but will acknowledge having certain symptoms or difficulties. Others may deny having any problems. Rather than trying to convince clients about having a psychiatric disorder, the clinician should seek to understand how clients perceive their own difficulties, and strive to emulate their language when discussing problems in order to develop and maximize rapport. Most clients can be engaged and helped to work on treatment issues if approached in this manner.

Similarly, when exploring the client's understanding of medication and treatment, the clinician should avoid attempting to correct or educate the client at this stage, maintaining focus instead on evaluating the client's perceptions. Exploring and understanding client perceptions about symptoms, diagnoses, medication and treatment facilitate the creation of treatment plans that correspond to clients' views of themselves and their world.

Physical health

It is important to conduct a careful evaluation of physical health, because clients with psychosis often neglect their health. In addition, the consequences of substance abuse, both direct and indirect, may include a range of health problems. An example of the direct effects of substance misuse on health is the effect of alcohol on liver functioning, which in severe cases can interfere with the client's ability to metabolize psychotropic medications. An example of the indirect effects of substance misuse on health is risky sexual behaviour, such as unprotected sexual contact with multiple partners. Clients may engage in these risky behaviours in exchange for drugs or money to support their substance use. Research indicates that clients with dual disorders are at substantially increased risk of contracting infectious diseases such as hepatitis B, hepatitis C, and HIV and other sexually transmitted diseases (Carey et al, 1995, 1999b; Cournos and McKinnon, 1997; Grassi et al, 1999).

If health problems are not addressed, they can compromise the quality of clients' lives, inhibit their ability to participate in treatment, and increase their risk of premature death. The clinician should be aware of the client's medical history, based upon a chart review and available medical records. If the clinician discovers that the client has not undergone a physical examination in the past year, one should be arranged.

Psychosocial adjustment

In the FAI, assessment of psychosocial adjustment covers the broad areas of family functioning, friendship and romantic relationships, leisure and recreational activities, work, spirituality, financial matters and legal problems. Again, this is an overview of the most critical components of these domains. Understanding a client's psychosocial adjustment is particularly important to integrated treatment planning. First, difficulties in psychosocial functioning may be directly related to substance use; if so, they can provide clues as to mechanisms for control to be used in the treatment plan. For example, conflict with family members is a common consequence of substance misuse (Dixon et al, 1995; Kashner et al, 1991). Clients experiencing substance-related family conflict may be motivated to control their substance use in order to improve their family relationships.

Second, a review of psychosocial adjustment may yield information about the motivational factors that maintain a client's use of substances. For example, if a client reports spending a great deal of time with a close circle of friends, the clinician may explore whether drug or alcohol use is a shared activity among these friends, and whether ongoing substance use serves to maintain these relationships.

Third, the evaluation of psychosocial adjustment may provide insights into both clients' strengths and the potential resources available in their social network. These strengths can be capitalized upon when developing the treatment plan. For example, if the client expresses a strong desire to work, or describes strong family ties, treatment can focus on establishing patterns of reduced substance use which assist in securing and maintaining employment, or involving family members and supporting those relationships, respectively.

Finally, the review of psychosocial adjustment helps to identify areas of the client's life in which functioning needs improvement, independently of substance use. Integrated treatment implies that both substance misuse and psychosis demand treatment in context; it is worth bearing in mind that some areas of clients' lives may need support by virtue of vulnerabilities inherent in their mental illness, perhaps separate from substance-use problems. Once identified, these vulnerabilities can become focal points in treatment planning.

Substance use

The substance-use subsection of the FAI entails a summary of substance-use patterns, but also explores potential motivating factors for substance use, as perceived by the client. We recommend that this material be reserved for review at a time when a good working relationship between the client and the clinician has become established, or at least is recognized as under way. This will lessen the likelihood that the client may feel threatened by a direct focus on issues of substance use, and increase the likelihood of an honest, fruitful discussion.

This section starts with questions regarding clients' patterns of substance use. When completed, information is accumulated regarding the type of substances clients prefer to use, the approximate frequency and regularity of use, and the situations in which use most commonly occurs. Note that accuracy with respect to amounts of substances used is not considered primary to this analysis.

Within this portion of the FAI, we administer the Time-Line Follow-Back, a standard instrument for evaluating the pattern of substance use over the previous 6 months (Fals-Stewart et al, 2000; Sobell et al, 1980). The use of the Time-Line Follow-Back assists with commonly found interview problems such as poor recall of substance use in the past 6 months as well as underreporting of most recent use.

Obtaining information about patterns of substance use is followed by obtaining information about motives for use. This part of the assessment represents clients' expressed perceptions of why they use substances as they do; however, it should be kept in mind that clients may be unable to identify or articulate all the reasons that they use. Motivational factors that are unidentified at the outset of treatment may contribute significantly to patterns of substance use, although these may become more evident over time.

There are a variety of different motives that are commonly associated with substance misuse in clients with psychosis (Addington and Duchak, 1997; Mueser et al, 1995; Noordsy et al, 1991; Test et al, 1989; Warner et al, 1994). Clients sometimes report using substances to alleviate troublesome symptoms, such as depression, anxiety, sleep disturbances or auditory hallucinations. Because substance use often occurs in a social setting, clients' use of alcohol or drugs may be related to social factors. Another commonly expressed motive for using substances is to combat boredom or anhedonia. Clients with psychosis frequently have limited past experience in and limited current resources for engaging in recreational pursuits. Substance use can be an easy, immediate and relatively predictable source of fun for them. Finally, clients with substance misuse sometimes appear to use because their addiction fills a void in their lives for meaning and purpose. For them, maintaining the routine in support of their addiction generates a sense of purpose, structures their time and gives them a reason to live.

In the final part of the substance-use section, the clinician evaluates the client's awareness of negative consequences associated with substance use, insight into having a substance-abuse problem, and motivation to work on substance abuse. When collecting this information, the clinician should avoid persuading the client about having a substance-use disorder; instead, the clinician should stay focused on collecting this information as it exists from the perception of the client.

Functional analysis

The culmination of the third step of assessment is the functional analysis. The goal of the functional analysis is to identify a tentative set of factors that are hypothesized to maintain the client's ongoing use of substances. To the extent that the client is abstinent, the functional analysis focuses on identifying those factors which maintain the abstinence as well as those factors which could precipitate a relapse. The functional analysis is like a set of working hypotheses which are used in treatment planning, but which are revised as necessary according to the client's subsequent progress within the context of that treatment plan.

The information relevant to the functional analysis is summarized in a payoff matrix, which the clinician completes according to the directions provided in the FAI. A payoff matrix uses a quadrant format within which the following four lists are grouped:

1. the perceived benefits to the client of using substances
2. the perceived disadvantages of using substances
3. the perceived advantages of not using substances
4. the perceived disadvantages of not using substances.

The primary assumption of a functional analysis is that human behaviour is maintained by a set of positive consequences for engaging in a behaviour and negative consequences for not engaging in it.

It is particularly important to identify the perceived costs of not using substances (i.e., what clients would have to give up if they stopped using), as the modification of these factors is often the focus of rehabilitation-based interventions for SMP. For example, clients whose substance use appears to be related to efforts to cope with symptoms, to facilitate socialization, or as a form of recreation, risk losing symptom control, social opportunities and recreational experiences. These clients may require assistance in developing alternative strategies to cope with symptoms, in creating new social outlets, and in pursuing different leisure and recreational activities.

Some clients may benefit from seeing the list of advantages and disadvantages of substance use compiled in the payoff matrix. Reviewing this list can serve to catalyse their motivation to cut down or stop using alcohol or drugs (Carey et al, 1999a; Prochaska and DiClemente, 1984; Zeidonis and Trudeau, 1997). However, the primary purpose of constructing a payoff matrix is not to motivate the client to stop using substances. Rather, a functional analysis is conducted in order to identify the factors most critical to sustaining ongoing substance abuse or posing an immediate risk of relapsing.

Step 4: treatment plan

The goal of treatment planning is to formulate a coherent set of actions to be taken by the treatment team, based upon information gleaned in the previous three steps, with the goal of improving clients' performance in areas of identified impairment. For severely mentally ill clients, treatment plans frequently need to address multiple impairments.

Treatment planning can be broken down into six steps:

1. evaluate pressing needs
2. determine client motivation to address problems
3. select target behaviours for change
4. determine interventions for achieving desired goals
5. choose measures to evaluate the effectiveness of the interventions
6. select follow-up times to review implementation of treatment plans and their success.

Each of these steps is discussed in turn below.

Evaluate pressing needs

In order to treat SMP successfully, it is helpful to achieve as much stability in clients' lives as possible. A number of identifiable pressing needs tend to present themselves in this population of clients. Common pressing needs include danger to self or others; housing instability or homelessness; shortage of food, money, or clothing; social network crises; acute or chronic medical problems; acute psychiatric symptoms; predatory behaviours (e.g., dealing drugs, stealing, or pressuring peers for money); acute intoxication; and legal problems.

Undoubtedly, resolution of these problems assists in attaining stability. However, delaying treatment of substance misuse until a client achieves a stable period is impractical, given the frequency with which such problems present themselves. Therefore, from the beginning of treatment, attention is given not only to the improvement of stability in clients' lives, but also to the treatment of substance use problems. Serious and acute pressing needs may occasionally take temporary precedence, but, in general, clinicians need to balance their emphasis on attaining stability with assisting in substance-misuse issues.

Determine client motivation to address problems

Integrated treatment for SMP is always geared to the client's motivational state. Effective treatment planning requires the clinician to establish clients' motivation to work on their problems with substance misuse and mental illness management.

In order to standardize the assessment of client's motivation to change their substance use behaviour, we have developed the Stages of Treatment Scale (SATS) (McHugo et al, 1995; Mueser et al, 1995). The SATS is an 8-point scale based on four stages of treatment: 1. engagement, 2. persuasion, 3. active treatment and 4. relapse prevention. Each stage of treatment is broken down into two substages. Behavioural anchors are used to describe the client's substance-use behaviour and involvement in treatment, so that reliable and objective ratings can be made. SATS ratings range from the low end of pre-engagement and engagement, characterized by little or irregular contact with a clinician, to the middle ranges of persuasion and active treatment, to the final stage of relapse prevention, in which the client has not met criteria for substance misuse for at least 6 months.

Like the Clinician Rating Scales for alcohol and drugs, the SATS is completed according to all available information, including client self-reports, observed behaviour, information from treatment providers, laboratory tests, and feedback from collaterals such as family members. Also like the Clinician Rating Scales, ratings are most accurate when they are completed after a discussion involving the whole treatment team, rather than a single clinician. Unlike the Clinician Rating Scales, which are based upon the client's worst period of substance use in the previous 6 months, the SATS is completed based upon the client's most recent substance use and involvement in treatment. This is done so that the treatment plan corresponds to the client's current level of participation in treatment. We recommend that SATS ratings be completed every 6 months.

Select target behaviours for change

When identifying targets for change, the clinician addresses the question, "What changes are necessary in order to decrease substance misuse or to minimize the chances of relapse into substance misuse?" Two factors need to be considered in order to answer this question: the individual client's stage of treatment (as determined by the SATS), and the functional analysis of substance use behaviours.

The client's stage of treatment has bearing on the selection of target behaviours since it reflects individuals' motivation to change their substance use behaviour. Target behaviours selected for change need to be consistent with client motivation.

In the engagement stage, clients do not have a working relationship with a clinician, and they are not motivated to change their substance use behaviour. Therefore, in the engagement stage, treatment goals primarily focus on establishing regular contact with clients and helping them meet their basic needs. In the persuasion stage, clients have regular contact with their clinicians, but they have only minimally invested in changing their substance use behaviour. In this stage of treatment, clients are often motivated to learn more and talk about their substance use, but they are not motivated to work on their substance-use problems. In active treatment, clients have begun to reduce their substance use, and are motivated to achieve further reductions or abstinence. In relapse prevention, when clients have not recently had problems related to substance use, there is motivation to keep the substance misuse in remission and to work on improving other areas of functioning.

Once target behaviours consistent with a client's stage of treatment are identified, a functional analysis of those factors believed either to maintain ongoing substance abuse (for clients in the engagement or persuasion stages) or threaten a worsening or relapse of substance abuse (for clients in active treatment or relapse prevention) can be considered. The functional analysis helps to select target behaviours that will control substance misuse mainly through indirect methods, such as providing clients with viable and less harmful methods for meeting their needs. Typically, substance use is only partially effective in enabling clients to meet their needs, so that treatment goals based on target behaviours identified by functional analysis can be implemented even when clients are not motivated to work directly on their substance misuse.

When selecting target behaviours for change, it is best for the clinician and the client to identify several targets, to break them down into small steps, and to select targets that elicit no resistance and offer high potential for success. Finally, it is best to limit the number of target behaviours selected for change to a small number.

In short, the process of identifying suitable target behaviours follows three steps. First, the problems that are preventing the person from progressing to the next stage of treatment need to be considered. Second, factors that maintain ongoing substance use or threaten a relapse are identified. Third, concrete changes or goals that would address these factors are specified.

Determine interventions for achieving desired goals

Once a suitable number of target behaviours for change have been selected, interventions for achieving the desired changes in these behaviours must be identified. When selecting treatment strategies to achieve specific goals, one must bear in mind that some methods are stage-specific, whereas others are not. For example, case management and family work are treatment modalities that can be provided at all stages of treatment. In contrast, motivational interviewing is most appropriate for the persuasion stage, and active treatment groups are most suitable for clients in the active-treatment or relapse-prevention stages. Table 10.1 provides a summary of the different stages at which different treatment modalities can be used. Sometimes clients may benefit from an intervention not usually provided at their stage of treatment. For example, clients in the persuasion stage occasionally benefit from attending a self-help group such as Alcoholics

Table 10.1   Potential interventions at different stages of treatment

	Stage of treatment			
	Engagement	*Persuasion*	Active *Treatment*	Relapse *Prevention*
Case management	×	×	×	×
Family work	×	×	×	×
Pharmacological treatment	×	×	×	×
Assertive outreach	×	×	×	
Coerced or involuntary interventions	×	×	×	
Residential programmes		×	×	
Motivational interviewing		×	×	
Persuasion groups		×	×	
Cognitive-behavioural counselling		×	×	×
Social skills training		×	×	×
Vocational rehabilitation		×	×	×
Active treatment groups			×	×
Self-help groups			×	×

Anonymous or Double Trouble. However, the summary of interventions for the different stages of treatment provides useful general guidance to clinicians for matching treatment to clients' motivational states.

Choose measures to evaluate the effectiveness of the interventions

When specific interventions have been selected to change targets, measures must be identified in order to determine their success in achieving the desired goals. Measures should be chosen that are objective, easy to observe (where possible), and clearly related to the target behaviour in question. Whenever possible, behavioural specificity of measures is desired. For example, the success of a sleep hygiene intervention for insomnia that leads to substance use might be measured by having clients log their daily substance use and sleep patterns.

Select follow-up times to review implementation of treatment plans and their success

Even the best of plans is ineffective without follow-up. In order to maximize the success of a treatment plan, efforts must be made for systematic follow-up to those plans, with modifications implemented as warranted. We recommend two types of follow-up to ensure effective treatment.

First, regular monitoring needs to be conducted to ensure that the interventions have been implemented as planned. Problems with successful implementation of an intervention should be identified and resolved as soon as possible. Treatment providers should monitor interventions for their clients with SMP on at least a weekly basis.

Second, review and evaluation of the entire treatment plan should be undertaken every 6 months. This is to determine the effectiveness of the overall plan, which may be successful in achieving goals, partially successful, or unsuccessful. Where the treatment plan has shortcomings, modifications can be made and further evaluations scheduled. Recall that information from the implemented treatment plan feeds back into prior steps in assessment. A careful analysis of the problems inherent in the treatment plan can provide information useful in reassessment of the client in terms of detection, classification, or subsequent functional assessment and analysis. These changes then affect the design of a subsequent treatment plan.

SUMMARY

We began this chapter with a review of common problems and obstacles to the assessment of substance misuse in persons with psychosis. Problems associated with the role of the clinician in the assessment process, the nature of psychosis and substance misuse, and systemic factors in the current mental health-care treatment system, as well as client-related issues, were identified and examined.

We presented a four-step assessment process, and explained the ongoing, continuous feedback loop involved in the assessment and treatment of SMP. The four steps include *detection* of substance abuse problems, *classification* of substance misuse, *functional assessment and analysis* of the client, and integrated *treatment planning*. Specific clinical recommendations and tools were provided for conducting these steps.

REFERENCES

Addington, J. and Duchak, V. (1997) Reasons for substance use in schizophrenia. *Acta Psychiatrica Scandinavica*, **96**: 329–333.

American Psychiatric Association (1994) *Diagnostic and Statistical Manual of Mental Disorders* (4th edn). Washington, DC, American Psychiatric Association Press.

Ananth, J., Vandewater, S., Kamal, M., Brodsky, A., Gamal, R. and Miler, M. (1989) Missed diagnosis of substance abuse in psychiatric populations. *Hospital and Community Psychiatry*, **40**: 297–299.

Barbee, J.G., Clark, P.D., Craqanzano, M.S., Heintz, G.C. and Kehoe, C.E. (1989) Alcohol and substance abuse among schizophrenic patients presenting to an emergency service. *Journal of Nervous and Mental Disease*, **177**: 400–407.

Bartels, S.J., Drake, R.E. and Wallach, M.A. (1995) Long-term course of substance use disorders in severe mental illness. *Psychiatric Services*, **46**: 248–251.

Carey, K.B. and Correia, C.J. (1998) Severe mental illness and addictions: assessment considerations. *Addictive Behaviors*, **23**: 735–748.

Carey, K.B., Purnine, D.M., Maisto, S.A., Carey, M.P. and Barnes, K.L. (1999a) Decisional balance regarding substance use among persons with schizophrenia. *Community Mental Health Journal*, **35**: 289–299.

Carey, M.P., Carey, K.B., Maisto S.A., Gleason, J.R., Gordon, C.M. and Brewer, K.K. (1999b) HIV-risk behavior among outpatients at a state psychiatric hospital: prevalence and risk modeling. *Behavior Therapy*, **30**: 389–406.

Carey, M.P., Weinhardt, L.S. and Crey, K.B. (1995) Prevalence of infection with HIV among the seriously mentally ill: review of research and implications for practice. *Professional Psychology: Research and Practice*, **26**: 262–268.

Cohen, M. and Klein, D.F. (1970) Drug abuse in a young psychiatric population. *American Journal of Orthopsychiatry*, **40**: 448–455.

Corse, S.J., Hirschinger, N.B. and Zanis, D. (1995) The use of the Addiction Severity Index with people with severe mental illness. *Psychiatric Rehabilitation Journal*, **19**: 9–18.

Cournos, F. and McKinnon, K. (1997) HIV seroprevalence among people with severe mental illness in the United States: a critical review. *Clinical Psychology Review*, **17**: 159–169.

Crowley, T.J., Chesluk, D., Dilts, S. and Hart, R. (1974) Drug and alcohol abuse among psychiatric admissions. *Archives of General Psychiatry*, **30**: 13–20.

Dixon, L., McNary, S. and Lehman, A. (1995) Substance abuse and family relationships of persons with severe mental illness. *American Journal of Psychiatry*, **152**: 456–458.

Drake, R.E. and Brunette, M.F. (1998) Complications of severe mental illness related to alcohol and other drug use disorders. In M. Galanter (Ed.), *Recent Developments of Alcoholism* (Vol. XIV, Consequences of Alcoholism, pp. 285–299). New York, Plenum.

Drake, R.E., Brunette, M.F. and Mueser, K.T. (1998) Substance use disorder and social functioning in schizophrenia. In K.T. Mueser and N. Tarier (Eds.), *Handbook of Social Functioning in Schizophrenia* (pp. 280–289). Boston, MA, Allyn & Bacon.

Drake, R.E., McHugo, G.J., Clark, R.E., Teague, G.B., Xie, H., Miles, K. and Ackerso, T.H. (1998) Assertive Community Treatment for patients with co-occurring severe mental illness and substance use disorder: A clinical trial. *American Journal of Orthopsychiatry*, **68**: 201–215.

Drake, R.E., Osher, F.C., Noordsy, D.L., Hurlbut, S.C., Teague, G.B. and Beaudete, M.S. (1990) Diagnosis of alcohol use disorders in schizophrenia. *Schizophrenia Bulletin*, **16**: 57–67.

Drake, R.E., Wallach, M.A. and Hoffman, J.S. (1989) Housing instability and homelessness among aftercare patients of an urban state hospital. *Hospital and Community Psychiatry*, **40**: 46–51.

Fals-Steward, W., O'Farrell, T.J., Freitas, T.T., McFarin, S.D. and Rutigliano, P. (2000) The Timeline Followback reports of psychoactive substance use by drug-abusing patients: psychometric properties. *Journal of Consulting and Clinical Psychology*, **68**: 134–144.

Fowler, I.L., Carr, V.J., Carter, N.T. and Lewin, T.J. (1988) Patterns of current and lifetime substance use in schizophrenia. *Schizophrenia Bulletin*, **24**: 443–455.

Fox, L. (1999) Missing out on motherhood. *Psychiatric Services*, **50**: 193–194.

Galletly, C., Field, C. and Prior, M. (1993) Urine drug screening of patients admitted to a state psychiatric hospital. *Hospital and Community Psychiatry*, **44**: 587–589.

Grassi, L., Pavanati, M., Cardelli, R., Ferri, S. and Peron, L. (1999) HIV-risk behavior and knowledge about HIV/AIDS among patients with schizophrenia. *Psychological Medicine*, **29**: 171–179.

Kashner, M., Rader, L., Rodell, D., Beck, C., Rodell, L. and Muller, K. (1991) Family characteristics, substance abuse and hospitalization patterns of patients with schizophrenia. *Hospital and community Psychiatry*, **42**: 195–197.

Kranzler, H., Bureleson, J., DelBoca, F., Babor, T., Korner, P., Brown, J. and Bohn, M. (1994) Buspirone treatment of anxious alcoholics. *Archives of General Psychiatry*, **51**: 720–731.

Lehman, A., Myers, C.J., Corty, E. and Thompson, J. (1994) Severity of substance-use disorders among people with psychoses. *Journal of Nervous and Mental Disease*, **182**: 164–167.

Linszen, D., Dingemans, P., Van derDoes, A.J.W., Scholte, P., Lenior, R. and Goldstein, M.J. (1996) Treatment, expressed emotion and relapse in recent onset schizophrenic disorders. *Psychological Medicine*, **26**: 333–342.

McHugo, G.J., Drake, R.E., Burton H.L. and Ackerson T.H. (1995) A scale for assessing the stage of substance abuse treatment in persons with severe mental illness. *Journal of Nervous and Mental Disease*, **183**: 762–767.

Mueser, K.T., Drake, R.E., Clark, R.E., McHugo, G.J., Mercer-McFadden, C. and Ackerson, T. (1995) *Toolkit for Evaluating Substance Abuse in Persons with Severe Mental Illness*. Cambridge, MA, Evaluation Center at HSRI.

Mueser, K.T., Drake, R.E. and Wallach, M.A. (1998) Dual diagnosis: a review of etiological theories. *Addictive Behavior*, **23**: 717–734.

Mueser, K.T., Noordsy, D.L., Drake, R.E. and Fox, M. (2002, in press) *Integrated Treatment for Dual Disorders: Effective Intervention for Severe Mental Illness and Substance Abuse*. New York, Guilford.

Mueser, K.T., Yarnold, P.R., Rosenberg, S.D., Swett, C., Miles, K.M. and Hill, D. (2000) Substance use disorder in hospitalized severely mentally ill psychiatric patients: prevalence, correlates and subgroups. *Schizophrenia Bulletin*, **26**: 179–192.

Noordsy, D.L., Drake, R.E., Biesanz, J.C. and McHugo, G.J. (1994) Family history of alcoholism in schizophrenia. *Journal of Nervous and Mental Disease*, **182**: 651–655.

Noordsy, D.L., Drake, R.E., Teague, G.B., Osher, F.C., Hurlbut, S.C., Beaudett, M.S. and Paskus, T.S. (1991) Subjective experiences related to alcohol abuse among schizophrenics. *Journal of Nervous and Mental Disease*, **179**: 410–414.

Pristach, C.A. and Smith, C.M. (1990) Medication compliance and substnce abuse among schizophrenic patients. *Hospital and Community Psychiatry*, **41**: 1345–1348.

Prochaska, J.O. and DiClemente, C.C. (1984) *The Transtheoretical Approach: Crossing the Traditional Boundaries of Therapy*. Homewood, IL, Dow-Jonew/Irwin.

Regier, D.A., Farmer, M.E., Rae, D.S., Locke, B.Z., Keithe, S.J., Judd, L.L. and Goodwin, F.K. (1990) Comorbidity of mental disorders with alcohol and other drug abuse: results from the Epidemiologic Catchment Area (ECA) study. *Journal of the American Medical Association*, **264**: 2511–2518.

Rosenberg, S.D., Drake, R.E., Wolford, G.L., Mueser, K.T., Oxman, T.E., Vidaver, R.M., Carrieri, K.L. and Luckoor, R. (1998) The Dartmouth Assessment of Lifestyle Instrument (DALI): a substance use disorder screen for people with severe mental illness. *American Journal of Psychiatry*, **155**: 232–238.

Schuckit, M. (1983) Alcoholism and other psychiatric disorders. *Hospital and Community Psychiatry*, **34**: 1022–1027.

Schuckit, M.A., Zisook, S. and Mortola, J. (1985) Clinical implications of DSM-III diagnoses of alcohol abuse and alcohol dependence. *American Journal of Psychiatry*, **142**: 1403–1408.

Schwab, B., Clark, R.E. and Drake, R.E. (1991) An ethnographic note on clients as parents. *Psychiatric Rehabilitation Journal*, **15**: 95–99.

Shaner, A., Khalsa, M.A., Roberts, L., Wilkins, J., Anglin, D. and Hsieh, S.C. (1993) Unrecognized cocaine use among schizophrenic patients. *American Journal of Psychiatry*, **150**: 758–762.

Shaner, A., Roberts, L.J., Eckman, T.A., Racenstein, J.M., Tucker, D.E., Tsuang, J.W. and Mintz, J. (1998) Sources of diagnostic uncertainty for chronically psychotic cocaine abusers. *Psychiatric Services*, **49**: 684–690.

Shea, S.C. (1998) *Psychiatric Interviewing: The Art of Understanding* (2nd edn). Philadelphia, W.B. Saunders.

Sobell, M.B., Maisto, S.A., Sobell, L.C., Copper, A.M. and Sanders, B. (1980) Developing a prototype for evaluating alcohol treatment effectiveness. In L.C. Sobell, M.B. Sobell and E. Ward (Eds), *Evaluating Alcohol and Drug Abuse Treatment Effectiveness* (pp. 129–150). New York, Pergamon.

Steadman, H.J., Mulvey, E.P., Monahan, J., Robbins, P.C., Appelbaum, P.S., Crisso, T., Roth, L.H. and Silver, E. (1998) Violence by people discharged from acute psychiatric inpatient facilities and by others in the same neighborhoods. *Archives of General Psychiatry*, **55**: 393–401.

Swartz, M.S., Swanson, J.W., Hiday, V.A., Borum, R., Wagner, H.R. and Burns, B.J. (1998) Violence and mental illness: the effects of substance abuse and nonadherence to medication. *American Journal of Psychiatry*, **155**: 226–231.

Swofford, C.D., Kasckow, J.W., Scheller-Gilkey, G. and Inderbitzin, L.B. (1996) Substance use: a powerful predictor of relapse in schizophrenia. *Schizophrenia Research*, **20**: 145–151.

Test, M.A., Wallish, L.S., Allness, D.G. and Ripp, K. (1989) Substance use in young adults with schizophrenic disorders. *Schizophrenia Bulletin*, **15**: 465–476.

Warner, R., Taylor, D., Wright, J., Sloat, A., Springett, G., Arnold, S. and Weinberg, H. (1994) Substance use among the mentally ill: prevalence, reasons for use and effects on illness. *American Journal of Orthopsychiatry*, **64**: 30–39.

Weiss, R.D., Najavits, L,M., Greenfield, S.F., Soto, F.A., Shaw, S.R. and Wyner, D. (1998) Validity of substance use self-reports in dually diagnosed outpatients. *American Journal of Psychiatry*, **155**: 127–128.

Yesavage, J.A. and Zarcone, V. (1983) History of drug abuse and dangerous behavior in inpatient schizophrenics. *Journal of Clinical Psychiatry*, **44**: 259–261.

Ziedonis, D. and Trudeau, K. (1997) Motivation to quit using substances among individuals with schizophrenia: implications for a motivation-based treatment model. *Schizophrenia Bulletin*, **23**: 229–238.

Ziedonis, D.M. and Stern, R. (2001) Dual recovery therapy for schizophrenia and substance abuse. *Psychiatric Annals*, **31**: 255–264.

Chapter 11

COGNITIVE-BEHAVIOURAL INTEGRATED TREATMENT APPROACH FOR PSYCHOSIS AND PROBLEM SUBSTANCE USE

Hermine L. Graham, Alex Copello, Max J. Birchwood, Jim Orford, Dermot McGovern, Jenny Maslin and George Georgiou

INTRODUCTION

The significance of the interrelationship between a person's drug/alcohol use and severe mental health problems is often overlooked, even in "integrated" treatment approaches. The quest for change in the treatment session tends to focus on one problem in parallel to the other. That is, individuals are taught particular strategies to improve management of their mental health difficulties and others to manage their problem substance use. Despite the fact that overlap exists between psychological treatment approaches for psychosis and problem substance use (i.e., cognitive approaches, motivational enhancing approaches, and relapse prevention), little has been done to combine and simplify them into a single strategy that can be used by clients to tackle both their difficulties simultaneously. The cognitive-behavioural integrated treatment (C-BIT) approach described in this chapter adapts standard techniques used in cognitive therapy for emotional disorders and draws together the key cognitive elements from a number of psychosocial approaches, so as to facilitate changes in the management of alcohol/drug use behaviour and psychosis. These include

Substance Misuse in Psychosis: Approaches to Treatment and Service Delivery.
Edited by Hermine L. Graham, Alex Copello, Max J. Birchwood and Kim T. Mueser.
© 2003 John Wiley & Sons, Ltd.

motivational approaches, relapse prevention for psychosis and substance use and social network approaches.

C-BIT is an approach that was specifically developed as part of the work of the COMPASS Programme in Birmingham, UK (as detailed in Chapter 7). It enables clinicians to put problematic substance use on the agenda on help clients think about the negative impact of problematic use on other areas of their life including mental health. It is designed to help clinicians (mental health/addiction) work in a structured but flexible way, collaboratively to tackle problematic drug/alcohol use. This chapter is not a clinician's manual but rather a description of the treatment approach. The C-BIT manual (Graham et al, unpublished) describes the full approach, but it should be accompanied by training.

The theoretical basis for the C-BIT approach is detailed in Chapter 5. The first part of this chapter will seek to set the scene by focusing on some of the important background factors to the treatment approach. The section entitled "Treatment overview" will outline the objectives of the treatment, its structure and the style of the approach. The second part of this chapter will provide a description of the approach with illustrative case examples. The final section will briefly outline the evaluation of this treatment approach.

Treatment overview

Objectives of treatment

The overall objective of the C-BIT approach is to negotiate and facilitate, with clients, some positive change in their problematic drug/alcohol use. In line with this, it encourages clients to develop "healthy" alternatives to drug/alcohol misuse. C-BIT is based on a "harm reduction" approach (Heather et al, 1993; Marlatt, 1998). Abstinence is not seen as the only possible goal. Problematic drug/alcohol use is seen as a pattern of substance use and its related negative consequences that interferes with clients' well-being and achievement of self-identified goals. The aim is to help clients achieve their self-identified goals within their spiritual and cultural frame of reference. The aims of C-BIT are thus threefold. First, it aims collaboratively to identify and challenge unhelpful unrealistic beliefs about drugs or alcohol that maintain problematic use, and replace them with more adaptive beliefs that will lead to and strengthen behavioural change. Second, it seeks to facilitate an understanding of the relationship between problem substance use and mental health problems. Third, it teaches specific skills for controlling and self-managing of substance use and the early warning signs of psychosis that it may trigger/exacerbate, and for developing social support for an alternative lifestyle.

Structure

C-BIT is structured in the sense that it provides a systematic method for clinicians to address their clients' alcohol/drug use. However, it is also flexible, as it allows clinicians to conduct this work in the time available to them and over whatever period is appropriate for the clients. The approach consists of the following core components; an assessment phase (screening and assessment), four treatment phases (engagement and building motivation to change; negotiating some behaviour change; early relapse prevention; and relapse prevention and relapse management) and two additional treatment components (skills building and working with families and social network members). The two additional treatment components are designed to be used in parallel with the treatment phases where appropriate.

The four treatment phases can be moved through sequentially. However, it is also possible that a client may relapse following a long period of non-problematic use/abstinence, and then the appropriate earlier phase will need to be revisited. For the majority of clients whose motivation will fluctuate, the time spent in each treatment phase of C-BIT will vary. It is important to emphasize that due to the C-BIT harm reduction philosophy it is not necessary with all clients to move through all the phases. A "successful outcome" can be achieved during any of the four treatment phases and can be defined as the client's achieving the harm reduction goal.

The treatment phases are constructed in such a way as to allow clinicians to address some aspect of a client's drug/alcohol use in whatever time is available. The four treatment phases in C-BIT roughly correspond to the four stages in the 'stages of treatment' as described by Mueser et al (1998) (i.e., engagement, persuasion, active treatment, and relapse prevention). These stages represent the extent to which a client is engaged in the treatment/change process. Table 11.1 serves as a guide to determine how engaged in treatment the client is and which C-BIT interventions are most likely to be useful at a given point.

Treatment style

The style of C-BIT is based on that utilized within cognitive therapy (e.g., Beck, 1976; Padesky and Greenberger, 1995; Salkovskis, 1996). It involves a *collaborative relationship* with clients, working in partnership with the clinician to tackle the problems they are experiencing. The approach is non-judgemental and embraces a relationship which is built on *empathy, warmth, trust, and positive regard* (Rogers, 1991). The style is non-confrontational. It seeks to encourage clinicians to adopt a motivational/educational role where *Socratic questioning and guided discovery* are used to encourage clients to re-evaluate the beliefs they hold and consider or discover alternative

Table 11.1 Phases of treatment, definitions and C-BIT interventions

Phase	Definition	Goal	Intervention
Engagement	Client does not have regular contact with keyworker and does not discuss alcohol/drug use. For example; *"it's up to me if I want to smoke cannabis—and I don't want to talk about it."*	To establish a working alliance with the client and be able to discuss alcohol/drug use and any problems it may be causing.	Treatment phase 1 and assessment phase (skills building/working with families/social network members where appropriate)
Negotiating behaviour change	Client has regular contact with key worker but does not want to work on reducing problematic alcohol/drug use. For example: *"My alcohol use is not a problem so why should I cut down."*	To develop the client's awareness of problems associated with alcohol/drug use and build motivation to change.	Treatment phase 2 (skills building/working with families/social network members where appropriate)
Early relapse prevention	Client is motivated to change problematic alcohol/drug use (as indicated by serious attempts at reduction for at least 1 month but less than 6 months). For example; *"Using crack has caused me a lot of problems, so I have to stop using."*	To help client further reduce alcohol/drug use and, if possible, attain abstinence.	Treatment phase 3 (skills: building/working with families/social network members where appropriate)
Relapse prevention/ management	Client has not experienced problems related to alcohol/drug use for at least 6 months or is abstinent. For example; *"Since I've cut down I'm not hearing voices—I want to get on with my life."*	To maintain awareness that relapse could happen and to extend recovery to other areas (such as mental health, social, relationships, work).	Treatment phase 4 (skills building/working with families/social network members where appropriate)

ways of thinking about their alcohol or drug use and coping with their difficulties (Padesky and Greenberger, 1995). Such a style is more likely to lead to positive change than direct confrontation (Miller and Rollnick, 1991).

The C-BIT approach, particularly treatment phases 1 and 4, was designed within an "integrated shared-care" service level approach, as described in Chapter 7, and is best implemented within such a context.

C-BIT CORE COMPONENTS

The following is a description of the core components of the C-BIT approach. Illustrative clinical examples are used throughout.

Assessment phase: screening and assessment

The assessment phase of C-BIT has three main aims. First, it aims to assess the types of substances used and the pattern of use, and to determine whether there are problems related to drug/alcohol use which pose a risk to mental health and well-being. Second, it aims to serve as a guide to planning the most appropriate treatment approach and treatment goals. Third, it aims to begin to engage clients in discussing their substance use and increase their awareness of the problems caused by their pattern of use, particularly their mental health. The assessment phase includes a semistructured clinical interview (Table 11.2), standardized substance use assessment and screening tools, and some guidelines on case formulation and how to use the outcome of assessments in treatment planning. The assessment is not intended to serve as a stand-alone assessment, but rather one that should form part of a fuller on-going assessment process. The assessment phase can be carried out during any C-BIT treatment phase as appropriate, but ideally during C-BIT treatment phase 1.

If problematic drug/alcohol use has been identified, the clinician proceeds with case formulation and treatment planning. The aim of a case formulation (see Chapter 5) is to understand or generate hypotheses about how a client's problems developed and are maintained, and the relationship between the various problems a client might have (particularly drug/alcohol use and mental health problems) (Beck et al, 1993). It also serves as a guide to appropriate treatment planning (Liese and Franz, 1996). A number of key factors are taken into consideration when planning treatment and deciding on the most appropriate intervention. These include the case formulation, the stage of change the client is in (Prochaska et al, 1992), the stage of engagement with treatment, self-identified goals and concerns, short and longer-term treatment needs, and the client's overall needs as recorded in the care plan.

Table 11.2   Clinical assessment of drug/alcohol use (for more information, see Glass, 1991; Beck et al, 1993)

- **Current functioning**
  Information should initially be gathered about current mood, sleeping patterns, appetite/eating patterns, concentration, general motivation and level of interest, daily activities/employment, social support, physical health, suicidal ideation/self-harm behaviours, and medication.
- **Typical (e.g., past week) use and current use (e.g., previous day) for each substance**
  This includes *pattern of use* (e.g., types of substances used; cost, quantity, frequency and pattern of use; route of use; triggers and moderators of use; and social network substance use), *effects of use, and problems related to use* (e.g., withdrawal symptoms and problems in the following domains: mental health/psychotic symptoms, financial/debts, social/relationships, physical/ health, housing, legal/forensic, occupational, child care, aggression, narrowing of usual repertoire of behaviours, activities and types of substances used).
- **Reasons for using and beliefs about the use of the substance**
  (e.g., pleasure, social/cultural, coping). To help identify key beliefs about alcohol/drug use, questions such as "What usually goes through your mind just before you use?" are included.
- **Drug/alcohol use history**
  As well as a brief developmental and family background history, this includes age of first use of each substance and how substance use progressed over time, periods of abstinence and treatment.
- **Assessment of the relationship between substance use and mental health**
  The focus is on whether the mental health problems/symptoms exist in the absence or presence of substance use, and includes assessing whether clients' reasons for using substances are related to their mental health problems/symptoms or their experience of taking medication, etc.
- **Motivation to change and goals**
  That is, whether clients perceives their use as problematic and their motivational stage of change.

Treatment phase 1: engagement and building motivation to change

Engagement strategies

The goal of the first treatment phase is simply to establish a working alliance with the client and begin to discuss alcohol/drug and associated problems. The key C-BIT engagement strategies fall into the categories of assertive outreach, attitudinal and motivational approaches.

Assertive outreach or assertive community treatment approaches have been described (e.g., Stein and Test, 1980; Mueser et al, 1998; Hemming et al, 1999). Clients with severe mental health problems become the responsibility of a team with no policy for case closure. The follow-up is therefore persistent. Within such an assertive approach, the inclusion of the treatment of substance use can be readily integrated. During the early stages of engagement, an emphasis is placed on practical assistance with everyday tasks, without focusing initially on the drug/alcohol use in an attempt to develop a collaborative working alliance. In addition, the extended hours of the team enables a rapid response for crisis intervention, but clear boundaries are important so that clients are not continually "bailed out" without facing some of the negative consequences of problematic drug/alcohol use. Symptom stabilization through medication adherence is a standard practice, and this in itself may modify reasons for using substances as a coping strategy. Psychological interventions (e.g., Birchwood and Tarrier, 1994; Kingdon and Turkington, 1994; Fowler et al, 1995; Kemp et al, 1996) are utilized to assist in medication adherence and for direct treatment of psychotic symptoms.

Clinicians are encouraged to step back, and readjust attitudes and goal posts to ensure they do not become discouraged and despondent when clients successfully make changes and then relapse or lapse. Adopting a long-term perspective within the team toward the change process enables clinicians to begin to empathize with clients' struggle to change, and helps them remain optimistic.

Initial motivational approaches to establish or improve engagement include identifying "motivational hooks". These are any goals that problematic drug/alcohol use has prevented the attainment of. The use of such hooks mobilizes motivation to make changes in substance use. Examples include getting a job, learning to drive, going on a holiday, starting a relationship, living independently, making friends, going out socially, having more disposable income, not being in debt, not being admitted to a psychiatric hospital, and appropriate reduction of medication.

Putting drug/alcohol use on the agenda

The aim here is to shift the focus and increase awareness of the impact of the negative aspects of problem substance use. It is often the case that the individual has disregarded, ignored, minimized, or simply traded these negative consequences for the positive benefits of the substance. Initially, clients are helped to talk about the positive aspects of substance use by the use of reflective listening so that clients feel more able to be open and honest. For example: "What do you enjoy about crack use?"; "When you drink, how do you find it helps you?". Through a Socratic questioning style, the focus is shifted to the problems associated with drug or alcohol use and the cognitive distortions that maintain problematic substance. For example: "What sorts of difficulties or problems has your alcohol use caused you?" or indirectly: "You seem to be getting into debt recently. What do you think has changed? What sorts of things are you spending more money on now?" (Beck

ADVANTAGES-DISADVANTAGES ANALYSIS

Name: _____ *Ray* _____
Date: _____ *10th Nov 1999* _____
Behaviour: ___*Smoking crack-cocaine*_____

	Ads (FOR)	DisAds (AGAINST)
SHORT TERM	• *Enjoy the buzz it gives me* • *Makes me feel relaxed and light* • *Made new friends*	• *Can end up spending all my money on it* • *Dealers can be a bit rough if I can't pay them* • *Family don't like me smoking...causes arguments*
LONG TERM	• *? Enjoy the buzz*	• *Health will get worse* • *Won't be able to buy anything else for myself* • *Will lose my family*

Self-motivational Statements:
Concern: My crack use is putting me in a lot of debt and causing problems with my family.
Intent to change: *I think I need to think about cutting down before it really gets out of hand.*

Figure 11.1   A typical advantages-disadvantages analysis

et al, 1993; Miller and Rollnick, 1991). These positive and negative aspects of substance use are recorded in the form of an advantages-disadvantages analysis (Figure 11.1). The main concerns and the client's desire to reduce the level of concern are then summarized and utilized as self-motivational statements of concern and intent to change.

Building on motivation for change

To move the client further forward in the change process, the clinician seeks to focus the client's attention on what could be gained and lost from changing the drug/alcohol use; that is, the "decisional balance", the part of the client that wants to change in opposition to the factors that prevent the client from making changes (Miller and Rollnick, 1991). This can be recorded on a decisional balance worksheet so that it can be revisited in future sessions (see Figure 11.2).

Once the pros and cons of change have been elicited from the client, the clinician can begin to tip the motivational balance in favour of change.

DECISION BALANCE SHEET

Name: _____ Tony _____
Date: _____ 18ᵗʰ July 1999_____
Behaviour: _____ Reduce Drinking _____

	'PROS' (FOR)	'CONS' (AGAINST)
SHORT TERM	• Use money to buy things I want e.g. radio/stereo • Learn how to drive • When I'm drinking I don't eat properly • Drinking can make me have hallucinations	• The friends I have and the people I live with all drink like I do • I have always enjoyed drinking with my mates
LONG TERM	• I'll be much healthier • I can look after myself better • Find a job	• ?

Figure 11.2   A typical decisional balance

Motivational (revisiting self-motivational statements of concern and intent to change) and cognitive (identifying and modifying cognitive distortions/positive reasons for use/substance-related beliefs) techniques are used. The aim is to increase and build up the client's awareness of/focus on the difficulties that drug/alcohol causes on the one hand as against the positive, immediate, but only short-term benefits of use on the other. For example, if a client's substance-related belief is that *"cannabis stops my voices"*, this can be re-evaluated and modified by the "three question technique" (i.e., *"What is the evidence for that belief?"*, *"Are there times when that is not the case?"*, *"If there are times when that is not the case, then what are the implications?"*). The resultant modified belief, it is anticipated, would be more realistic, accurate, and in accord with the evidence and thus would enhance motivation/awareness of the need for change. For example, *"I guess after one or two joints they do seem to stop for a while, but if I smoke any more it makes the voices seem worse"*.

Dealing with resistance

It is not uncommon that resistance is initially encountered when the issue of alcohol or drug use is raised with a client who is not well engaged in the change process. Resistance from clients is said to come about because the clinicians are not matching their approach to the stage of the client or are being too confrontational (Miller and Rollnick, 1991). In accord with ideas from motivational interviewing, the C-BIT approach encourages clinicians to use the following strategies to work with resistance. First, they should reflect the client's ambivalence. For example, *"You don't think you are drinking too much but at the same time you are worried about the long-term effect on your health"*. Second, they should move the focus away from the problematic issue and come back to it at a later stage from a slightly different angle. For example,*"Rather than labelling your drinking as a problem, let's just focus on the positive things you were telling me about your drinking right now and the concerns you have for your health in the long term."* Third, they should roll with resistance rather than fighting against it or opposing it. For example *"From what you have said, I can see why you feel the way you do about drinking and don't feel your drinking is too much."* Finally, clinicians are encouraged to go back, if necessary, to using one of the earlier engagement strategies.

Identifying social networks supportive of change

As substance use increases in severity, individuals' energy, activities, social networks, and relationships can be seen to revolve increasingly around their drug and/or alcohol use, as outlined in Chapter 3. Clients may hold the belief that *all* the people they know use drugs/alcohol. Such a belief may also be one of the reasons cited for continued problematic use. However, this belief may not be completely true. It is possible that a substance-using social group becomes one in which a more favoured identity and social acceptance can be found more readily, in contrast to difficulties which may be experienced in conventional society where societal norms are less accepting of apparently odd or bizarre behaviour. Hence, if significant changes are to be made in drinking or drug use, contact and reliance on drinking and drug-using peers must be reduced, particularly in the early stages of the change process. Attention therefore needs to be paid to the development of a replacement "healthy" social network. Its aim is to fulfil the positive functions of a social network without encouraging the harmful use of substances, and to support positive changes in drug/alcohol use and lifestyle (e.g., Drake et al, 1993; Galanter, 1993, 1999; Copello et al, 2002). In essence, it provides social support for the new way of thinking about the substance and behaviour change.

There are several ways identified within the C-BIT approach that clinicians can use to help clients increase social support for change. These include re-engagement with members of a client's social network who are supportive of change. The networks of many clients are quite limited, and so it may be necessary to facilitate the broadening of their social networks by helping them to meet new people who might support efforts to change. Clients are

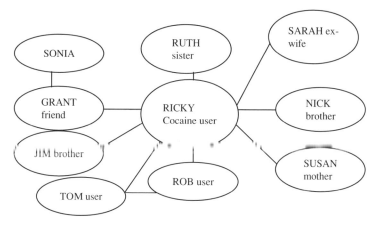

Figure 11.3   Ricky's social network map

also encouraged to identify supportive persons in their networks who are prepared to be involved in the treatment sessions, a practice used in other interventions (e.g., Copello et al, 2002).

Ricky is a 25-year-old man who uses cocaine and suffers from manic depression. Figure 11.3 shows that there are a significant number of people represented in his network. Some of the people, such as Tom and Rob, are drug users themselves and therefore may not be able to support change for Ricky. However, Ricky is close to his brother Jim and his friend Grant, and it may be possible to engage one of them in supporting his efforts to give up cocaine. This can be achieved either by inviting them to the sessions or by making sure that Ricky seeks their support and help between sessions.

Finances/money management

Clients may find that they are spending a significant proportion of their income on drugs/alcohol, making it extremely difficult for them to change substance use behaviour. For example, the availability of money may trigger cravings for them to use (especially on pay day). Alternatively, the lack of money may lead clients into a vicious cycle of debt, with dealers preventing them from spending money on non-drug/alcohol related activities or extracting themselves from a drug/alcohol-using lifestyle.

Strategies used to improve money management are included within C-BIT to facilitate the change process. These include identifying alternative activities or things to spend money on, developing budgeting skills, and having benefits paid directly into bank/building society/post office accounts. For some clients, the ability to budget on a weekly basis is too difficult, and they will tend to spend the majority of their money on the day they are paid, or dealers will control their finances. At this stage, appointeeships may need to be considered (Roberts et al, unpublished).

Treatment phase 2: negotiating some behaviour change

Identifying and setting achievable harm reduction goals

Treatment phase 2 seeks to help clinicians negotiate with clients and achieve some change in alcohol/drug-using behaviours. In addition, it aims to target alcohol/drug-related beliefs in order to increase clients' awareness of the problematic links between their mental health and substance use. The changes sought are based on the harm reduction philosophy (Heather et al, 1993). Complete abstinence at this stage is viewed as probably unrealistic and not necessary. Clients are more willing to think about change and more likely to succeed if changing alcohol/drug use behaviour feels achievable. Clients at this stage are engaged in a goal-setting exercise that involves identifying a goal, the steps needed to achieve it, and a problem-solving approach to any obstacles that may prevent goal attainment.

Roan is 28 years old and has a diagnosis of schizophrenia. He uses ecstasy and cocaine on an occasional and recreational basis at the weekends within the gay club culture. He is aware that he typically becomes depressed and, at times, paranoid, and he does not function too well during the week after he has used these drugs. However, he says that he feels a "normal" part of the gay scene when he uses and is more accepted by his partner. He also says he has a "good time" when he is using, and finds having mental health problems demoralizing. Roan says that he wants "just to get on with his life" (i.e., get a job). Roan did not see his use of drugs as a problem and did not really want to change his pattern of use. However, he began to realize that it affected his ability to function during the week after he had used. To enable him to set achievable harm reduction goals, the following goal setting and problem-solving exercise was done.

Identify longer-term goal in terms of alcohol/drug use behaviour or general goals

Roan had identified his longer-term goal as getting on with his life and getting a job. By re-evaluating his positive beliefs about drug use, Roan was able to begin to see that using on weekends affected his ability to function properly during the week, and that this would in turn affect his ability to work.

Write down where the client is now in terms of alcohol/drug use behaviour

Roan stated that he was using two ecstasy tablets and £50 worth of cocaine on two nights during the weekend.

Identify the client's harm reduction steps, that is, the areas where he could make some changes to his alcohol/drug-using behaviour that would have a positive impact on his life

Roan concluded that he could take five steps to achieve his goal:

Step 1: Cut down his drug use by going clubbing only on one night of the weekend

Step 2: When he went clubbing, use later on in the night to reduce further his drug use

Step 3: Go clubbing less often (i.e., every two weeks/monthly) and try to enjoy it without using drugs

Step 4: Get back into a work routine

Step 5: Get a job.

Identify what the client could do to achieve each of these goals

Step 1: go clubbing on a Saturday night rather than on a Sunday, so that he would not feel as bad on Monday morning. Go out with friends who do not use drugs on a Sunday (e.g. cinema, bowling, restaurant).

Step 2: spend more time with friends at the club who don't use.

Step 3: modify and re-evaluate his belief: "Everyone at the club is using, and I'll feel left out if I don't use", and tell myself: "Not everyone is using. I can spend more time with my friends who don't use and still have a good time."

Step 4: do some voluntary work on two days of the week (Wednesday and Thursday).

Step 5: look for a part-time job.

Identify any obstacles that might prevent goal attainment and identify strategies to overcome these obstacles

Obstacle: Wanting to achieve my goal immediately.
Strategy: Tell myself to take one step at a time.
Obstacle: If I use more drugs or go clubbing on more nights than I planned, I'll feel that I'm a failure.
Strategy: Tell myself that if I have a slip or a setback, it doesn't mean that I have failed. I can learn from the experience and do things differently next time.

Working with resistance to goal setting

When trying to set harm reduction goals, it is common to experience some resistance and find that clients may still be unwilling to make any positive change in alcohol/drug use. There may be several reasons they give for not wanting to make any changes. Thus, clinicians are encouraged to remain optimistic, take a long-term perspective, and directly address these reasons and negotiate with the clients some behaviour change in relation to alcohol/drug use. Some common reasons clients give for not wanting to change are as follows: *"I don't need to change—I enjoy using and it's not really a problem"; "There is no point in trying to change—I've tried before and failed"; "I get bored if I'm not using"; "Everyone I know uses, especially all my friends, so it is hard not to use."* Some strategies that are used to overcome resistance include the following:

- Emphasizing that any goals set will be realistic and achievable.
- Remaining optimistic and taking a long-term perspective on achieving change.
- Reviewing the client's decisional balance and all the factors listed as reasons "for" change.
- Setting up behavioural experiments to test beliefs that prevent clients from wanting to change (e.g., *"There is no point in trying to change—I've tried before and failed and so I'll fail again"*).
- Using cognitive strategies (e.g., recognizing cognitive distortions, three question technique, and reviewing evidence for and against beliefs) to re-evaluate and modify beliefs that prevent clients from wanting to change (e.g., *"I don't want to stop using cannabis; I enjoy it and I can control it"*).

Strategies to increase awareness of problematic links between mental health and substance use

The underlying philosophy of the C-BIT approach is that the substance-related beliefs of problematic substance users are linked with their experience of psychosis. Generally speaking, problematic substance use is maintained by positive links between mental health experience and alcohol/drug use. For example, substance-related beliefs may be that *"alcohol helps to reduce anxiety"*, that *"cannabis helps relaxation and sleep"*, or that *"crack-cocaine has a positive effect on mood and does not really worsen psychotic symptoms"*. Therefore, clients do not see any reason to change their use. Although clients' may have some evidence to support these positive beliefs about the effects of alcohol/drug use on mental health, this is perceived within C-BIT as only a *"snapshot"* of what actually happens when alcohol/drugs are used. Thus, these beliefs are actually viewed as cognitive distortions that allow clients to convince themselves that it is acceptable to keep using. Therefore, the challenge here is for clinicians to help clients look at the fuller picture, almost like pressing the "fast forward" button on a video player. That is, clinicians must stress the effects of drug/alcohol use on mental health and well-being not just immediately, but one hour later, later still in the day, the next day, the rest of the week, and so on. Thus, one aim at this stage is for clinicians to mobilize motivation for change by helping clients to see that problematic alcohol/drug use adversely affects mental health and well-being.

Two key strategies are employed: *re-evaluating and modifying beliefs, and provision of educational information*. Standard cognitive therapy techniques are employed to re-evaluate and modify positive beliefs about the impact of alcohol/drug use on clients' mental health (as outlined in treatment phase 1).

For example, Daniel believes that "alcohol helps reduce my stress and nervousness". The cognitive distortions in this belief are overgeneralization and the all-or-nothing thinking style.

Clinician: Daniel, you've said that you have found that alcohol helps your stress and nervousness. What evidence do you have to support that belief?

Daniel: After I drink, I feel relaxed and the tension that I had been feeling goes away.

Clinician: Are there times when that is not the case?

Daniel: No, it always helps to reduce my stress and nervousness.

Clinician: Daniel, tell me about a recent time when you had a drink. You mentioned that you had a drink last night. Tell me about last night... for about how long did you feel relief of your tension, nervousness, and stress following your drinking session?

Daniel: Well, I felt relief for most of the evening and then I fell asleep.

Clinician: How did you feel in the morning?

Daniel: I actually felt guilty because I was disappointed in myself for drinking and felt that I had let you down again.

Clinician: Daniel, it sounds as if you didn't feel very relaxed in the morning.

Daniel: No, I didn't. I felt quite anxious and edgy, and a bit depressed that I had failed again.

Clinician: So, from what you are saying it sounds as if there are times when after a drinking session you feel some relief for a few hours, but then you can actually end up feeling quite nervous and edgy. If there are times when alcohol doesn't alleviate your tension and stress but actually can set it off, then what are the implications?

Daniel: Probably it's fairer to say that alcohol helps my stress and anxiety for a short while, but then it becomes a bit of a vicious circle and I feel worse the next day. Then I am more likely to feel depressed and feel like ending it all and to call the team in a crisis.

In addition, the provision of educational information serves to provide clients with more accurate information/facts about the actual effects that the substances used have on their mental health and the effectiveness of medication, this may help clients to re-evaluate any distortions in their residual substance-related beliefs.

Treatment phase 3: early relapse prevention

By this treatment phase, clients will be aware of some of the difficulties as-sociated with their drug or alcohol use and will have begun to re-evaluate some of their distorted positive substance-related beliefs. They will also have identified a goal to change their substance use and made some pos-itive change in alcohol/drug-using behaviour. However, clients may feel that their alcohol/drug use is out of their control, find themselves slipping back to using, and feel unable to identify the chain of events that led to using again. Thus, the clinician's aim in this treatment phase is twofold; first, to help clients identify activating stimuli/high-risk situations and substance-related beliefs that trigger a desire to use and maintain a vi-cious cycle of problematic use, and, second, to facilitate the generation of a relapse-prevention plan and strengthen commitment to change. The re-lapse cycle and prevention plan is formulated with the cognitive model of problem substance use (Beck et al, 1993; Liese and Franz, 1996), and it incorporates the standard principles of relapse prevention (Marlatt and Gordon, 1985; Marlatt and Barrett, 1994).

The link between thoughts, feelings and subsequent behaviour (i.e., alcohol/drug use) is explained with the cognitive model. Clinicians elicit a client's chain of events that led to problematic substance use. This is done by closely examining the client's description of a recent occasion of using alcohol/drugs, particularly after a period of abstinence or after hav-ing made some positive changes to drug/alcohol use, according to the following guidelines:

- To identify activating stimuli/high-risk situations, *ask clients where they were, who they were with, how they were feeling, what they were doing before they used. Also ask, "What situations/things (internal and external) usually make you feel like using?"*
- To identify alcohol/drug beliefs, *ask, "What was going through your mind at that time (just before you got the urges/cravings to use)?"*
- To identify automatic thoughts, ask, *"What thoughts popped into your head?"*
- To identify facilitative/permission beliefs, ask *"What did you say to your self that convinced you that it was OK to use or gave you permission to use?"*
- To identify instrumental strategies, *ask, "How did you think/decide you would be able to get alcohol/drugs?"*

Irene has a long history of heavy drinking. She drinks in a binge pattern and has had a number of periods of abstinence, the longest lasting about 8 months. After a recent binge, she said she cannot understand why she started drinking again. When Irene is drinking heavily, her life becomes chaotic and she stops taking her medication. Often the result is that she becomes quite paranoid and disinhibited, and hears voices telling her to kill herself. On some occasions, this had led to her going into hospital, and she doesn't want to go back to hospital. Therefore, a brief explanation is given of relapse prevention and the cognitive model of substance use. It is suggested that there are strategies that will help her to recognize the chain of events that has led to her drinking binges in the past, and that will put her in the driving seat to manage her drinking and psychotic relapses. The clinician suggested that they try to map out the chain of events that led to her last two binges, using the guidelines outlined above. For Irene, both relapses were then mapped out on a relapse cycle of problem substance use worksheet (see Figure 11.4).

Relapse prevention: helping clients manage substance use

The chain of events that contribute to the problematic pattern of alcohol/drug use forms the basis for the development of a relapse-prevention plan, that is, a plan of action that enables clients to self-manage substance use. This is done by encouraging replacement of alcohol/drug-related beliefs with more realistic beliefs about alcohol/drugs emphasizing control, and by learning new coping skills and making lifestyle changes (Beck et al, 1993; Liese and Franz, 1996). A relapse-prevention plan should address the cognitive, behavioural, and social factors that have maintained clients' problematic use of alcohol/drugs.

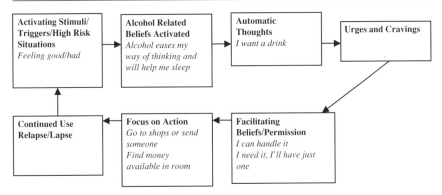

Figure 11.4   Irene's relapse cycle of problem alcohol use

Relapse prevention: including social network member(s)

Clients are encouraged to include, wherever possible, members of the social network in preventing/managing relapses. This ensures that clients have shared their decision to make a positive change in alcohol/drug use with someone else, and it will provide an additional incentive to maintain the changes achieved. It is fundamental that clinicians provide psycho-educational information regarding the ideas and concepts that are part of relapse prevention (that is, that lapses and relapses are common, particularly during the early stages, and do not denote "weakness") to those who will be involved in providing support.

Developing a relapse-prevention plan for substance use

The relapse-prevention plan of each client will be different because the chain of events and beliefs held about alcohol and drug use is unique to each individual. The clinician then seeks, with the client and others who are willing to provide support, to identify the key events in the relapse, cycle that have significantly contributed to past relapses and to generate alternative beliefs/ways of coping. The cognitive model of control is used (Beck et al, 1993; Liese and Franz, 1996).

It is important for a relapse-prevention plan to be rehearsed and updated on a regular basis to ensure that it can be used effectively should the need arise. Clients are also encouraged to carry a written summary of their relapse-prevention plan on a flashcard that can be referred to quickly. Two important additional areas that need to be addressed when developing a relapse-prevention plan are coping with cravings and the abstinence/rule violation effect. Three strategies are utilized to cope with cravings and

Irene's Relapse-Prevention Plan Summary (see also Figure 11.5)
Social network support: Bob, Karen, brother, Alcoholics Anonymous
(AA) meetings and Sponsor, key worker, and mental health team.

Activating stimuli: high/low moods
Safe situations: how I can keep my mood on an even keel:

1. Make simple plans.
2. Take each day as it comes.
3. Take medication regularly.
4. Spend time with friends Bob and Karen who don't drink.
5. Go to AA meetings and get a sponsor.
6. Talk through the things that worry me with my friends, brother, and
   mental health team.

Alcohol-related belief: "Alcohol eases my way of thinking and helps me
to sleep."
New control belief: "Alcohol eases my way of thinking by helping me to
sleep, but in the morning I feel panicky and nervous, and find it hard
to think rationally."
Permission belief: "I can handle it."
Deny permission belief: "I tell myself I can handle alcohol, but this is
false—I can't handle it. Once I get a taste of it, I am beaten."

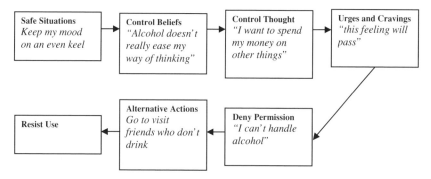

Figure 11.5 Irene's diagramatic relapse-prevention plan

urges; *provision of psychoeducational information about the nature of cravings
and urges, both cognitive (e.g., positive talk, re-evaluating substance-related beliefs, and imagery) and behavioural (e.g., counting, avoidance, relaxation, and
distraction).* As part of the abstinence violation effect, people engage in
particular distorted styles of thinking and feeling which may serve to increase the risk of a return to previous problematic patterns of use. *For*

example, "I've blown it"; "I knew I wouldn't be able stop." Clients may then give themselves permission to keep on using by thinking, *for example, "I've messed up already so I might as well keep going."* In such instances, cognitive restructuring strategies are used to help clients generate more helpful way of perceiving lapses and relapses.

Treatment phase 4: relapse prevention and relapse management

To ensure that clients have strategies in place both to manage better the use of alcohol/drugs and to prevent relapses to psychosis, clinicians aim to work collaboratively in order to develop comprehensive relapse-prevention/relapse-management plans with their clients, thus building on the work done in treatment phase 3 (early relapse prevention). This plan incorporates both substance use and psychosis. Some strategies included in this process are *inclusion of social network member(s), identifying a relapse signature, and development and use of a comprehensive relapse-prevention/management plan* (Marlatt and Gordon, 1985; Liese and Franz 1996; Plaistow and Birchwood, 1996; Weiss et al, 1999; Birchwood et al, 2000).

Identifying relapse signatures to psychotic relapses and the role of substance use

During this treatment phase, clinicians work with clients and their social network members to map out the chain of events that led to relapses to acute psychosis and the relationship between these events, alcohol/drug use, and medication adherence. The techniques that are described here are similar to the ones utilized in treatment phase 3 for substance use. A cognitive-behavioural relapse-prevention package for psychosis (e.g., Plaistow and Birchwood, 1996; Birchwood et al, 2000) is a useful template. The following guidelines are used to identify psychotic relapse signatures (i.e., idiosyncratic patterns of symptoms occurring within a particular time period that serve as early indicators of impending psychotic relapse):

- Introduce clients to examples of early warning signs of psychotic relapse (i.e., changes in thinking/perception, feelings, and behaviour that indicate impending psychotic relapse) (Birchwood et al, 2000).
- Ask clients to review the most recent episode when they experienced a relapse to psychosis or were admitted to hospital.
- Identify any noticeable changes in perceptions, thoughts, feelings, and behaviours, using the examples of early warning signs of psychotic relapse as a prompt.

- Identify any particular stressful events or factors that may have triggered these changes. Prompt clients with open-ended questions about any stressful or unusual events, worries, or concerns they may have had around that time.
- Identify through discussion the chain of external events and internal events (i.e., relapse signature) that preceded clients becoming psychotic/being admitted to hospital. Divide events into three stages: early, middle, and late.
- Find out whether this is the general chain of events leading up to clients becoming unwell. You can do this by asking about another recent occasion and the first time they became unwell or were admitted.

To identify the role/impact of alcohol/drug use on clients' psychotic relapse signature, the following process is used:

- Explore the role of alcohol/drug use within clients' relapse signature, by identifying the points along the chain of events at which they used alcohol/drugs. You can do this by asking clients directly whether they used during this episode and at which points they used.
- Identify the clients' patterns of use by asking what they used, how much they used, how often they used, where they used, and whom they used with.
- It is also important to identify the reasons why clients used alcohol/drugs at each point and what were their beliefs about using the substance (e.g., was it to increase pleasure, to socialize, or to cope?).

The role of medication adherence in a client's psychotic relapse is identified by using a similar strategy. Table 11.3 illustrates a relapse signature.

Developing a comprehensive relapse-prevention/relapse-management plan

The comprehensive relapse-prevention/relapse-management plan should incorporate the relapse-prevention plan identified in treatment phase 3, with reference to the role of substance use within the psychotic relapse signature. The plan needs to include a number of practical, simple strategies that the clients can use should they begin to experience a relapse to acute psychosis. These can incorporate personal coping strategies, social network support, accessing mental health services, and treatment interventions. The following areas are addressed within the comprehensive relapse-prevention/management plan: *managing early warning signs and the role of alcohol/drug use, medication adherence, and specific skills.* Clients are encouraged to learn to self-regulate substance use in relation to their mental state. The client's relapse signature is broken down into three stages that

Table 11.3   Rose's psychotic relapse signature and role of alcohol/cannabis

---

Stopped taking medication
Feeling odd
Thinking I am no good (boyfriend doesn't like me, I'm to blame for car accident)
Bad things always happen to me
Worry, and feel frustrated, angry, scared, sad, and edgy
Spend a lot of time alone
Difficulty getting to sleep
Racing thoughts
Arguing with boyfriend
Continued use of alcohol and cannabis (belief: cannabis and alcohol help me relax, and cannabis will help me sleep)

Thinking that everyone blames me and is against me
Feeling paranoid
Hear a faint voice
Sleep for only a few hours
Take some of my medication for a few days
Stay in bedroom a lot
Shout at boyfriend
Smoke more cannabis to help me sleep

Feel very paranoid (everyone, especially boyfriend, against me)
Voices get louder
Can't sleep
Lock myself in flat
Small reduction in alcohol use
Smoke more cannabis to help me relax
Screaming at voices

---

correspond, respectively, to the warning signs that occur earliest in the relapse signature, those that occur in the middle, and those that occur just prior to the psychotic relapse. The aim of developing a comprehensive relapse-prevention plan is to help your client have in place appropriate alternative coping strategies at each of the three stages.

The following process is used to develop a comprehensive relapse-prevention plan or "relapse drill":

- With the client and social network member(s), review the client's relapse signature and break it into three stages: early, middle, and late.
- Go through each of the early warning signs listed in the relapse signature and identify alternative "healthy" coping responses that can be included in the plan, as well as strategies the client has found helpful in the past. These should be listed on a comprehensive relapse-prevention/management summary in a column entitled "relapse drill" alongside the "relapse signature" (see Figure 11.6).

Support network : Mum, Key worker, Jo	
Relapse signature	**Relapse drill**
Early stage	
Stopped taking medication	Take medication regularly.
	Remind myself: "The cost of taking meds is putting on a bit of weight and feeling drowsy sometimes. However, the benefits are that I don't get worrying thoughts about Tania, I can sleep and I won't end up in hospital".
Feeling odd	Key worker to check I am taking it.
Thinking I am no good (boyfriend doesn't like me, I'm to blame for car accident)	Call mother and key worker, talk over worries and coping with fears.
▓ ▓▓▓ ▓▓▓▓▓▓▓ ▓▓▓▓▓▓▓ ▓ ▓▓▓ ▐ ▓▓ ▓▓▓	
Worry, and feel frustrated, angry, scared, sad, and edgy	Use relaxation techniques.
Spend a lot of time alone	
Difficulty getting to sleep	
Racing thoughts	
Arguing with boyfriend	Stay at Mum's if I am arguing a lot with boyfriend.
Continued use of alcohol and cannabis	Safe Situation: Go out and visit Jo.
Belief: "cannabis and alcohol help me to relax and cannabis will help me sleep"	Control Belief: "cannabis and alcohol only help for a little while and then I only feel worse".
Middle Stage	
Thinking that everyone blames me and is against me	Increase contact with services.
Feeling paranoid	Discuss feelings and thoughts.
Hear a faint voice	Use distraction (Walkman).
Only sleep for a few hours	
Take some of my medication for a few days	Take extra medication as prescribed.
Stay in bedroom a lot	See my psychiatrist and keyworker.
Shout at boyfriend	
Smoke more cannabis to help me sleep	Safe Situation: Stay at Mum's and stop cannabis use.
	Control belief: "cannabis is NOT helpful at this stage".
Late Stage	
Feel very paranoid (everyone, especially boyfriend, against me)	Ring key worker/emergency contact number.
Voices get louder	Tel: xxx xxxx
Can't sleep	Ask for respite/hospital.
Lock myself in flat	
Small reduction in alcohol use	
Screaming at voices	

Figure 11.6   Example of Rose's comprehensive relapse prevention management plan summary

- Agree with all involved an overall policy of how to respond to early warning signs/relapse and their roles in this response.
- When drug/alcohol use is identified in the relapse signature, refer back to the client's substance use relapse-prevention plan and include the strategies already identified (safe situations and control/deny permission beliefs) in the "relapse drill". Encourage the client to distinguish

between the types of substances used and to decide whether it is better to abstain or reduce use at key points along the relapse signature.

- Include in the "relapse drill" strategies already identified to increase medication adherence.
- Identify any additional skills/coping strategies the client may need to increase the chances of being able to cope with early warning signs.

Relapse-prevention plans have been likened to fire drills, because they are plans that are put in place to be preventative and need to be practised even in the absence of any early warning signs. Therefore, to ensure that clients use their plan effectively, clinicians are encouraged to ensure that clients practise, refine, and update their relapse drill in conjunction with the support person. Figure 11.6 provides an example of a relapse drill which could be simplified for clients to use.

EVALUATION OF THE C-BIT APPROACH

As outlined in Chapter 7, the C-BIT approach is in the process of being evaluated in a large, community-based mental health treatment service (Northern Birmingham Mental Health Trust [NBMHT]) within an integrated-shared care service model. The study is based on a quasi-experimental design. The five Assertive Outreach Teams in NBMHT were randomly assigned to one of two conditions: training plus support, or control (standard practice). The three teams in the former condition were all trained to use the C-BIT approach and provided with treatment manuals and resource materials. In addition, a member of staff from the COMPASS Programme was allocated to each of the three teams in the "trained plus support" condition. The role of this staff member is to model the skills within C-BIT, while working clinically alongside the Assertive Outreach Team, and support the staff in implementing the approach. After 18 months, the two teams in the "control" condition will also receive the training and support. The study aims to answer two main questions. First, can integrated treatment delivery be achieved within the existing Assertive Outreach Teams? Second, once integrated treatment is achieved, does it have a positive impact on clients? Outcome evaluation will focus on a number of domains, including substance-use behaviour and beliefs, mental health, level of engagement, satisfaction with life, personal and social functioning, and resource use. A range of standardized assessment tools are being used to obtain this information from clients, key workers, and case notes/records. Exposure and fidelity to the treatment approach are also being measured within this study. Measures are also included to assess the extent to which the treatment approach has been adopted by the team and incorporated into team discussions.

The study includes all clients in the Assertive Outreach Teams who, at the start of the evaluation, had both a severe mental health problem (i.e., by ICD-10 criteria, schizophrenia, schizotypal, delusional disorder, or major mood (affective) disorder) and problems with drug/alcohol use (i.e., ICD-10 abuse/dependent use). Clients who met the criteria were asked for consent to be engaged in the evaluation. Clients in both study conditions were then interviewed prior to the intervention (i.e., "training plus support"). They are being followed up at 6-month intervals over the study period, allowing for a comparison between clients in the two study conditions.

REFERENCES

Beck, A.T., Wright, F.D., Newman, C.F. and Liese, B.S. (1993) *Cognitive Therapy of Substance Misuse*. New York, Guilford.

Beck, A.T. (1976) *Cognitive Therapy and the Emotional Disorders*. New York, International Universities Press.

Birchwood, M. and Tarrier, N. (1994) *Psychological Management of Schizophrenia*. London, Wiley.

Birchwood, M., Spencer, E. and McGovern, D. (2000) Schizophrenia: early warning signs. *Advances in Psychiatric Treatment*, 6: 93–101.

Copello, A., Orford, J., Hodgson, R., Tober, G. and Barrett, C. on behalf of the UKATT research team (2002) Social behaviour and network therapy: key principles and early experiences. *Addictive Behaviors*, 27: 345–366.

Drake, R.E., Bebout, R.R. and Roach, J.P. (1993). A research evaluation of social network case management for homeless persons with dual disorders. In: M. Harris and H.C. Bergman (Eds.), *Case Management for Mentally Ill Patients: Theory and Practice*, pp. 83–98. Pennsylvania, Harwood Academic Publishers.

Fowler, D., Garety, P. and Kuipers, E. (1995) *Cognitive Behaviour Therapy for Psychosis*. Chichester, Wiley.

Galanter, M. (1993) Network therapy for substance abuse: a clinical trial. *Psychotherapy*, 30: 251–258.

Galanter, M. (1999) *Network Therapy for Alcohol and Drug Abuse*. New York, Guilford.

Glass, I.B., Farrell, M. and Hajek, P. (1991) Tell me about the client: history-taking and formulating the case. In I.B. Glass (Ed.), *International Handbook of Addiction Behaviour*. London, Tavistock/Routledge.

Graham, H., Copello, A., Birchwood, M., Orford, J., McGovern, D., Atkinson, E., Maslin, J. Mueser, K., Preece, M., Tobin, D. and Georgiou, G. (Unpublished) *Cognitive Behavioural Integrated Treatment (CBIT): An Approach for Working with Your Clients Who Have Severe Mental Health Problems and Use Drugs/Alcohol Problematically*. Northern Birmingham Mental Health Trust.

Heather, N., Wodak, A., Nadelman, E. and O'Hare, P. (1993) *Psychoactive Drugs and Harm Reduction from Faith to Science*. London, Whurr.

Hemming, M., Morgan, S. BO'Halloran, P. and O'Halloran (1999). Assertive outreach: implications for the development of the model in the United Kingdom. *Journal of Mental Health*, 8: 141–147.

Kemp, R., Hayward, P., Applewaite, G., Everitt, B. and David, A. (1996) Compliance therapy in psychotic patients. A randomised controlled trial. *British Medical Journal*, 312: 345–349.

Kingdon, D.G. and Turkington, D.G. (1994) *Cognitive-Behavioural Therapy of Schizophrenia*. Hove, Psychology Press.

Liese, B.S. and Franz, R.A. (1996) Treating substance use disorders with cognitive therapy. In P. Salkovskis (Ed.), *Frontiers of Cognitive Therapy*. New York, Guilford.

Marlatt, G.A. and Barrett, K. (1994) Relapse prevention. In M. Galanter and H.D. Kleber (Eds), *Textbook of Substance Abuse Treatment*. Washington, DC, American Psychiatric Press.

Marlatt, G.A. and Gordon, J.R. (1985) *Relapse Prevention. Maintenance Strategies in the Treatment of Addictive Behaviours*. London, Guilford.

Marlatt, G.A. (1998) Highlights of harm reduction. In G.A. Marlatt (Ed.), *Harm Reduction: Pragmatic Strategies for Managing High Risk Behaviours*. New York, Guilford.

Meyers, R.J., Dominguez, T.P. and Smith, J.E. (1996). Community reinforcement training with concerned others. In V.B. Van Hasselt and R.K. Hersen (Eds.), *Sourcebook of Psychological Treatment Manual for Adult Disorders*. New York, Plenum.

Miller, W.R. and Rollnick, S. (1991) *Motivational Interviewing: Preparing People to Change Addictive Behaviour*. London, Guilford.

Mueser, K.T., Drake, R.E. and Noordsy, D.L. (1998) Integrated mental health and substance abuse treatment for severe psychiatric disorders. *Journal of Practical Psychiatry and Behavioural Health*, May: 129–139.

Padesky, C. and Greenberger, D. (1995) *Clinician's Guide to Mind Over Mood*. New York, Guilford.

Plaistow, J. and Birchwood, M. (1996) *Back in the Saddle*. Early Intervention Service, North Birmingham Mental Health Trust.

Prochaska, J.O., DiClemente, C.C. and Norcross, J.C. (1992) In search of how people change: applications to addictive behaviours. *American Psychologist*, **47**: 1102–1114.

Roberts, L.J., Shaner, A. and Eckman, E. (Unpublished) *Substance Abuse Management Module (SAMM): Skills Training for People with Schizophrenia Who Are Also Addicted to Drugs and Alcohol*. West Los Angeles VA Medical Center and the Department of Psychiatry and Biobehavioral Sciences, UCLA.

Rogers, C.R. (1991) *Client Centered Therapy: Its Current Practice, Implications and Theory*. London, Constable.

Salkovskis, P. (1996) Preface. In P. Salkovskis (Ed.), *Frontiers of Cognitive Therapy*. New York, Guilford.

Stein, L.I. and Test, M.A. (1980) An alternative to mental hospital treatment. I. Conceptual model, treatment program and clinical evaluation. *Archives of General Psychiatry*, **37**: 392–7.

Weiss, R.D., Najavits, L.M. and Greenfield, S.F. (1999) A relapse prevention group for patients with bipolar and substance use disorders. *Journal of Substance Abuse Treatment*, **16**: 47–54.

Chapter 12

RELAPSE PREVENTION FOR PATIENTS WITH BIPOLAR AND SUBSTANCE USE DISORDERS

Roger D. Weiss, Shelly F. Greenfield and Grace O'Leary

INTRODUCTION

In studies of community samples (Kessler et al, 1997; Regier et al, 1990) and treatment populations (Brady et al, 1991; Keller et al, 1986; Mirin et al, 1991; Ross et al, 1988; Rounsaville et al, 1991), a high rate of co-occurrence of bipolar disorder and substance use disorders has been consistently demonstrated. The National Institute of Mental Health Epidemiologic Catchment (ECA) study (Regier et al, 1990) found that bipolar disorder was the Axis I disorder associated with the greatest risk of having a co-occurring substance use disorder. In fact, an individual with bipolar disorder is six times more likely to have a substance use disorder than the general population. People diagnosed with bipolar I disorder (i.e., those who have been hospitalized for mania) had an even higher risk of having a substance use disorder—nearly eight times more likely than the general population.

Studies of clinical populations have also shown higher rates of comorbidity between bipolar disorder and substance use disorders. The prevalence rate of substance use disorders determined from surveys of patients being treated with bipolar disorder is 21–31% (Brady et al, 1991; Hasin et al, 1985; Keller et al, 1986; Miller et al, 1989; Reich et al, 1974). Additionally, patients seeking substance abuse treatment have an elevated rate of bipolar disorder (Hesselbrock et al, 1985; Mirin et al, 1991; Ross et al, 1988; Rounsaville et al, 1991).

Substance Misuse in Psychosis: Approaches to Treatment and Service Delivery.
Edited by Hermine L. Graham, Alex Copello, Max J. Birchwood and Kim T. Mueser.
© 2003 John Wiley & Sons, Ltd.

There is some evidence that the co-occurrence of bipolar disorder and substance use disorders worsens prognosis. Patients with bipolar disorder and substance use disorders have demonstrated an increased likelihood of rapid cycling and a slower time to recovery from bipolar episodes (Keller et al, 1986). Bipolar disorder patients with comorbid substance use disorders also have higher rates of suicide attempts than non-substance-abusing bipolar disorder patients (Feinman and Dunner, 1996; Morrison, 1974). Patients with bipolar disorder who have co-occurring substance use have higher rates of hospitalization (Brady et al, 1991; Feinman and Dunner, 1996; Goldberg et al, 1999; Reich et al, 1974) and a greater likelihood of medication non-compliance (Goldberg et al, 1999; Keck et al, 1997; Maarbjerg, 1988) than their non-substance-using counterparts. Finally, in a 4-year prospective study of 75 patients who recovered from an index manic episode, Tohen et al (1990) revealed that a history of alcoholism was a predictor of poor outcome for the course of bipolar disorder, as evidenced by a shorter time to relapse and poor psychosocial outcome.

Although patients with bipolar disorder and coexisting substance use disorders have an especially poor prognosis, few studies of treatment for this population have been conducted. To date, only three, open pharmacologic trials with a total sample size of 24 patients have been conducted (Brady et al, 1995; Gawin and Kleber, 1984; Nunes et al, 1990). One double-blind, placebo-controlled study of lithium in adolescents with bipolar disorder and substance dependence (Geller et al, 1998) found that treatment with lithium was an effective treatment for both disorders. Moreover, despite a great deal of research interest in psychotherapeutic approaches for bipolar disorder (Bauer et al, 1998; Frank et al, 1994, 2000; Miklowitz and Goldstein, 1990; Miklowitz, 1996; Miklowitz et al, 1996, 2000) and substance use disorders (Crits-Christoph et al, 1999; Najavits and Weiss, 1994; Onken et al, 1993; Project MATCH Research Group, 1997), no studies have specifically targeted patients with this combination of disorders. For this reason, our group at McLean Hospital and Harvard Medical School developed and piloted a manual-based group psychotherapy, "integrated group therapy" (IGT), for patients with co-occurring bipolar and substance use disorders. The following sections of this chapter will review

1) the theory and rationale for developing IGT for this particular patient population
2) the development of the treatment, including characteristics of patients and therapists
3) the structure and content of the therapy sessions
4) specific session topics
5) results from a pilot study of IGT
6) a case example to illustrate patients' experience of IGT.

IGT FOR CO-OCCURRING BIPOLAR AND SUBSTANCE USE DISORDERS

The theory and rationale behind the development of IGT

Several studies of group therapy combined with pharmacotherapy have demonstrated promising results for the treatment of bipolar disorder (Bauer et al, 1998; Cerbone et al, 1992; Davenport et al, 1977; Graves, 1993; Kripke and Robinson, 1985; Reilly-Harrington et al, 1999; Volkmar et al, 1981; Wulsin et al, 1988). Group therapies for patients with bipolar disorder exhibit common characteristics, including education about the disorder and the importance of disease acceptance despite the desire to deny it; a setting where patients can share their experiences and offer mutual support; discussions of medications and compliance; and discussions about difficulties in interpersonal relationships. Substance use has not been a central point of emphasis in these previous studies, and only one study (Kripke and Robinson, 1985) mentioned alcohol use; one study (Graves, 1993) excluded patients with substance use disorders. Additionally, manuals were not developed or employed in any of the earlier studies. Bauer et al (1998) described a structured, manual-based group psychotherapy that was utilized in two treatment programmes for patients with bipolar disorder. The therapy was well-tolerated, could be administered effectively, and helped patients achieve the goals of the group. This manual-based treatment, however, did not emphasize issues related to substance use.

The rationale for developing a specific treatment for patients with co-occurring bipolar and substance use disorders is multifactorial. Bipolar disorder has certain characteristics that would theoretically make these patients especially suitable for a specific treatment intervention. First, there is some evidence that patients diagnosed with bipolar disorder are at higher risk of using alcohol or drugs when hypomanic or manic than when depressed (Weiss et al, 1988, Zisook and Schuckit, 1987). Second, patients with bipolar disorder differ from those with unipolar depression in that substance use and noncompliance with medication regimens in the former group are often related to their *positive* attitudes towards their hypomanic symptoms. In a study by Jamison et al (1979), for example, patients with bipolar disorder were more likely to comply with medications because they feared depression rather than mania. Additionally, studies conducted by our group of patients hospitalized for cocaine dependence reported that the majority of patients with bipolar spectrum disorder who were interviewed claimed to use cocaine primarily when hypomanic, in part to enhance their endogenous symptomatology (Weiss et al, 1986, 1988). We decided to offer a separate group for bipolar disorder rather than a heterogeneous group including schizophrenia, because, unlike the latter group, when patients with bipolar disorder are in remission from a bipolar episode, they may experience few symptoms. Indeed, this absence of symptoms can be a major reason for medication non-compliance (Jamison et al, 1979).

The use of treatment manuals is widespread in the field of psychiatric research. Treatment manuals are believed to assist the therapist by providing a theoretically based rationale for a set of therapeutic techniques, a detailed description of techniques, and a logical organization of treatment content. Treatment manuals also provide a documented treatment that can be replicated in future studies, thereby enhancing the rigour of treatment outcome research (Rounsaville et al, 1988). While manuals for relapse prevention of substance use disorders exist (Carroll et al, 1991, 1998; Daley, 1986; Wanigaretne et al, 1990), we were unaware of manuals that had been developed for the specific purpose of treating patients with coexisting substance use and bipolar disorders.

The development of an *integrated* treatment of the two disorders was our primary objective. The treatment of patients with concomitant disorders often occurs in either sequential (e.g., patients receive substance abuse treatment, after which they are treated for bipolar disorder) or parallel (patients simultaneously receive treatment for each disorder at two different clinics) fashion (Weiss and Najavits, 1998a). Many researchers and clinicians have recommended integrated treatment of patients with substance use and bipolar disorders; that is, treatment of both disorders at the same time in the same setting by the same clinicians who are familiar with both disorders (Mueser et al, 1992). This treatment approach has been advocated for a number of years, but there have been relatively few empirical studies of integrated treatment for patients with co-occurring substance use and other psychiatric disorders (Carroll et al, 1995; Drake et al, 1993; Hellerstein et al, 1995; Kofoed et al, 1986; Lehman et al, 1993; Najavits et al, 1996).

Several reasons can be given for the development of a manual based on a relapse-prevention approach. First, this cognitive-behavioural treatment modality, which seeks to prevent relapse through the use of self-control strategies, skill training, identification of high-risk situations, impulse control, advantage-disadvantage analysis, and lifestyle changes, has been used with some success in the treatment of patients with a variety of substance use disorders (Carroll et al, 1994; Project MATCH Research Group, 1997). Second, the flexibility of relapse-prevention therapy and its adaptability for a variety of populations (Carroll et al, 1991) is an advantage; relapse-prevention techniques have been directly modified for use with certain other Axis I disorders (Gossop, 1989). Third, relapse-prevention treatment addresses some of the major issues that patients with both substance use disorders and bipolar disorders frequently face, including ambivalence about complying with treatment; coping with high-risk situations; self-monitoring of drug craving, moods, and thought patterns; and altering lifestyle to improve self-care and develop better interpersonal relationships. Finally, Cochran (1984) has provided empirical evidence of the potential utility of a cognitive-behavioural intervention for patients with bipolar disorder. She found that a six-session course of modified cognitive-behavioural treatment significantly enhanced lithium compliance in 14 patients with bipolar disorder, when compared with an equal number of patients who did not receive this treatment. Basco and Rush (1996) have published a cognitive-behavioural manual for the treatment of patients with bipolar disorder, although it is not specifically tailored for patients with coexisting substance use disorders. Miklowitz et al (2000) have demonstrated that patients with bipolar disorder who received pharmacotherapy plus a manual-based, family-focused treatment, consisting of education about bipolar disorder, communication training, and problem-solving skills training, had a longer delay in mood disorder relapses than patients with bipolar disorder who received pharmacotherapy plus a standard community care treatment. None of these treatments, however (Basco and Rush, 1996; Cochran, 1984; Miklowitz et al, 2000), was designed specifically to address issues associated with bipolar disorder and co-occurring substance use disorder.

Development of the treatment

The development of IGT and the associated manual involved an iterative process. IGT was conducted three times: once by the senior investigator (RDW), once by one of the collaborators (SFG), and once by a PhD-level psychologist. The manual was modified as the result of feedback from therapists, patients, and investigators, who all evaluated each session's strengths and weaknesses, and a thorough review of the manual by two outside expert consultants. Structured, open-ended interviews were conducted with all subjects after they completed IGT to elicit their opinions about the treatment and their suggestions for future groups.

Structure of group sessions

The major goals of the group programme are to educate patients about the nature and treatment of their two illnesses; to help patients gain further acceptance of their illnesses; to help patients offer and receive mutual social support in their effort to recover from their illnesses; to help patients desire and reach a goal of abstinence from substances of abuse; and to help patients comply with the medication regimens and other treatments recommended for their bipolar disorder.

The group therapy consists of 20 hour-long, weekly sessions, each devoted to a particular topic. Several topics of particular importance are repeated, but most are covered in one session. Each session consists of several fundamental components. The group begins with a "check-in", in which group members report how they are progressing with the major goals of treatment. During this part of the session, all members report on their past week's experience regarding drug and alcohol use, mood, and medication compliance. The patients have approximately 2 min each for the check-in reports. After a review of the previous week's session, the therapist introduces the current group topic. The therapist uses a combination of didactic presentation and group discussion. The manual provides the therapist with guidelines for conducting each discussion.

Each session is designed to function independently so that the treatment can be carried out in an "open" format. With this format, patients can enter the group at any time. The group sessions, therefore, cycle, rather than building on the previous sessions. An open format is desirable because one of the problems intrinsic to patient recruitment for group therapy is the fact that a therapy group needs a critical mass of patients in order to begin. Recruited patients may lose interest in the group if the period of time from initial recruitment until the actual start of the group is lengthy.

Session topics and descriptions

"It's Two Against One, But You Can Win." After reviewing the relationship between substance use disorders and bipolar disorder, the session emphasizes the potential of certain drugs to trigger manic or depressive episodes. The potential negative effects of substance use on medication adherence, as well as the effect of manic or depressed thinking on judgement, including attitudes toward substance use (Beck et al, 1993), are highlighted. The session also discusses the similarity between addictive, depressive, and manic thinking (such as irrationality and failure to consider the consequences of one's actions).

"Identifying and Fighting Triggers." (Two sessions.) The nature of high-risk situations or "triggers" is presented to the group. Patients are taught about both internal (irritability, depressed mood) and external (seeing one's drug dealer) triggers. Patients are asked to identify major triggers for their substance use, depression, and mania. Coping strategies are reviewed, including the use of the "3 A's": *avoiding* triggers when possible, avoiding facing triggers while *alone*, and distracting oneself with *activities*.

"Managing Bipolar Disorder Without Abusing Substances." (Two sessions.) The concepts of depressive thinking and manic thinking are reviewed. The discussion also focuses on the characteristics of depressive and manic thinking, such as irrationality, difficulty in prioritizing, and pathological pessimism/optimism. Patients are taught to cope with mood changes by stressing both behavioural methods (e.g., recognizing and fighting the desire to "give up") and the importance of reporting early mood changes to one's psychiatrist.

"Dwelling with Friends and Family Members." (Two sessions.) This module is designed to help patients understand the common difficulties that people diagnosed with bipolar disorder and substance use disorders commonly encounter in their relationships with family members and friends. By hearing what other group members have experienced, the patients are helped to put their own experiences into perspective. They are helped to identify ways in which family relationships can be improved. Since patients often report that their families have "given up" on them, this topic commonly invokes more affect, especially sadness, than any other session. The therapist tries to help patients to accept what they can and cannot expect from their friends and family members.

"Denial, Ambivalence, Admitting, and Acceptance." This session reviews the concepts of denial, ambivalence, admitting, and acceptance. Patients are educated about the common occurrence of ambivalent feelings towards sobriety and bipolar disorder treatment. Nonetheless, patients are told that while it is helpful to recognize feelings of ambivalence, acting on these feeling by using substances or stopping bipolar disorder treatment can be very detrimental. Identification of their ambivalent feelings and early manifestations of denial are taught to the patients.

"Reading Your Signals: Recognizing Early Signs of Trouble." This session discusses typical early warning signs of relapse to mania, depression, and substance abuse. Patients are taught to monitor their moods and their desire for substance use as a way of identifying these early warning signs. This session also reviews the concept of the "abstinence violation effect", and discusses the difference between a "lapse" (slip) and a relapse (Marlatt and Gordon, 1985).

"Refusing Alcohol and Drugs." Skills for refusing drugs and alcohol are discussed in this session. Patients are told that they need to know what to say if someone offers them a drink or a drug. Emphasis is placed on the idea that alcohol and drug refusal skills are the last line of defence against using. Thus, avoiding high-risk situations and seeking out others for support can help reduce the likelihood of being offered drugs or alcohol.

"Using Self-Help Groups." Self-help groups for addiction and for bipolar disorder are both discussed. Both the positive and the negative experiences

patients have encountered in self-help groups are reviewed. Much of this group is dedicated to a discussion of how patients can overcome common problems that individuals with co-occurring substance use and bipolar disorders face when attending addiction self-help groups. For example, other self-help group attendees may tell patients that they should stop taking prescribed medications, arguing that their psychiatric symptoms are merely a result of their substance use. This session focuses on how to distinguish between the good and the bad advice emanating from self-help groups. Emphasis is placed on the importance of seeking professional opinions when dealing with psychiatric issues.

"Taking Medication." (Two sessions.) This session discusses taking medication for both bipolar disorder (such as mood stabilizers) and substance use disorder (such as naltrexone or disulfiram). The group focuses on the difficulties that patients have had with medication and endeavours to generate solutions to these problems. Commonly discussed problems include ambivalence about one's need to take medication at all, the stigma associated with taking psychotropic medications, physical and psychological side effects, and disagreements with one's prescribing psychiatrist.

"Recovery Versus Relapse Thinking." The difference between the types of thinking processes that are likely to lead to recovery as opposed to relapse is the focus of this session. The concept of "may as well" thinking is reviewed ("I may as well use" or "I may as well stay in bed all day", for example). This is contrasted with a recurring theme of the group, that "it matters what you do"; that is, it matters whether one decides to use substances or not, and whether one takes medication or not.

"Taking Care of Yourself." Two aspects of self-care are discussed in this group: sleep hygiene and human immunodeficiency virus (HIV) risk behaviours. Sleep disturbances are common in substance use disorders and they can increase the risk of relapse to bipolar disorder (Goodwin and Jamison, 1990). Concrete skills for establishing a healthy sleep pattern are reviewed. The increased likelihood of HIV-related risk behaviours associated with both bipolar disorder and substance use disorder is also reviewed. Experience with IGT has demonstrated that by incorporating the discussion of HIV risk into a general discussion of self-care, patients are willing to discuss this very sensitive topic more openly.

"Balancing Recovery with the Rest of Your Life." This group reviews two common problems associated with patients' attempts to balance early recovery with other important areas of their lives. Patients are often busy with other life obligations, thus leaving little time for their treatment. In contrast, others spend so much time on treatment that they may lose touch with the rest of their lives. The latter situation may cause patients to resent treatment, and some may precipitously stop all treatment as a result. The different

stages of treatment and recovery are reviewed, and the discussion includes ways to recognize an imbalance between recovery and the rest of one's life. Potential strategies to overcome this lack of balance are reviewed.

"Getting Support from Other People for Recovery." This group emphasizes the importance of developing healthy relationships and avoiding difficult ones (e.g., relationships with active substance users). The concept that people who develop healthy relationships are more likely to have successful recovery than are those who remain involved in their old, troubled relationships is discussed. Involvement in self-help groups, therapy groups, and the use of supportive friends and family members are discussed as methods for creating supportive relationships.

"Weighing the Pros and Cons of Recovery." This session encourages patients to discuss both the positive and negative aspects of their substance use disorder and bipolar disorder. The similarities between addictive thinking and bipolar disorder thinking are emphasized. The concept of "hanging up your disease" is taught as a way of challenging this type of thinking. Addictive thoughts, such as "It's okay to get high", are compared to a telephone salesperson trying to sell people something that they do not want; patients are taught to "hang up" rather than engage in this internal discussion.

"Taking the Group with You." This session discusses how patients can continue their recovery successfully after completing the group. Several guidelines to help patients maintain recovery successfully after completing the group are offered. These include building up other supports, either through individual or group therapy, or self-help groups; continuing to review session materials even after the group has ended; and identifying the recovery thoughts and recovery strategies that specifically work well for them.

"Stabilizing Your Recovery: Thinking Through Your Decisions." Difficulties in early recovery from bipolar and substance use disorders are discussed. These include resolving problems resulting from patients' recent acute episode, such as debts from a manic spending spree; trying to break long-standing addictive habits; and difficulties associated with long-standing poor decision-making. The concept of "thinking through solutions" is highlighted to aid people to identify problems and devise better solutions. Patients are taught to think through the consequences of their behaviour, and to discuss their decisions with other people who are supportive of their recovery.

While many different topics are discussed in the group sessions, several major themes have been identified. The first is "the central recovery rule", and is discussed in every group: "Don't drink, don't use drugs, and do take your medication as prescribed, no matter what." This rule is held up as an example of "recovery thinking", which is contrasted with "relapse thinking", whereby patients give themselves permission to abuse substances in certain situations, such as feelings of depression, conflict with a family member, or feeling that they need to "reward" themselves.

The aforementioned concept of "may as well" thinking is also discussed regularly as an example of relapse thinking, and is contrasted with the idea that "it matters what you do". This pattern of thinking is discussed with respect to both substance abuse and bipolar disorder. For example, some patients may question the need for taking medications as prescribed if they continue to experience mania or depression; patients may then think about discontinuing their medications. This type of decision-making will surely lead to an exacerbation of the patient's problems. Discussing "may as well" thinking is an example of our adaptation of the abstinence violation effect (see Marlatt and Gordon [1985] for the treatment of substance abusers) to bipolar disorder. This is one example of how the themes of recovery and relapse that are shared by both disorders are discussed in an integrated fashion.

A PILOT STUDY OF INTEGRATED GROUP THERAPY

Over the past several years, under the auspices of the National Institute on Drug Abuse Behavioral Therapies Development Program, we have developed IGT and studied its efficacy. Our initial pilot study (Weiss et al, 2000) was an attempt to demonstrate that IGT is a feasible treatment, that patients would attend these groups and find them helpful, that therapists could conduct the treatment successfully, and that patients who attended the IGT had better outcomes than did patients who did not attend IGT.

Characteristics of the patient population

Adults between the ages of 18 and 65 who had current diagnoses of both bipolar disorder and psychoactive substance use disorder, according to the *The Diagnostic and Statistical Manual of Mental Disorders* (4th edn) (*DSM-IV*) (American Psychiatric Association, 1994), were recruited in sequential blocks, either for IGT or for monthly assessments only (non-IGT). There was no random assignment, but subjects could not choose one condition or the other. Rather, they were recruited in blocks for only one condition.

Subjects for the study were recruited while inpatients at McLean Hospital (Belmont, MA, USA), but they did not enter the study until after discharge. The inclusion criteria for the study included:

1) current diagnoses of bipolar disorder and substance dependence based on a trained interviewer's administration of the Structured Clinical Interview of the DSM-IV (First et al, 1994)
2) substance use within the 30 days prior to admission to the hospital
3) current treatment with a mood stabilizer and written consent for study clinicians to contact the subject's pharmacotherapist, for both data collection and emergency purposes (e.g., if a patient arrived at a group session manic or suicidal)
4) the ability to give informed consent.

Patients were excluded from the trial if they

1) had a medical condition that would prevent regular group attendance
2) had a psychiatric disorder that was organic in nature or had mental retardation
3) were planning to live in a residential treatment setting in which substance use was monitored and restricted.

Subjects could be involved in concurrent psychosocial treatment without restrictions.

Characteristics of the therapists

Therapists who conducted the group met the following criteria: a master's or doctoral degree in an area that included training in psychopathology (e.g., MSW, PhD, MD), at least 1 year of experience in a general psychiatric setting, at least 1 year of substance use disorder treatment experience, and at least 1 year of group therapy experience. The therapists were supervised weekly by the senior author, based on videotaped group sessions.

Results

We recruited 45 patients either for IGT or for monthly assessments only (non-IGT). The IGT patients were assessed at baseline, each month during treatment, and monthly for 3 months after treatment completion. The non-IGT group cohort participated in six monthly evaluations, which were identical to those received by the IGT subjects.

Substance use data were collected as part of the monthly assessments. The assessment instruments included:

1) the Addiction Severity Index (ASI), Fifth Edition (McLellan et al, 1992a), a measure of drug-related problem severity

2) the Timeline Followback (Sobell and Sobell, 1992), a measure that uses a calendar to determine actual days of use

3) urine toxicology screens and breath alcohol assessments.

Mood symptoms were measured with the Young Mania Rating Scale (YMRS) (Young et al, 1978) and the Hamilton Rating Scale for Depression (HAM-D) (Hamilton, 1960).

Medication compliance was assessed with a structured interview regarding medication compliance (Weiss et al, 1998b). Subjects were asked to rate how often they had taken their medications as prescribed in the previous month by using a 5-point scale ranging from "not at all" to "100% of the time". Involvement in non-study treatments was tracked monthly with the Treatment Services Review (McLellan et al, 1992b) to monitor treatments likely to be attended by this patient population.

Outcomes

Several promising outcomes emerged from this study. Patients who received IGT had significantly greater improvement in the ASI drug composite score and significantly more months of abstinence from drugs and alcohol than did the group that did not receive IGT. Patients enrolled in IGT also had significantly greater improvement in manic symptoms (as measured by the YMRS) than did the non-IGT group. Changes in HAM-D scores, however, were not significantly different in the two cohorts. The IGT patients also demonstrated better medication compliance than the non-IGT patients. Although many patients participated in non-study treatments, no significant differences were found between the IGT and the non-IGT cohorts (Weiss et al, 2000).

While encouraging, these results do raise questions about the effective components of IGT. The improvement by the IGT group may be attributable to the specific content of the therapy, but there may also be a nonspecific therapeutic value of gathering diagnostically homogeneous patients together each week to share their experiences. Although we posit that integrating the treatment of bipolar disorder and substance dependence into a unified approach is a critical therapeutic element in IGT, randomized trials will provide a needed test of this hypothesis. We are currently conducting such a trial, comparing IGT with group drug counselling (Mercer et al, 1994) that focuses on substance use outcomes alone.

CASE EXAMPLES

The following case report illustrates a patient's experience with IGT.

Clarence, a 25-year-old, single, unemployed man, was admitted to an in-patient psychiatric unit for the treatment of manic symptoms, including racing thoughts, pressured speech, increased energy, irritability, and diminished sleep for 1 week. Clarence had been diagnosed with bipolar disorder when he was 20 years old. He admitted that he stopped taking his prescribed dosages of valproate 2 weeks prior to admission because he "missed the highs". Clarence said he was attempting to modulate his mood with daily use of marijuana, a pattern that began in the months preceding the onset of his first episode of mania. He also admitted that he smoked marijuana four times per week even when his mood was stabilized and euthymic. Clarence has had eight hospitalizations in the past 5 years, and each admission was secondary to a manic episode precipitated by medication non-compliance and subsequent attempts to control his mood with marijuana. During each hospitalization, Clarence was restarted on valproate and his manic symptoms resolved.

Clarence was concerned because his parents threatened to evict him from their home if he did not stop smoking marijuana, take his medication as prescribed, and return to one of the four psychiatrists he has seen over the past 5 years. Clarence admitted that he "fired" psychiatrists when they questioned him about his substance use or recommended medications that might make him "fat and bald". He had alienated several friends and his significant other with his erratic behaviour and heavy use of marijuana. He had never had individual or group treatment for either disorder.

Clarence was evaluated for the IGT and met criteria for bipolar disorder and marijuana dependence. He signed the informed consent form and was enrolled in the study.

Clarence gave his "check-in" at the beginning of each group session. At the beginning of each of the first three group sessions, Clarence admitted that he had used marijuana three times per week with people he knew. He had also "forgotten" some doses of valproate each week. In the first three sessions, he learned how substance dependence and bipolar disorder affect each other in negative ways. He realized that regular contact with his friends was a trigger (high-risk situation) for marijuana use. Clarence developed a plan in which he would spend more time with friends who do not use drugs. He decided to join a gym so he would have an alternative to spending time with people who use marijuana.

At each check-in for the next four group sessions, Clarence reported a gradual decline in marijuana use from three times per week to no more than one time per week. He was still missing his valproate doses to achieve a "small high". He admitted that he had been feeling sad because his parents no longer trusted him; he said he often thought about stopping his medications altogether and returning to daily marijuana use. During the group discussion, Clarence learned how these depressive thoughts could lead to relapse. He heard the experience of another group member, Sonia, whose similar thinking caused several relapses. Sonia said she learned to call her supports when she was sad. She said regular contact with supportive friends and family was one factor that had helped her remain abstinent for the previous 5 weeks. Sonia also shared feelings of sadness because her own parents treated her much as Clarence's parents treated him. Although their relationship was often difficult, Sonia and her parents improved their communication because she included them in her support group.

At the subsequent four group sessions, Clarence expressed the feelings of anger he experienced because he felt "saddled" with the diagnoses of bipolar disorder and marijuana dependence. He admitted that he was having difficulty saying "no" to a friend with marijuana, and he smoked marijuana once to ameliorate these angry feelings. He also missed doses of valproate one or two times per week and skipped a meeting with his psychiatrist.

After hearing the similar experiences other patients had in managing difficult feelings and a subsequent desire to use substances, Clarence shared his experience of eight hospitalizations and how he had denied the seriousness of his bipolar disorder and his marijuana dependence. In the past, within weeks of discharge, he had always convinced himself that he was fine but a little "dull"; he rationalized his non-compliance with medication by thinking that marijuana was "more natural" than valproate. The group learned how to acknowledge their feelings (such as Clarence's anger) about these disorders and to manage them by different means. Clarence learned ways to say "no" to people who might offer him marijuana; the group also discussed the importance of supports and the use of self-help groups. Clarence decided to attend a self-help meeting in his neighbourhood.

Clarence reported compliance with his medication at the next two sessions because he was not losing his hair, and regular exercise at the gym was helping to prevent significant weight gain. He discussed his history of "firing" former psychopharmacologists and was working with his current psychiatrist to help prevent that situation from occurring in the future. At the 14th session, he said he had decided to spend his 26th birthday with his significant other, his parents, and some friends he made at self-help groups to prevent thinking that he "may as well" get high to celebrate the occasion. He noted feeling more confident in his ability to manage thoughts of using marijuana or discontinuing medications.

After a group session emphasizing the importance of good sleep hygiene to prevent a bipolar episode, Clarence made modifications to his bedtime. Since he had not smoked marijuana during the 4 weeks prior to this group session, he found it easier to regulate his sleep cycle because he was no longer staying out all night, smoking marijuana. After the 16th session, he began looking for a part-time job because group members were concerned that he had nothing else in his life at that time, other than recovery.

Clarence reported abstinence from marijuana at each of the last four group sessions. He had not missed a dose of valproate in 5 weeks. In these final groups, he and the other group members were reminded of the importance of support networks, compliance with medications, and the need to identify problems (such as arguments with parents and cutting back on recovery work) and to "think through solutions" to discover what recovery thoughts and recovery plans worked well for the each individual. At the termination of the group sessions, Clarence had achieved 8 weeks of sobriety.

At a 3-month follow-up visit, Clarence reported that he had smoked marijuana twice in one week during the last month. He had reported complete abstinence from marijuana during the first and second month follow-up telephone calls. He noticed symptoms of depression prior to using marijuana but he did not seek help from his psychiatrist until his friend spoke to him about changes in his mood. Sertraline was added to his medication regimen during an emergency visit with his psychiatrist. The addition of an antidepressant to the mood stabilizer, and an increase in self-help group attendance helped him resolve the problem quickly.

This case illustrates a man with bipolar disorder and substance use disorder who committed to a 20-week group therapy that integrated a treatment that was relevant to both his mood disorder and his substance dependence. With both regular group attendance and employment of skills learned in the group, Clarence achieved abstinence and medication compliance for the first time since he had been diagnosed with bipolar disorder. Three months after group treatment, he did return to marijuana use, but Clarence's marijuana use was significantly less than it had been in the past. His relationship with a supportive friend led to a rapid identification of the problem, intervention from his psychiatrist, and, ultimately, a positive outcome.

CONCLUSIONS

In this chapter, we have presented information about the unique issues facing patients diagnosed with bipolar and substance use disorders and the subsequent development of an IGT for patients with these co-occurring disorders. Preliminary results have shown that IGT may cause a significant reduction in substance use as well as a significant reduction in manic symptoms. Currently, our group is undertaking a randomized, controlled study in which we are comparing IGT with a group therapy that focuses on drug use but does not attempt to integrate the treatment of the two disorders. In this manner, we plan to continue in the process of developing and testing specific effective treatment protocols for this challenging patient population.

REFERENCES

American Psychiatric Association. (1994) *Diagnostic and Statistical Manual of Mental Disorders* (4th edn). Washington, DC, American Psychiatric Association.

Basco, M.R. and Rush, A.J. (1996) *Cognitive-Behavioral Therapy for Bipolar Disorder*. New York, Guilford.

Bauer, M., McBride, L., Chase, C., Sachs, G. and Shea, N. (1998) Manual-based group psychotherapy for bipolar disorder: a feasibility study. *J Clin Psychiatry*, **59**: 449–455.

Beck, A.T., Wright, F.D., Newman, C.F., and Liese, B.S. (1993) *Cognitive Therapy of Substance Abuse*. New York, Guilford.

Brady, K., Casto, S., Lydiard, R.B., Malcolm, R. and Arana, G. (1991) Substance abuse in an inpatient psychiatric sample. *American Journal of Drug and Alcohol Abuse*, **17**: 389–397.

Brady, K.T., Sonne, S.C., Anton, R. and Ballenger, J.C. (1995) Valproate in the treatment of acute bipolar affective episodes complicated by substance abuse: a pilot study. *Journal of Clinical Psychiatry*, **56**: 118–121.

Carroll, K.M. *A Cognitive-Behavioral Approach: Treating Cocaine Addiction.* (1998) National Institute on Drug Abuse (NIH Publication No. 98-4308). Washington, DC, US Government Printing Office.

Carroll, K.M., Rounsaville, B.J., Gordon, L.T., Nich, C., Jatlow, P., Bisighini, R.M. and Gawin, F.H. (1994) Psychotherapy and pharmacotherapy for ambulatory cocaine abusers. *Archives of General Psychiatry*, **51**: 177–187.

Carroll, K.M., Rounsaville, B. and Keller, D. (1991) Relapse prevention strategies for the treatment of cocaine abuse. *American Journal of Drug and Alcohol Abuse*, **17**: 249–265.

Carroll, K.M., Rounsaville, B.J., Nich C., Gordon, L. and Gawin, F. (1995) Integrating psychotherapy and pharmacotherapy for cocaine dependence: results from a randomized clinical trial. In National Institute on Drug Abuse Research Monograph 150, pp. 19–35. Washington, DC.

Cerbone, M.J.A., Mayo, J.A., Cuthbertson, B.A. and O'Connell, R.A. (1992) Group therapy as an adjunct to medication in the management of bipolar affective disorder. *Group*, **16**: 174–187.

Cochran, S.D. (1984) Preventing medical noncompliance in the outpatient treatment of bipolar affective disorders. *Journal of Consulting and Clinical Psychology*, **52**: 873–878.

Crits-Christoph, P., Siqueland, L., Blaine, J., Frank, A., Luborsky, L., Onken, L.S., Muenz, L.R., Thase, M.E., Weiss, R.D., Gastfriend, D., Woody, G.E., Barber, J.P., Butler, S.F., Daley, D., Salloum, I., Bishop, S., Najavits, L., Lis, J., Mercer, D., Griffin, M.L., Moras, K. and Beck, A.T. (1999) Psychosocial treatments for cocaine dependence: National Institute on Drug Abuse Collaborative Cocaine Treatment Study. *Archives of General Psychiatry*, **56**: 493–502.

Daley, D. (1986) *Relapse Prevention Workbook: For Recovering Alcoholics and Drug Dependent Persons*. Holmes Beach, FL, Learning Publications.

Davenport, Y.B., Ebert, M.H., Adland, M.L., and Goodwin, F.K. (1977) Couples group therapy as an adjunct to lithium maintenance of the manic patient. *American Journal of Orthopsychiatry*, **47**: 495–502.

Drake, R.E., McHugo, G.J. and Noordsy, D.L. (1993) Treatment of alcoholism among schizophrenic outpatients: 4-year outcomes. *American Journal of Psychiatry*, **150**: 328–329.

Feinman, J.A. and Dunner, D.L. (1996) The effect of alcohol and substance abuse on the course of bipolar affective disorder. *Journal of Affective Disorders*, **37**: 43–49.

First, M.B., Spitzer, R.L., Gibbon, M. and William, J.B.W. (1994) *Structured Clinical Interview for Axis I DSM-IV Disorders—Patient Edition* (SCID-I/P, Version 2.0). New York, Biometrics Research, New York State Psychiatric Institute.

Frank, E., Kupfer, D.J., Ehlers, C.L., Monk, T.H., Corne, S.E., Carter, S. and Frankel, D. (1994) Interpersonal and social rhythm therapy for bipolar disorder: integrating interpersonal and behavioral approaches. *Behavior Therapist*, **17**: 143–149.

Frank, E., Swartz, H.A. and Kupfer, D.J. (2000) Interpersonal and social rhythm therapy: managing the chaos of bipolar disorder. *Biological Psychiatry*, **48**: 593–604.

Gawin, F.H. and Kleber, H.D. (1984) Cocaine abuse treatment: open pilot trial with desipramine and lithium carbonate. *Archiver of General Psychiatry*, **41**: 903–909.

Geller, B., Cooper, T.B., Sun, K.A.I., Zimmerman, B., Frazier, J., Williams, M. and Heath, J. (1998) Double-blind and placebo-controlled study of lithium for adolescent bipolar disorders with secondary substance dependency. *Journal of the American Academy of Child and Adolescent Psychiatry*, **37**: 171–178.

Goldberg, J., Garno, J., Portera, L., Kocsis, J. and Whiteside, J. (1999) Correlates of suicidal ideation in dysphoric mania. Journal of Affective Disorders, **56**: 75–81.

Goodwin, F.K. and Jamison, K.R. (1990) *Manic-Depressive Illness*. New York, Oxford University Press.

Gossop, M. (ed.). (1989) *Relapse and Addictive Behavior*. London, Tavistock/Routledge.

Graves, J.S. (1993) Living with mania: a study of outpatient group psychotherapy for bipolar patients. *American Journal of Psychotherapy*, **47**: 113–126.

Hamilton, M. (1960) A rating scale for depression. *Journal of Neurology, Neurosurgery and Psychiatry*, **23**: 56–62.

Hasin, D., Endicott, J. and Lewis, C. (1985) Alcohol and drug abuse in patients with affective syndromes. *Comprehensive Psychiatry*, **26**: 283–295.

Hellerstein, D., Rosenthal, R. and Miner, C. (1995) A prospective study of integrated outpatient treatment for substance-abusing schizophrenic patients. *American Journal of Addiction*, **4**: 33–42.

Hesselbrock, M., Meyer, R. and Keener, J. (1985) Psychopathology in hospitalized alcoholics. *Archives of General Psychiatry*, **42**: 1050–1055.

Jamison, K.R., Gerner, R.H. and Goodwin, F.K. (1979) Patient and physician attitudes toward lithium: relationship to compliance. *Archives of General Psychiatry*, **36**: 866–869.

Keck, P., McElroy, S., Strakowski, S., Bourne, M. and West, S. (1997) Compliance with maintenance treatment in bipolar disorder. *Psychopharmacology Bulletin*, **33**: 87–91.

Keller, M.B., Lavori, P.W., Coryell, W., Andreasen, N.C., Endicott, J., Clayton, P.J., Klerman, G.L. and Hirschfeld, R.M. (1986) Differential outcome of pure manic, mixed/cycling, and pure depressive episodes in patients with bipolar illness. *Journal of the American Medical Association*, **255**: 3138–3142.

Kessler, R.C., Crum, R.C., Warner, L.A., Nelson, C.B., Schutenberg, J. and Anthony, J.C. (1997) Lifetime co-occurrence of DSM-III-R alcohol abuse and dependence with other psychiatric disorders in the National Comorbidity Survey. *Archives of General Psychiatry*, **54**: 313–321.

Kofoed, L., Kania, J., Walsh, T., and Atkinson, R.M. (1986) Outpatient treatment for patients with substance abuse and coexisting psychiatric disorders. *American Journal of Psychiatry*, **143**: 867–872.

Kripke, D.F. and Robinson, D. (1985) Ten years with a lithium group. *McLean Hospital Journal*, **10**: 1–11.

Lehman, A., Herron, J. and Schwartz, R. (1993) Rehabilitation for young adults with severe mental illness and substance use disorders: a clinical trial. *Journal of Nervous and Mental Disease*, **181**: 86–90.

Maarbjerg, K., Aagaard, J. and Vestergaard, P. (1988) Adherence to lithium prophylaxis. I. Clinical predictors and patient's reasons for nonadherence. *Pharmacopsychiatry*, **21**: 121–125.

Marlatt, G.A. and Gordon, J.R. (1985) *Relapse Prevention: Maintenance Strategies in the Treatment of Addictive Behaviors*. New York, Guilford.

McLellan, A.T., Alterman, A.I., Cacciola, J. and Metzger, D. (1992b) A new measure of substance abuse treatment: initial studies of the Treatment Services Review. *Journal of Nervous Mental and Disease*, **180**: 101–110.

McLellan, A.T., Kushner H., Metzger, D., Peters, R., Smith, I., Grissom, G., Pettinati, H. and Argeriou, M. (1992a) The Fifth Edition of the Addiction Severity Index. *Journal of Substance Abuse Treatment*, **9**: 199–213.

Mercer, D., Carpenter, G., Daley, D., Patterson, C. and Volpicelli, J. (1994) *Addiction Recovery Manual*. Treatment Research Unit, University of Pennsylvania.

Miklowitz, D.J. (1996) Psychotherapy in combination with drug treatment for bipolar disorder. *Journal of Clinical Psychopharmacology* **16** (Suppl 1): 56S–66S.

Miklowitz, D.J., Frank, E. and George, E.L. (1996) New psychosocial treatments for the outpatient management of bipolar disorder. *Psychopharmacology Bulletin*, **32**: 613–621.

Miklowitz, D.J. and Goldstein, M. (1990) Behavioral family treatment for patients with bipolar affective disorder. *Behavior Modification*, **14**: 457–489.

Miklowitz, D.J., Simoneau, T.L., George, E.L., Richards, J.A., Kalbag, A., Sachs-Ericsson, N. and Suddath, R. (2000) Family-focused treatment of bipolar disorder: 1-year effects of a psychoeducational program in conjunction with pharmacotherapy. *Biological Psychiatry*, **48**: 582–592.

Miller, F.T., Busch, F. and Tanenbaum, J.H. (1989) Drug abuse in schizophrenia and bipolar disorder. *American Journal of Drug and Alcohol Abuse*, **15**: 291–295.

Mirin S.M., Weiss, R.D., Griffin, M.L., and Michael, J.L. (1991) Psychopathology in drug abusers and their families. *Comprehensive Psychiatry*, **32**: 36–51.

Morrison, J.R. (1974) Bipolar affective disorder and alcoholism. *American Journal of Psychiatry*, **131**: 1130–1133.

Mueser, K.T., Bellack, A.S. and Blanchard, J.J. (1992) Comorbidity of schizophrenia and substance abuse: implications for treatment. *Journal of Consulting and Clinical Psychology*, **60**: 845–856.

Najavits, L.M., Weiss, R.D. and Liese, B.S. (1996) Group cognitive-behavioral therapy for women with PTSD and substance use disorder. *Journal of Substance Abuse Treatment*, **13**: 13–22.

Najavits, L.M. and Weiss, R.D. (1994) The role of psychotherapy in the treatment of substance use disorders. *Harvard Review of Psychiatry*, **2**: 84–96.

Nunes, E.V., McGrath, P.J., Wager, S., Quitkin, J.M. (1990) Lithium treatment for cocaine abusers with bipolar spectrum disorders. *American Journal of Psychiatry*, **147**: 655–657.

Onken, L.S., Blaine, J.D. and Boren, J.J. (1993) *Behavioral Treatments for Drug Abuse and Dependence*. Rockville, MD, US Department of Health and Human Services.

Project MATCH Research Group. (1997) Matching alcoholism treatments to client heterogeneity: Project MATCH posttreatment drinking outcomes. *Journal of Studies in Alcoholism*, **58**: 7–29.

Regier, D.A., Farmer, M.E., Rae, D.S., Locke, B.Z., Keith, S.J., Judd, L.L. and Goodwin, F.K. (1990) Comorbidity of mental disorders with alcohol and other drug abuse: results from the Epidemiologic Catchment Area (ECA) study. *Journal of the American Medical Association*, **264**: 2511–2518.

Reich, L.H., Davies, R.K. and Himmelhoch, J.M. (1974) Excessive alcohol use in manic-depressive illness. *American Journal of Psychiatry*, **131**: 83–86.

Reilly-Harrington, N.A., Alloy, L.B., Fresco, D.M. and Whitehouse, W.G. (1999) Cognitive styles and life events interact to predict bipolar and unipolar symptomatology. *Journal of Abnormal Psychology*, **108**: 567–578.

Ross, H.E., Glaser, F.B. and Germanson, T. (1988) The prevalence of psychiatric disorders in patients with alcohol and other drug problems. *Archives of General Psychiatry*, **45**: 1023–1031.

Rounsaville, B.J., Anton, S.F., Carroll, K., Budde, D., Prusoff, B.A. and Gawin, F. (1991) Psychiatric diagnoses of treatment-seeking cocaine abusers. *Archives General Psychiatry*, **48**: 43–51.

Rounsaville, B.J., O'Malley, S., Foley, S., and Weissman, M.M. (1988) Role of manual-guided training in the conduct and efficacy of interpersonal therapy for depression. *Journal of Consulting and Clinical Psychology*, **56**: 681–688.

Sobell, L.C. and Sobell, M.B. (1992). Timeline followback: a technique for assessing self-reported alcohol consumption. In R. Litten and J. Allen (Eds), *Measuring Alcohol Consumption*, pp. 41–72. New York, Human Press.

Tohen, M., Waternaux, C.M. and Tsuang, M.T. (1990) Outcome in mania: a 4-year prospective follow-up of 75 patients utilizing survival analysis. *Archives of General Psychiatry*, **47**: 1106–1111.

Volkmar, F.R., Bacon, S., Shakir, S.A. and Pfefferbaum, A. (1981) Group therapy in the management of manic-depressive illness. *American Journal of Psychotherapy*, **35**: 226–234.

Wanigaretne, S., Wallace, W., Pullin, J. Keaney, F. and Farmer, R. (1990) *Relapse Prevention for Addictive Behaviours*. Oxford, Blackwell Scientific.

Weiss, R.D., Griffin, M.L., Greenfield, S.F., Najavits, L.M., Wyner, D., Soto, J.A. and Hennen, J.A. (2000) Group therapy for patients with bipolar disorder and substance dependence: results of a pilot study. *Journal of Clinical Psychiatry*, **61**: 361–367.

Weiss, R.D., Mirin, S.M., Griffin, M.L., and Michael, J.L. (1988) Psychopathology in cocaine abusers: changing trends. *Journal of Nervous Mental and Diseases*, **176**: 719–725.

Weiss, R.D., Mirin, S.M., Michael, J.L., and Sollogub, A. (1986) Psychopathology in chronic cocaine abusers. *American Journal of Drug and Alcohol Abuse*, **12**: 17–29.

Weiss, R.D. and Najavits, L.M. (1998a) Overview of treatment modalities for dual diagnosis patients: pharmacotherapy, psychotherapy, twelve-step programs. In H. Kranzler and B. Rounsaville (Eds), *Dual Diagnosis: Substance Abuse and Comorbid Medical and Psychiatric Disorders*, pp. 87–105. New York, Marcel Dekker.

Weiss, R.D., Najavits, L.M., Greenfield, S.F., Soto, J.A., Shaw, S.R. and Wyner, D. (1998b) Validity of substance use self-reports in dually diagnosed outpatients. *American Journal of Psychiatry*, **155**: 127–128.

Wulsin, L., Bachop, M. and Hoffman, D. (1988) Group therapy in manic-depressive illness. *American Journal of Psychotherapy*, **42**: 263–271.

Young, R., Biggs, J., Ziegler, V., and Meyer, D. (1978) A rating scale for mania: reliability, validity, and sensitivity. *British Journal of Psychiatry*, **133**: 429–435.

Zisook, S., and Schuckit, M.A. (1987) Male primary alcoholics with and without family histories of affective disorder. *Journal of Studies in Alcoholism*, **48**: 337–344.

Chapter 13

FAMILY INTERVENTION FOR SUBSTANCE MISUSE IN PSYCHOSIS

Christine Barrowclough

INTRODUCTION

The efficacy of family interventions for people with schizophrenia is now well established, with a number of controlled trials having consistently demonstrated the superiority of family intervention over routine care in terms of relapse outcomes (Mari and Streiner, 1997). However, there are few reports of family intervention which address the particular issues arising in families where a member has a substance misuse problem in addition to the psychosis, and, to date, no published evaluations of family work in such contexts. This chapter attempts to review the limited literature available about family issues with clients experiencing substance misuse and psychosis (SMP), before describing a family treatment approach focusing on drug and alcohol problems in psychosis clients.

There is much evidence that stress and burden are associated with caring for a person with severe mental illness (Barrowclough et al, 1996). However, there has been little investigation into those carers who have the additional strain of dealing not only with schizophrenia but also with substance misuse. The few available reports tend to come from the USA, and the indications are that family stress has a high prevalence in the households of clients with SMP. In a small survey of 25 inpatients with SMP, Alterman et al (1980) reported that family problems were evident in half the cases. In another very small US sample of 22 families (Sciacca and Hatfield, 1995), many relatives of persons with a dual disorder reported being significantly troubled by difficulties, the most salient of which were

Substance Misuse in Psychosis: Approaches to Treatment and Service Delivery.
Edited by Hermine L. Graham, Alex Copello, Max J. Birchwood and Kim T. Mueser.
© 2003 John Wiley & Sons, Ltd.

patient denial of the problem and patient decline in health. These concerns are likely to lead to both frustration and anger with the patient's attitude and behaviour, and also anxiety about their well-being. Such conflicting emotions are suggested in the descriptive account of carers of people with SMP reported by Mueser and Gingerich (1994). Further evidence of family stress in this context comes from a case note study of 121 persons admitted to hospital with a schizophrenia diagnosis (Kashner et al, 1991). This showed that those with a substance abuse problem were nearly four times as likely to have family members with "severely disturbed affect". The latter was considered to be present if there was evidence of refusal to discuss the patients' problems, or severe family conflict, or cynicism, hopelessness and pessimism. This finding is consistent with the report that SMP clients expressed lower levels of satisfaction with their families than clients with just a psychiatric disorder alone (Dixon et al, 1995). The latter study looked at 179 patients with a DSM-III-R Axis I current primary mental disorder, of whom 101 had a current additional psychoactive substance use disorder, and concluded that "inner-city mentally ill patients with a co-morbid substance use disorder perceive lower levels of family satisfaction than comparable patients with severe mental illness only", and "Of note patients with a comorbid use disorder did not report less frequent family contacts, which made their family potentially no less available" (p. 457).

The family problems in SMP households have important implications. Not only is such stress likely to affect the well-being of the carers and compromise their long-term ability to support the client, but it may also have an impact on the course of the illness itself and on outcomes for the client. Many studies have found that high expressed emotion (EE) in carers—a measure of the patient-directed affect and behaviour—is associated with an increased risk of relapse (Butzlaff and Hooley, 1998). Although little is known of the reasons why some carers develop high EE attitudes, a consistent finding in the literature is that high-EE relatives tend to assume that clients can control their problematic behaviour and symptoms (e.g., Brewin et al, 1991; Barrowclough et al, 1994; Lopez et al, 1999). On these grounds, Turner (1998) suggests that high EE will be prevalent in families where there is a substance-abusing individual, especially since dominant societal attitudes in Western culture tend to blame substance abusers for their behaviour. If this prediction is correct, we would expect to see raised levels of high EE in SMP households, and hence such patients would have additional relapse risks.

THE MANCHESTER DUAL DIAGNOSIS INTERVENTION STUDY

The Manchester Dual Diagnosis study (Barrowclough et al, 2001) was a randomized, controlled trial designed to evaluate of the effectiveness of a treatment programme with schizophrenia patients who had either drug or alcohol use problems. The aim of this trial was to investigate whether the programme of interventions had a beneficial effect on illness and substance use outcomes over and above that achieved by routine care. This chapter will focus mainly on the family intervention component of the programme. However, since we first present details of the study design and the full treatment programme, the reader will hopefully be able to place the family work in context.

Inclusion criteria for the study were as follows.

1. a non-affective psychotic disorder: schizophrenia or schizoaffective disorder according to ICD-10 and DSM-IV criteria
2. meeting DSM-IV diagnostic criteria for substance dependence or misuse
3. in current contact with mental health services
4. age 18–65 years
5. a minimum of 10 h face-to-face contact with the carer per week
6. no evidence of organic brain disease, significant concurrent medical illness or learning disability.

A final sample of 36 patient–carer dyads took part in the study. Thirty-three (92%) of the patients were male, and they were mainly young (mean age 31.1 years; SD 9.69) with an established illness history (mean illness duration 8.4 years; SD 8.44). In the total study sample, 19 patients had both drug and alcohol misuse, 11 alcohol only and 6 drugs only. Fifteen patients used only one substance (11 alcohol only, 3 cannabis only, and 1 amphetamines only). For the remaining 11 single-drug users, 10 used cannabis and alcohol, and 1 heroin and alcohol. All other patients (10) had polydrug use. The drug used by most patients was cannabis (22 patients), followed by amphetamines (10), cocaine (4) and heroin (4). The demographic characteristics of the sample would seem to be in accord with gender and age biases found in larger studies: substance use in schizophrenia (as in the general population) is more likely to be found in young males (e.g., Mueser et al, 1990). Similarly, the substance use profile of the study sample matches the type of substance use most prominent with schizophrenia patients. A recent review of prevalence studies for substance use in schizophrenia (Blanchard et al, 2000) reports cannabis to be the most frequently used drug. Alcohol use frequently occurs with drug use, and multiple substance use is common. Alcohol is also the most frequently found substance of abuse in this population (Smith and Hucker, 1994).

The planned intervention period was 9 months with sessions taking place in the carers' and patients' homes, except where clients expressed a preference for a clinic-based appointment (one individual cognitive-behavioural therapy [CBT] intervention, no carer interventions). All patients in the study (treatment and control groups) were allocated a family support worker from the voluntary carers' organization Making Space. The services of this support worker included information, benefits advice, advocacy, emotional support, and practical help. The frequency and nature of support worker contact was decided by mutual agreement between carer and support worker. For clients in the treatment group, the intervention attempted to integrate three treatment approaches: motivational interviewing (MI), individual CBT, and family or carer intervention (FI). In the absence of empirical data of treatment efficacy in the area, or clear theoretical models of why substance disorders develop and are maintained in psychosis patients, the rationale for this treatment synthesis was based on a number of a priori assumptions detailed elsewhere (Barrowclough et al, 2000). Briefly, there was firstly the expectation that the majority of patients would be unmotivated to change their substance use at the outset; hence, interventions to enhance motivation would be necessary. Secondly, it was felt that symptomatology might be implicated in the maintenance of substance use while, in turn, the drug and alcohol use might exacerbate symptoms; thus, psychological interventions to address symptoms would be important. Thirdly, it was thought that family factors might have a bearing both on symptomatology and continuation of drug or alcohol use; hence, the need for family interventions. Thus, we assumed an underlying model for the maintenance of the problem whereby motivation to use substances, symptomatology, and environmental stress in the social milieu were locked in an iterative and mutually reinforcing process.

OVERVIEW OF THE INTERVENTION

The intervention began with the MI phase, which consisted initially of five weekly sessions designed to assess then enhance the patient's motivation to change. With the introduction of the individual CBT at week 6 (or earlier if appropriate) the MI style was integrated into subsequent CBT sessions. Where clients remained unmotivated or ambivalent about substance use, motivational work was continued. "Booster" motivational work was appropriate if problems with client commitment became apparent at a later stage in the intervention. Once client commitment was obtained, changes in substance use were negotiated on an individual basis and might involve reduction, stabilization or abstention. The individual CBT took place over approximately 18 weekly sessions, followed by six sessions every 2 weeks. This phase included a detailed assessment of psychotic symptoms, techniques to reduce the severity and distress of persistent positive symptoms, and techniques to enhance self-esteem and improve depressed mood, as well as interventions to improve knowledge and understanding of the illness and the medication. Relapse-prevention strategies were used both for psychotic symptoms and to maintain changes in substance use.

After assessment of both patient and carers, shared goals were generated that become the focus of conjoint patient/family sessions. The family intervention consisted of 10–16 sesssions, and some of which took the form of integrated family/patient sessions and some of which might involve family members alone. Details of the motivational and individual CBT components have been given elsewhere (Barrowclough et al, 2000; Haddock et al, 2002). The remainder of this chapter will focus on describing the family intervention in more detail.

CHARACTERISTICS OF CARERS IN THE STUDY

To give a context to the family intervention, some descriptive statistics about the carers in the study may be helpful. Twenty-seven were female and 9 male; and the mean age was 51 years (SD 12.12). In terms of relationships, the majority (24, 67%) were parents, 6 (17%) were partners, and the remainder consisted of sibling (1), grandparent (1), landlady (2) and ex-partner (2). Of the 32 households who consented to undergoing Camberwell Family Interviews, which were assessed for EE (Vaughn and Leff, 1976), 66% (21/32) were rated high EE. In terms of subjective burden or distress, 53% (19/36) fulfilled criteria for "caseness" on the 28-item General Health Questionnaire (GHQ) (Goldberg and Williams, 1988). In summary, the profile of these families fulfilled the predictions of the available literature on this area reviewed earlier: by and large, they were a highly stressed group of people who were predominantly high EE status.

FAMILY INTERVENTION

The family intervention was strongly influenced by the motivational component of the programme. In working with people's motivation to change their substance use, we adopted the stages of change model developed by Prochaska and DiClemente (1986). The model describes how in the process of change people pass through states or stages of readiness, ranging from precontemplation (clients do not perceive themselves as having a problem or needing to make a change), contemplation (both considering change and rejecting it), preparation/action (being motivated to make change), and maintenance (taking steps to keep up the change). Motivation is conceptualized as an internal state of readiness which can be influenced by external factors. One way of influencing change readiness is by the therapist's style of interviewing, and "MI" (Miller and Rollnick, 1991) was used in this study to facilitate increased motivation for change. The importance of this intervention component was borne out by the characteristics of the sample. With the University of Rhode Island Change Assessment

Scale (McConnaughy et al, 1983), 78% (28/36) of the sample were found to have low motivation at pretreatment assessment, defined as being "pre-contemplative" or "contemplative". The key concepts employed in this style of interviewing are as follows: ambivalence is normal, resolving ambivalence is the key to change, responsibility for problems and their consequences is left with the client, and change efforts are not started before clients have committed themselves to particular goals and strategies.

A key underlying assumption of the family intervention was that patients' motivational state as regards changing their substance use could be influenced by the family environment. The intervention sought to promote a family response that was consistent with the MI style and the stages of change model. Hence, the aspects of such a response would be as follows: responsibility for problems and their consequences needs to be left with the client, confrontation about substance use may create more resistance to change, and family help will be most effective when it matches the stage of change of the client. It should be emphasized that the stress reduction approach of the generic family intervention model (Barrowclough and Tarrier, 1992) and motivational enhancement approaches were in complete concordance. The approaches shared a common framework about the kind of help from family members that was likely to be most effective. Take, for example, patients who are, at best, only at the "contemplative" stage of change. The family intervention in such cases might be directed at helping relatives to appreciate that attempts, on the one hand, to try to make people change their substance use or, on the other hand, to buffer the consequences of the use would be counterproductive. If responsibility for change is to be left with the patient, the family may need to embrace the deliberate strategy of not persuading, cajoling, or even encouraging clients to stop drinking or using drugs. This approach was promoted in the educational and subsequent interventions as an active and positive strategy of detachment, rather than a passive and negative way of behaving. It emphasized that the family need to leave it up to the client to make changes.

However, at the same time, it is good to communicate personal feelings about substance use; and to set boundaries and limits on the extent to which family members will tolerate the substance abuse having adverse consequences on the family life. Such limits would include not rescuing clients from the consequences of drug/alcohol use— for example, not bailing them out financially if they blow their money on drugs/alcohol—not covering up for their periods of drunkenness; and establishing reasonable house rules about acceptability of behaviour with age-appropriate sanctions that the relative is willing to carry through if rules are broken. For patients who have accepted the need to cut down or abstain from using substances and who have started to make change, the emphasis on client responsibility would also endorse the relative supporting changes once they have happened, but not the relative attempting to initiate change.

The general approach to cognitive-behavioural family intervention used in the study has been documented (Barrowclough and Tarrier, 1992). It begins with a detailed assessment of family problems and needs elicited from structured interviews, supplemented where appropriate by question-naires. Following from this assessment, a collaborative problems and needs list is formulated, which would typically include:

1. issues concerning the relatives' understanding of the illness
2. relatives' distress
3. coping difficulties
4. dissatisfaction with particular aspects of the patient's behaviour
5. restrictions and hardships that the relative is suffering as a consequence of the illness.

Additionally, family strengths would be highlighted. With the problem list as a guide, the interventions to address the family needs are then structured around three components:

1. education
2. stress management and coping strategies
3. goal setting to promote patient and relative change.

In the study, using the motivational framework, problems associated with substance use were identified in the assessment phase, highlighted in the problem formulation, and addressed in each of the intervention compo-nents. An outline of these adaptations of the family intervention is given below.

EDUCATION

Brief family educational interventions alone have no effects on patient be-haviour and do not appear to effect long-term changes in family well-being or relatives' management strategies (see Barrowclough and Tarrier, 1992: Chapter 5, for a brief review). It is argued that they are best construed as setting the scene for bringing about family change (Smith and Birchwood, 1987). In CBT terms, they attempt to begin to "socialize" the family into the stress-vulnerability model of psychotic illness. A simple model of psy-chosis is presented whereby enduring biological vulnerability may be ex-acerbated by environmental stress. The aim is to communicate to families, on the one hand, a sense of realism about the long-term risks of contin-ued problems and illness exacerbations and, on the other hand, a sense of optimism. Such optimism is derived from an understanding that in working together it may be possible to improve the course of the illness and improve patient functioning by taking illness (vulnerability) and environmental (stress) factors into account. Information that is incorporated into this framework includes details of the patient's illness symptoms (positive and negative), the causes of psychosis, treatment and the role of medication, the course and prognosis, and the role of the social environment, including how their own behaviour may influence outcomes. The content of sessions is modified to accommodate the relatives' current understanding and models of illness. There is also flexibility about which family members attend, although, invariably, patients would be encouraged to attend some of the sessions to enable them to contribute to describing the experience of psychosis. An interactive and collaborative style is used, acknowledging the relatives' viewpoint while sensitively working to offer alternative explanations where appropriate.

In assessing the relatives' understanding of substance use in schizophrenia, the Knowledge About Schizophrenia Interview (KASI) (see Barrow-clough and Tarrier, 1992) was modified for SMP families by the addition of sections asking about relatives' understanding of drug and alcohol issues. As with other sections of the KASI, the questions attempt to assess how helpful or unhelpful the beliefs they hold are likely to be—in this context, in terms of supporting a motivational approach. "Helpful" information and beliefs which might be targetted at the information sessions include beliefs likely to lead to a less blaming attitude. These are ones which associate the substance use more with the illness and less with factors personal to the patients themselves, and which acknowledge that it is difficult for patients to change without help from others and exceptional effort on the patients' part. Hence, the ideas incorporated in the educational sessions on substance use include the following:

- Substance use in schizophrenia is very common.
- Drugs and alcohol in themselves cannot cause schizophrenia.
- Drugs and alcohol use can sometimes worsen symptoms and have a negative effect on the illness, but this needs to be balanced by the patient's perspective of the positive effects. Such positive, or at least "benign", reasons why patients abuse substances are that they help to socialize, help to cope with symptoms, give pleasure—and patients do not have many pleasure opportunities—and ameliorate the negative effects of medication.
- Substance use is not completely under the patient's control—change can be made, but this requires exceptional and long-term effort on the part of the patient.

- An understanding of the stages of change model and a person's current position in the change cycle will determine the kind of support that is most helpful. When people are currently not ready for change, persuasion serves only to set their minds against change.
- Change is not an all-or-none process, and it is usual for people to go through a cycle of cessation and relapse, back to thinking about change, and then preparing for change, several times before achieving permanent abstinence.
- The education sessions also emphasize helpful strategies. The general message is that the best strategies for helping patients are non-confrontational, non-critical, and non-intrusive; do not require self-sacrifice on the relative's part; and focus on positives rather than negatives. In place of arguments, basic house rules about acceptability, with sanctions that can be followed through if rules are broken (such as taking drugs at home), are suggested as an alternative.
- Similarly, not rescuing patients from the consequences of drug/alcohol use (e.g., not covering up for their drunkenness, not doing things they themselves are unable to do because of drugs/alcohol) is stated to be the best policy.
- Making time for oneself is prioritized, while it is emphasized that sacrificing one's own well-being to the problem is unlikely to help anyone in the long term.

One or two educational sessions were dedicated to communicating these ideas to the relatives. The precise content would be determined by the KASI assessment and other information about the relatives' viewpoints. The style of information giving would be as interactive as possible.

As noted earlier, these points of information were viewed as setting the scene for exploring possible ways the family might change their responses to substance misuse. Since many of the ideas were new and did not fit their personal models of construing the substance use, the information alone was not expected to change beliefs or behaviours. Care had to be taken not to give families the impression that there was implicit criticism of their current perspective or behaviour. The commitment and experience of the carers and their enormous contribution to supporting the well-being of the patients were frequently acknowledged. Engagement and then collaboration were key strategies for the intervention. Common problems associated with the substance use identified time and again in the education sessions were as follows:

1. relatives tending to blame patients for making their problems worse through substance misuse
2. relatives underestimating the patient's symptomatology in relation to schizophrenia and tending to attribute all the problems to the substances

3. relatives being reluctant to stand back and leave responsibility for change with clients, feeling that this would be tantamount to condoning substance use.

STRESS MANAGEMENT

While the education sessions offered information, ideas and general advice, the stress management component of the intervention aimed to introduce change and thereby to reduce intrafamilial stress in the household. It focused directly on the situations associated with stress, and it attempted to conduct a cognitive-behavioural assessment of these situations, and from this assessment collaboratively to explore ways of reducing stress. The transactional model of stress was used to conceptualize problems in the household whereby stress was seen as a transaction between the patients' symptoms and behaviours and the relatives' attempts to cope with these problems. Without denying the very real problems relatives often have to deal with—disturbed behaviours, behavioural deficits, and, in this context, problems associated with drugs and alcohol use—the model underlined the importance of the relatives' reactions in determining stress responses: how the relatives construe situations and what they do about them may not only fail to resolve the problem but also serve to maintain or exacerbate it. Examples here in the context of substance misuse in psychosis would be the relatives' attempts to deal with a patient's excessive drinking through verbal persuasion not to drink or through arguments when the patient returns to the house intoxicated. Such attempts to reduce the drinking, although well intended, may fail to have an impact on the drinking, or may, in fact, indirectly increase the patient's motivation to drink where alcohol is used to cope with the patient's stress, or where arguments against drinking increase the patient's resistance to change as suggested by the motivational model. Moreover, given that the relatives' energies are invested in non-productive attempts to change the patient's behaviour, they are likely to become more frustrated, dissatisfied with the patient and stressed themselves in the long term.

In collaborating with family members on how best to deal with stressful situations, it is helpful to look at stress-reduction techniques as having two forms. If we view the difficulties as a transaction between the problem itself and how the relative appraises or responds to it, it follows that there are two possible avenues to reducing the stress response. The first is to ameliorate the problem itself through interventions that would decrease or eradicate the problem behaviour. These might focus mainly on working with the patient through psychological approaches to symptom management, or, in the case of dual diagnosis, through motivational work on substance use. The second avenue is to help the relative to manage negative emotions, thoughts and behaviours associated with or triggered by the patient's problems. Interventions might include reappraising the patient's behaviour, helping relatives to increase the time spent on their own interests, and using anxiety-reduction techniques such as relaxation or challenging negative thoughts. In practice, most interventions involve both problem-based coping and emotion-focused coping, and take into account the particular family situation.

The following case example illustrates some of the issues outlined above.

The patient, Susan, is a woman in her late twenties with a 6-year history of psychosis. There have been frequent hospital admissions, and she has persistent paranoid ideas. Susan's fears make it difficult for her to go out. She has a group of local friends who drink quite heavily and smoke cannabis. She lives with her mother, who, at assessment, believed that her daughter's illness was caused and maintained by drug use. Her mother goes to great lengths to try to find occupation and distraction for her daughter in order to keep her safe at home and away from her friends. As a consequence, the mother's life is very restricted. She has given up her job and has become isolated, not wanting to leave her daughter alone in the house. Despite these sacrifices, the daughter does meet her friends and uses cannabis several times a week, spending all her benefit income on drugs. This is the source of arguments between mother and daughter, and the mother suffers considerable financial hardship since Susan pays nothing towards her keep.

One of the issues targeted in the education sessions was the need for Susan to take sole responsibility for the drug use. In a gentle, non-confrontational manner, the stage-of-change model was used to help the mother see that Susan was only at the beginning of the contemplative (or "thinking") stage. Susan was just beginning to think about some of the negative aspects of cannabis use (such as the costs and fears of long-term health problems), but still, in Susan's eyes, the good things about smoking cannabis outweighed the bad. In other words, Susan was not ready for change. However, the mother's actions assumed that Susan was ready. Hence, her mother was getting very frustrated when her attempts to help Susan not to use drugs met with resistance and did not have any impact on the problem.

In the stress management sessions, her mother was encouraged to reappraise the help she was giving Susan in the light of the stages-of-change model. Through such a guided discovery process, she was helped to see that there were more disadvantages than advantages in maintaining this role of attempting to control the substance use. For example, the surveillance of Susan's behaviour and the arguments did not affect the drug use. The arguments might be increasing Susan's resistance to change. At the same time, there were personal costs for the mother in terms of deterioration in her social life, finances and mood as a consequence of her sacrifices. In joint sessions with Susan, it was agreed that the mother should experiment in leaving Susan alone some days and monitoring the consequences. This required some gentle challenging of the mother's catastrophic beliefs about what might happen if her daughter were left to her own devices, alongside some help in learning how to distract herself from her own anxious thoughts. At the same time, the mother was encouraged to set some clear limits about Susan's behaviours associated with the drug use. Susan agreed not to smoke cannabis in the house, and her mother made it clear that she would not provide Susan with cigarettes or money once she had run out of her benefits money. She also began to ask Susan for a contribution to her keep.

The first stress management session in this intervention was attended by the mother alone. Once the mother's permission was obtained to try out these new strategies, Susan attended and was encouraged to contribute to the planning. As in most similar situations, Susan was fully aware of her mother's stress and hardship, and welcomed the opportunity to attempt to resolve some of the conflict and support her mother. Moreover, the negative impact of increased financial constraints arising from her mother's demands for more money from her helped to increase Susan's ambivalence about her cannabis use. It was important that this was highlighted in subsequent individual sessions with Susan, in which it was attempted to enhance her motivation to reduce substance use.

One of the difficulties encountered in the study was the resistance of family members to reducing the amount of control they perceived themselves to have over the substance use. The way this control was exerted was through methods such as managing patients' money, searching the house for drugs and disposing of any found, expressing dissatisfaction with their drug use, or attempting to keep patients occupied in the hope that they would not feel the need to seek out substances. Although by their own admission the substance use remained problematic, family members had real concerns over what might happen if they released this control. Getting the family to see new ways of coping as "experiments" did facilitate change, which could be reinforced when they found that releasing "control" did not have obvious adverse effects. Moreover, the patients themselves often encouraged these changes, expressed a desire to help the relatives have more time for themselves, and offered reassurance that the controls were unlikely to influence their own substance-using behaviour.

A CONSTRUCTIONAL APPROACH TO PROBLEMS: GOAL SETTING

The chief aim of the goal-setting component in the family intervention is to improve the social functioning of the family members (Barrowclough and Tarrier, 1992). With the format of goal planning and seeing the whole family together, the aim is to teach the family a constructional approach to the problems of family members. This entails seeing problems as needs which might best be met through promoting positive behaviour change. An indirect aim is to reduce family stress by directing their attempts to assist the patient at methods which are constructive and have a high chance of success, hopefully replacing previous unsuccessful attempts which focused on trying to eradicate problem behaviours. In the context of families facing substance misuse in psychosis, this emphasis was very important and helped to counter the feeling that, by suggesting they left responsibility for substance use with the patient, they were being asked to do nothing. It was presented as an opportunity to channel all the carers' efforts to help into plans which might promote positive client behaviours (rather than in fruitless arguments and frustrated attempts to control the substances).

This component was closely linked to individual CBT patient sessions and was a forum for addressing problem areas identified as common to both patients and relatives during the initial problem identification and formulation stage. Additionally, it offered the opportunity for families to assist with patient plans and goals developed in the individual sessions.

The chief assessment tool is a strengths/problems/needs list, which identifies, on the one hand, a person's abilities, interests and resources, and, on the other hand, difficulties, issues or problems (Table 13.1). By combining the individual and the family work, the common problem areas identified were highlighted, and both family members and the patient were encouraged to contribute further items.

In the strengths/needs list shown in Table 13.1, the asterisked items formed part of the original joint problem list, while the other items were elicited through later assessments and discussions. As may be seen from the example, the assessment tries to identify issues that may benefit from co-joint working. The problems are translated into needs that are responses to the question, "If the problem were resolved, what would the person be doing?" Working on the needs of all family members prevents undue "pathologizing" of the patient's problems, and encourages joint working.

Once the list is constructed, the needs are reviewed and rank-ordered by the family in terms of priority and being realistic to achieve in the short term. It is important that all the patient needs are of relevance to patients, or the exercise may be construed as critical of them and one-sided, and be unlikely to achieve change. Relevance may be achieved by restructuring a problem which is a priority to the relative so it has increased patient relevance. For example, Linda was very dissatisfied with Paul's inactivity, while it is the boredom that Paul finds unacceptable; hence, the two may be linked to a common goal. Similarly, while Linda feels that Paul pays too little towards his keep while frittering money away on drink and amphetamines, Paul

Table 13.1 Example of strengths/needs list for a man (Paul) using amphetamines and living with his mother (Linda) and younger brother (Keith)

Strengths	Problems/issues/areas for change	Needs
Paul's interests/abilities: music, driving, TV, books, seeing friends, playing football, cycling, cooking skills, computer skills, enjoys helping others	Linda has a restricted social life	Linda needs to increase social activities away from family
	*Linda tends to do all the domestic chores; Paul would like to be more independent	Linda and Paul need to plan to share some domestic tasks
Linda's interests/abilities: job (nursing), reading, walking, dressmaking, cooking, seeing family	Paul has difficulty in going out alone	Paul needs to increase his confidence in getting out
	*Paul spends a lot of time inactive and is bored	Paul needs to increase his interests and activites
Resources: close, caring family; other relatives want to help; Linda has local friends	*Paul and Linda argue about money	Paul and Linda need to resolve money issues
	Linda and Paul feel Keith misses out on time with the family	Paul and Linda needs to find ways of spending more time with Keith

* These items formed part of the original joint problem list. Other items were elicited through later assessments and discussions.

is upset by the arguments. While, for Linda, the issue is about feeling overburdened with housework when Paul seems to have nothing to do, the issue for Paul is autonomy. Needs are by no means independent, and clear links between needs may be used to advantage: for example, Paul's inactivity might be addressed by his doing things outside the house, or even doing things outside the house while spending more time with his brother.

After identifying the need, the strengths list is scanned for approaches that might be used to meet the need; a goal is specified in clear behavioural terms (and possibly broken down into easily attainable steps); and patients' and relatives' participation in the goal step is reviewed, whether this be an active, facilitating, or passive role, the last being desirable if the relative's response is intrusive or fosters dependency. At further sessions, the goal is reviewed.

A potential problem in the goal-planning sessions was that the family members might easily fall back into the old arguments about drinking and drug use. Hence, it was helpful to raise that potential difficulty at the beginning of sessions, and to encourage agreement that drug and alcohol issues per se would not be discussed (although associated problems such as finances might well be on the agenda).

OUTCOMES AND CONCLUSIONS FROM THE STUDY

The full results of the study have been reported elsewhere (Barrowclough et al, 2001), but there is now good evidence for the efficacy of the combined programme into which the family intervention was integrated. The study demonstrated that an intensive treatment programme incorporating a family intervention resulted in significant improvement in the main outcome of patients' general functioning (General Assessment of Functioning [GAF] scores) when compared with treatment as usual. There were also significant benefits to patients in terms of some secondary outcomes, including a significant reduction in positive symptoms, a reduction in symptom exacerbations, and an increase in days abstinent from drugs and alcohol averaged over the 12-month period. Thus, the advantage of treatment was evident in terms of both symptomatic improvement and a reduction in substance use.

The relatively small sample size is a limitation of the study, and a key issue is the potential generalizability of the findings to other schizophrenia patients with substance use. Certainly, the demographic characteristics of the sample would seem to be in accord with the gender and age biases found in larger studies: substance use in schizophrenia (as in the general population) is more likely to be found in young males. Similarly, as noted earlier, the substance use profile of the study sample matches the type of substance use most prominent among schizophrenia patients. Hence, there is some evidence that our patient group was representative of other schizophrenia sufferers with substance use problems.

Little information is available to indicate what percentage of schizophrenia patients with substance use have contact with families, or whether family contact patients have a different profile of substance use from those without. Our clinical observations suggested that the levels of substance use may be lower in patients living with or in close contact with relatives. This may arise when relatives control substance use in the ways we have described. Although this control may have short-term benefits in terms of less substances consumed, the situation may inadvertently contribute to decreasing the patient's readiness to change, simply because the negative consequences of substance consumption are limited or buffered by the well-meaning attempts of the family to protect the patient from the harmful effects of increased use. Certainly, feelings of frustration over failed attempts to persuade the patient to change were very prevalent among family members. Carer assessments indicated that there were high levels of stress in the households. This suggested not only that carer well-being was compromised by the "double burden" of schizophrenia and substance use, but also that an adverse social environment was a contributory factor to symptom exacerbations in the patients.

The study reported here has demonstrated that it is possible to improve the illness course and reduce substance use in SMP clients through a multi-component psychological and psychosocial intervention. Although the indications are that such multifaceted treatments may be required to have an effective impact on the complex and challenging problems of this client group, longer-term research is needed to examine the relative efficacy of different components of integrated interventions. Further studies are also required to examine the long-term outcomes and cost benefits of such treatment programmes.

ACKNOWLEDGEMENTS

This work was supported by the West Pennine, Manchester and Stockport health authorities; Tameside and Glossop NHS Trust R & D Support funds; and Making Space, the organization for supporting carers and sufferers of mental illness. The author acknowledges the contributions of the research team and the therapists involved in the trial described here, including Gillian Haddock, Nicholas Tarrier, Shôn Lewis, Jan Moring, Rob O'Brien, Nichola Schofield, John McGovern, and Ian Lowens.

REFERENCES

Alterman, A.I., Erdlen, F.R., McLellan, A.T. and Mann, S.C. (1980) Problem drinking in hospitalised schizophrenic patients. *Addictive Behaviour*, 5: 273–276.

Barrowclough, C. and Tarrier, N. (1992) *Families of Schizophrenic Patients: Cognitive Behavioural Intervention*. London, Chapman & Hall.

Barrowclough, C., Tarrier, N. and Johnston, M. (1994) Attributions, expressed emotion and patient relapse: an attributional model of relatives' response to schizophrenic illness. *Behaviour Therapy*, 25: 67–88.

Barrowclough, C., Tarrier, N. and Johnston, M. (1996) Distress, expressed emotion and attributions in relatives of schizophrenic patients. *Schizophrenia Bulletin*, 22: 691–701.

Barrowclough, C., Haddock, G., Tarrier, N., Lewis, S., Moring, J., O'Brien, R., Schofield, N. and McGovern, J. (2001) Randomised controlled trial of motivational interviewing and cognitive behavioural intervention for schizophrenia patients with associated drug or alcohol misuse. *American Journal of Psychiatry*, 158: 1706–1713.

Barrowclough, C., Haddock, G., Tarrier, N., Moring, J., Lewis, S. (2000) Cognitive behavioural intervention for individuals with severe mental illness who have a substance misuse problem. *Psychiatric Rehabilitation Skills*, 4: 216–233.

Blanchard J.J., Brown S.A., Horan W.A. and Sherwood A.R. (2000) Substance use disorders in schizophrenia: review, integration and a proposed model. *Clinical Psychology Review*, **20**: 207–234.

Brewin, C.R., MacCarthy, B., Duda, K. and Vaughn, C.E. (1991) Attributions and expressed emotion in the relatives of patients with schizophrenia. *Journal of Abnormal Psychology*, **100**: 546–554.

Butzlaff, R.I. and Hooley, J.M. (1998) Expressed emotion and psychiatric relapse: a meta-analysis. *Archives of General Psychiatry*, **55**: 547–552.

Dixon, L., McNary, S., and Lehman, A. (1995) Substance abuse and family relationships of persons with severe mental illness. *American Journal of Psychiatry*, **152**: 456–458.

Goldberg, D. and Williams, P.A. (1988) *A Users' Guide to the General Health Questionnaire*. Windsor, NFER-Nelson.

Haddock, G., Barrowclough, C. and Moring, J. (2002) Cognitive behaviour therapy for patients with co-existing psychosis and substance use problems. In Morrison, A.P. (Ed.), *A Casebook of Cognitive Therapy for Psychosis*. Hove, Brunner-Routledge.

Kashner, T.M., Rader, L.E., Rodell, D.E., Beck, C.M., Rodell, L.R. and Muller, K. (1991) Family characteristics, substance abuse, and hospitalisation patterns of patients with schizophrenia. *Hospital and Community Psychiatry*, **42**, 195–197.

Lopez, S.R., Nelson, K.A., Snyder, K.S. and Minz, J. (1999) Attributions and affective reactions of family members and course of schizophrenia. *Journal of Abnormal Psychology*, **108**: 307–314.

Mari, J. and Streiner, D.L. (1997) Family intervention for those with schizophrenia. In C. Adams, J. Anderson, De Jesus J. Mari (Eds), *Schizophrenia Module of the Cochrane Database of Systematic Reviews*. Available in the Cochrane Library, the Cochrane Collaboration, Issue 3. Oxford: Update Software. London, BMJ Publishing Group.

McConnaughy, E.A., Prochaska, J.O. and Velicer, W.F. (1983) Stages of change in psychotherapy: measurement and sample profiles. *Psychotherapy: Theory, Research and Practice*, **20**: 368–375.

Miller, W.R. and Rollnick, S. (1991) *Motivational Interviewing: Preparing People to Change Addictive Behaviour*. New York, Guilford Press.

Mueser, K.T., Yarnold, P.R., Levinson, D.F., Singh, H., Bellack, A.S., Kee, K., Morrison, A.L. and Yaddalam, K.G. (1990) Prevalence of substance abuse in schizophrenia: demographic and clinical correlates. *Schizophrenia Bulletin*, **16**, 31–56.

Mueser, K.T. and Gingerich, S. (1994) Alcohol and drug abuse. In *Coping with Schizophrenia: A Guide for Families*. Oakland, New Harbinger Publications.

Prochaska, J.O. and DiClemente, C.C. (1986) Towards a comprehensive model of change. In W.R. Miller and N. Heather (Eds), *Treating Addictive Behaviours: Processes of Change*. New York, Plenum.

Sciacca, K. and Hatfield, A.B. (1995) The family and the dually diagnosed patient. In A.F. Lehman and L.B. Dixon (Eds), *Double Jeopardy: Chronic Mental Illness and Substance Use Disorders*. New York, Harwood Academic Publishers.

Smith, J. and Birchwood, M. (1987) Education for families with schizophrenic relatives. *British Journal of Psychiatry*, **150**: 645–652.

Smith, J. and Hucker, S. (1994): Schizophrenia and substance abuse. *British Journal of Psychiatry*, **165**: 13–21.

Turner, S.M. (1998) Comments on expressed emotion and the development of new treatments for substance abuse. *Behaviour Therapy*, **29**, 647–654.

Vaughn, C.E. and Leff, J.P. (1976) The measurement of expressed emotion in the families of psychiatric patients. *British Journal of Social and Clinical Psychology*, **129**: 125–137.

Chapter 14

START OVER AND SURVIVE: A BRIEF INTERVENTION FOR SUBSTANCE MISUSE IN EARLY PSYCHOSIS

David J. Kavanagh, Ross Young, Angela White, John B. Saunders, Natalie Shockley, Jeff Wallis and Anne Clair

Over the last decade, brief intervention for alcohol problems has become a well-validated and accepted treatment, with brief interventions frequently showing equivalence in terms of outcome to more extended treatments (Bien et al, 1993). A recent review of these studies found that heavy drinkers who received interventions of less than 1 h were almost twice as likely to moderate their drinking over the following 6–12 months as did those not receiving intervention (Wilk et al, 1997). Some studies have used motivational interviewing (MI) strategies (Monti et al, 1999); others have simply given information and advice to reduce drinking (Fleming et al, 1997). Leaflets or information on strategies to assist in the attempt or follow-up sessions are sometimes provided (Fleming et al, 1997). In general practice research, provision of one or more follow-up sessions increases the reliability of intake reductions across studies (Poikolainen, 1999).

After a review of the existing research (Kavanagh, 1995), we initially designed a 6-month intervention for substance misuse in psychosis (Substance Treatment Options for Psychosis [STOP]; Kavanagh et al, 1998), and applied it to 10 patients. The intervention began during inpatient treatment for an acute episode, and involved the components described in Table 14.1. It strongly emphasized engagement, distinguishing initial engagement in sessions and establishment of a therapeutic alliance from collaborative development of substance use goals. MI strategies

Substance Misuse in Psychosis: Approaches to Treatment and Service Delivery.
Edited by Hermine L. Graham, Alex Copello, Max J. Birchwood and Kim T. Mueser.
© 2003 John Wiley & Sons, Ltd.

Table 14.1   Components of Substance
Treatment Options in Psychosis (STOP)

Engagement in sessions
Information about substances and symptoms
Development of a substance intake goal
Reduction of exposure to high-risk situations
Reduction of sequelae from symptoms
Development of alternate activities
Cognitive therapy for substance expectancies
Applied relaxation
Assertive substance refusal
Impulse control
Relapse prevention

(Miller and Rollnick, 1991) were used to enhance motivation to change substance use. Once an attempt to modify use was planned, the intervention focused on strategies to maximize the likelihood of successful control of both the substance use and psychiatric symptoms. Participants had an average of 11 sessions over 17 weeks.

The most striking finding from our STOP intervention was the high degree of variability in the responses of individual patients. Where the psychosis or substance use had produced significant cognitive deficit, there was little treatment progress (cf. Green, 1996). Not only was there little retention from previous sessions but also working memory was so poor that MI was very difficult (even with the extensive use of written summaries and visual aids). In contrast, we were surprised to find that others undertook sustained reductions in consumption of some substances after very brief discussion about its effects on their psychotic symptoms. These patients were at an early episode, and were using at levels that were similar to their social group. Overall, two of the 10 single cases were substantially improved at 6 months and a further five had variable improvement (improving on some substances only, or having periods of control and of uncontrolled use). These results led us to have some confidence that a brief motivational intervention might be effective in changing substance use by at least some people with psychosis.

Our interest in relatively brief intervention also stemmed from our investigation of current practices in managing the combination of mental health and substance misuse in the health services across our state (Kavanagh et al, 2000). We surveyed 380 staff from mental health services and 112 from alcohol and drug services in urban and regional settings, some of which were in remote and sparsely populated areas. A range of needs for increased facilities and services for people with substance misuse and mental disorders was reported, and significant problems in coordinating care across the services were identified. Staff of each service said that limited access to training and consultation in the area covered by the other service was a significant problem for their management of this population.

A separation between alcohol and drug services and mental health services has long been known to be a significant problem for the management of their co-occurrence (Ridgely et al, 1990). The essence of the problem is a need to develop an integrated approach to the two closely interrelated problems (Minkoff, 1989)—a need that cannot fully be met with parallel treatment. Current evidence on treating the combination of substance misuse and psychosis (SMP) clearly supports the view that integrated treatment by a single therapist has more favourable outcomes than parallel or sequential treatment (Drake et al, 1998).

In the short term, there seems little chance of organizational change to create a single integrated service. Furthermore, the high rate of substance misuse in treated populations (Mueser et al, 1990) suggests that the development of some small specialist teams will be grossly insufficient to address the problem alone. Training and supporting staff in the existing mental health services to address SMP appears critical to successful integration of its management into standard care, and specialist staff probably are most appropriately used as consultant supervisors (Kaner et al, 1999). Since staff of mental health services are more likely to have the primary management responsibility for people with psychosis, they will usually be delivering the intervention. The extent of additional time the intervention requires is likely to be a significant barrier to its use (Kavanagh et al, 1993), given high caseloads and other demands on time. A wider range of new skills and greater level of required expertise also represent significant challenges for dissemination, and substantially increase the amount of training and supervision that is required (Kavanagh, 1994; Kavanagh et al, 1993). However, a brief motivational intervention is likely to be easily integrated in routine clinical practice, and involves relatively circumscribed skills that have wide clinical application. Wide dissemination of training in screening for substance use and conducting brief interventions would also promote a greater awareness of the issue by mental health staff and would offer an intake route to more extensive intervention.

Our focus on brief intervention in early psychosis was only partly based on our clinical observations of greater benefit in this population. Substance misuse in people with psychosis is predicted by the same characteristics as in the general population, with young men being most likely to show these problems (Mueser et al, 2000). Early stages of psychosis therefore coincide with the period of greatest risk of substance misuse. Intervention in early psychosis appears to be critical to the prevention of long-term problems (McGorry et al, 1996). The first episodes present opportunities to retain family support, social networks, and educational and vocational opportunities, and to prevent recurrences of symptoms (Kavanagh and Mueser, 2001). The potential impact of interventions for people with SMP may be even greater than for those without substance misuse. Apart from an earlier age of onset, patients with SMP have initially better prognostic indicators on average than those without substance misuse (Andreasson and Allebeck, 1989; Arndt et al, 1992). However substance misuse significantly decreases the chance of full recovery from an initial psychotic episode, and produces poorer symptomatic and functional outcomes in the longer term than are seen in people without substance-related problems (Drake and Brunette, 1998). An early intervention for this group therefore has potential to affect subsequent outcomes significantly.

START OVER AND SURVIVE! (SOS)

Based on these considerations, we developed a relatively brief intervention that was appropriate for people with early psychosis and applicable to routine clinical practice. The approach was based on the STOP intervention, but reduced its duration and the number of components that participants received. The treatment was manualized for administration in controlled trials (Kavanagh et al, 1999b).

As in the STOP treatment, SOS was designed so that it could be started during an inpatient stay for acute exacerbation of psychotic symptoms, and delivered by primary mental health case workers in the unit as part of their total management of SMP. While this timing may not be critical to the success of the intervention, it does have some advantages. For example, it facilitates engagement in initial sessions at a stage where the person may not otherwise attend appointments, and it allows brief contacts at frequent intervals. For many participants, the inpatient stay provides a vivid example of the problems that are produced by their substance use (Walitzere et al, 1999). These advantages appear to outweigh the difficulties that acute symptoms produce for development of rapport and maintaining attention during sessions.

Like STOP, SOS emphasizes motivation enhancement (Miller and Rollnick, 1991), which has been shown to improve treatment adherence by patients with depression and cocaine dependence (Daley et al, 1998). The relatively gentle nature of this approach is likely to make it especially applicable to inpatients with an exacerbation of psychosis, who may respond to a strongly confrontative approach with confusion and distress. Clinical trials of psychological therapies for SMP that have not employed these strategies have not resulted in strong clinical outcomes (Hellerstein et al, 1995; Lehman

Table 14.2   Components of Start Over and Survive! (SOS)

Phase 1: Rapport building
Phase 2: Motivational interviewing
Phase 3: Planning for substance control
  • Contracting for start of the control attempt
  • Identification and problem solving high-risk situations
    in the short term
  • Acquisition of one skill (drug refusal or coping with symptoms)
Phase 4: Encouraging maintenance

et al, 1993). Uncontrolled studies suggest that approaches incorporating motivational components have more promise (Addington and el Guebaly, 1998; Drake et al, 1998; Kavanagh et al, 1998).

The SOS intervention is only brief in a relative sense, in that the first three phases of the intervention consist of 3 h of individual treatment (or 6–9 sessions) plus a 1-h session with relatives. Follow-up contact over the next 4 weeks totals about another 30 min. This duration is not brief in the same sense as a single 5–20-min session to advise a reduction in alcohol use (Bien et al, 1993), but it is brief in terms of typical durations of treatment for SMP (Drake et al, 1998). The frequency of the inpatient sessions is modified according to the mental state of the participant and the plan for discharge, with the full intervention normally being completed within 7–10 days. If a participant is discharged before the completion of SOS, the intervention is continued on an outpatient basis.

Components of SOS are displayed in Table 14.2. Phase 1, or rapport building, begins as soon as possible after admission and consists of 2–4 very brief contacts (2–10 min). These brief conversations aim to build rapport and engagement in discussions, and involve conversations with participants about their past and present interests and activities. In many cases, these discussions provide a basis for later discussions about the relationship of substance use to other goals, and sometimes they elicit pleasurable activities that may present an alternative to substance use. This phase continues until symptoms are stabilizing sufficiently for a more extended conversation and some rapport has been established. Further assessment of symptoms and substance use is then undertaken.

Phase 2 is delivered in sessions of 20–30 min, and involves motivational interviews (after Miller and Rollnick, 1991) that aim to facilitate participants' understanding of the current benefits and costs of their substance use, develop concern, and elicit commitment to change the nature and/or extent of their consumption. The style of interviewing is directive, but empathic and accepting. There is no attempt to confront the participant directly: instead, therapists join participants in a collaborative examination of the functionality of the substance use and its match with other beliefs and priorities. Information about substance effects is given in answer to questions or in response to expressed beliefs, and participants are encouraged to test overly positive expectations about the substances. Dissonance between life goals and outcomes of substance use, and between positive aspects of their self-image and themselves as a substance users are elicited, with monitoring to ensure that this does not produce high levels of distress. Self-efficacy about attempting substance control is fostered by eliciting memories of past successes in self-control and in other performance domains. The intervention continues at this phase until the participants decide to change the mode or extent of their substance use or 3 h is reached, and returns to this phase if motivation flags. While we typically advise abstinence from the problematic substances (Drake and Wallach, 1993), the goal that is selected by the participant is adopted as an initial starting point (abstinence, moderated use, or harm minimization from current use). This flexibility recognizes the positivity of any attempted change, and allows continuance of the therapeutic alliance.

Phase 3 usually involves two sessions of 20–45 min, and involves planning for substance control after discharge. The primary focus is on identifying and dealing with difficult situations for substance control that are expected to emerge in the month after discharge. Participants apply problem solving to minimize exposure to the situation and identify ways to avoid inappropriate substance use if the situation cannot be avoided (cf. Marlatt and Gordon, 1985). One of two specific skills are focused on, depending on the issue that participants see as most important in the early period after discharge. These are substance refusal and strategies to deal with symptoms without substance use.

Substance refusal has been incorporated in a number of other more extensive treatment approaches (Bellack and DiClemente, 1999), and skill deficits in this area do seem to be particularly important in early psychosis, when substance use is often within a social setting. A social skills approach is used (Liberman et al, 1986; Wallace and Liberman, 1985), in which the problem is discussed, the skill is modelled, and enactive practice with feedback follows. Symptom control often focuses on control of dysphoria, since this is the type of symptom that appears to be most strongly associated with substance use for self-medication (Mueser et al, 1998). Dysphoria also impedes the optimal application of skills by reducing motivation and impairing self-efficacy, presumably because of selective recall of negative performance and outcome information (Kavanagh, 1987, 1992; Kavanagh and Bower, 1985). Increasing pleasurable activities that are inconsistent with substance use can address both the dysphoria and the substance use (Azrin, 1976; Lewinsohn and Graf, 1973). The training of both substance refusal and relief of symptoms involves working through material in leaflets that includes an individualized application of the skill that is relevant to the likely challenges over the following 4 weeks. The skills training is intended to be introductory only, and to provide a basis for later relevant work in the community.

During this phase, we also ask participants to develop a safety plan in case their strategy for control of their substance use and symptoms runs into problems. While we attempt to convey confidence in their ability to maintain control, we discuss the fact that lapses can occur. We assist them to identify danger signals for incipient episodes (Birchwood, 1992), and to define a lapse in their substance use. An individualized plan is developed for these situations and is written on a leaflet that clients retain.

In cases where family members are in regular contact with the participant, they typically are extremely distressed, and sometimes are considering withdrawing support. SOS does not include a full family intervention, but all families are offered a single session during phases 2 or 3 in which relatives discuss the participant's problems and how they have coped with them. The history of both problems is articulated, and their interrelationship clarified. Family members are offered written information about psychosis, substance use and psychosis, how to obtain help from the health system, support services for families, and how family members can help with psychosis and substance use. Participants are not present at this session, because of their vulnerable mental state and the high degree of distress and anger that is frequently expressed. They are briefed about the session before and afterwards. A primary focus of the session is on how relatives might deal with future challenges, both the patient's problems and their own emotional reactions to the situation. In cases where relatives blame the participant for the psychotic episode or for associated behaviour, the therapist attempts to develop empathy for the participant and encourages family members to reattribute causation of problems to biochemical processes, external influences and skills deficits rather than to person variables. Likely motivations for the substance use, and similarities with their own motivations are elicited. If necessary, MI is applied to develop commitment to support participants in their attempt to address their problems.

Phase 4 of the intervention focuses particularly on the first 4 weeks after discharge, which encompasses the early phases of a substance control attempt, and represents a period when the participant is especially vulnerable to reversion to substance use. Unless there is full integration of inpatient and community staffing, it is also a period in which a therapeutic alliance is being re-established, and it may be a time when participants are awaiting contact by their case worker. We propose that the staff member who provided SOS on the ward should provide brief support by telephone over this period to ensure a smooth transition to community management of the psychosis and substance misuse. However, it is intended that ongoing support for substance control, problem solution and re-engagement after lapses will be provided in the context of later case management and follow-up assessments.

Phase 4 consists of 5–10-min weekly contacts with participants that may be in person or by telephone, together with brief telephone calls every 2 weeks to a carer where relevant. Contact with participants assesses their substance use, reinforces their motivation to stay in control of substance use and reviews the strategies discussed in the face-to-face sessions. It encourages them to predict difficult situations they may encounter in the following week, and develop a plan to address them. Telephone contact with carers aims to confirm participants' reports of substance use, and prompts carers to continue using functional coping strategies, to apply problem solving to challenging situations and to locate community assistance where required.

CURRENT PRACTICE

At present, the SOS intervention is being trialled in a series of outcome studies, prior to full implementation within the health service. Unfortunately, this means that SOS is not currently fully integrated with the overall mental health treatment being received by the patient, since the research staff do not currently have a full case management role by the service. A second therapist is therefore also involved in the mental health treatment. We attempt to minimize the negative effects of this "parallel" aspect to our current implementation, by;

1. involving the primary mental health worker in at least some of the sessions
2. having frequent discussions with case workers, both on the ward and in subsequent community management, requesting their support and continued implementation of the strategies
3. maintaining notes on the patient file regarding our contacts
4. attending discharge planning and case review sessions

At the next stage of implementation, we will train existing staff in the service to implement the SOS intervention in a fully integrated manner with other treatments.

CASE EXAMPLES

Two recent examples of the application of SOS to people we will call Pete and Brendan illustrate how the intervention is applied to specific problems.

At baseline, Pete, a 24-year-old single man living with his parents, became involved in the SOS programme during his second admission for schizophrenia. He met Composite International Diagnostic Interview (CIDI) criteria for alcohol abuse/dependence and cannabis abuse/dependence. Alcohol and drug screening on the DrugCheck (Kavanagh et al, 1999a) indicated moderate nicotine use, moderately high caffeine consumption (2 l Coca-Cola/day), daily use of cannabis (about two "cones"/day) up to 1 oz per week, and binge drinking every 2 weeks (total score of 20 on AUDIT).

Pete reported significant problems resulting from his alcohol use, including legal, interpersonal, psychological and emotional difficulties (total problem list score of 15). Of particular concern to Pete and his family were the impulsive, inappropriate, and at times aggressive behaviours that resulted from his binge drinking.

Pete completed the SOS programme over five sessions while in hospital. Although assessment indicated both cannabis and alcohol as being significant problem drugs for Pete, he felt that alcohol was causing him more difficulties. After building rapport, sessions focused on MI for alcohol use. Pete chose to work on reducing his alcohol consumption. Subsequent sessions targetted problem solving, with a focus on coping with symptoms and developing substance refusal skills. Initial follow-up calls indicated that Paul was not experiencing difficulties in cutting down his alcohol immediately after discharge. At 6 weeks and 3 months, Pete was using cannabis every 2 weeks, at a greatly reduced level compared with baseline (two "cones" per 2 weeks versus two "cones" per day at baseline), and reported no alcohol consumption at all since the previous assessment. Pete reported that he now considered his cannabis and nicotine use to be problematic.

At 6 months, Pete's cannabis use had decreased to one "cone" every 3–4 months. He reported experiencing one lapse with alcohol, during which he consumed approximately 36 standard drinks in a 12-h period, and experienced some alcohol-related problems at this time. Pete described an ongoing battle with cravings for alcohol; however, his readiness and confidence to maintain his reduced alcohol intake remained high. By this stage, Pete was no longer receiving any mental health follow-up.

At 24 months, Pete's pattern of greatly reduced substance use was well maintained. He stated that he had had one episode of cannabis use at a party (one "cone") during the previous year, and was now drinking monthly or less at occasional social events where he would consume approximately 5–6 standard drinks. Pete indicated that there had been no problems from his alcohol use. In addition, Pete reported an absence of mental health symptoms, and no hospital admissions. Collateral data obtained from his parents throughout the follow-up period were consistent with Pete's self-reported information. At 24 months, his parents reported that they felt that his alcohol and cannabis use was no longer of concern. Pete reported that he would now like to address his cigarette smoking, which had risen from 20 per day at baseline to 40 per day (12 mg) at 2 years.

A second case, conducted since the SOS study mentioned below, illustrates how the effects in some cases are less clear-cut. Brendan, a 21-year-old, single, apprentice painter, was admitted to hospital with his first acute psychotic episode, with symptoms of disorientation, social withdrawal, bizarre delusional beliefs (such as being responsible for the suicide of a rock star), blunted affect and thought disorder. The admission was preceded by heavy cannabis use and job instability. The differential diagnoses were schizophreniform psychosis, drug-induced psychosis, and psychotic depression, with suspected schizoid traits. Screening with the DrugCheck revealed moderate daily use of caffeine and nicotine; alcohol use 2–4 times/week plus twice a month binges of unknown quantity, during which he would become "very drunk"; and daily cannabis use of about three "cones" per day (up to 1 oz per week).

Brendan completed 3.5 h of therapy over six sessions of 20–60 min during a 10-day admission. He was initially keen to cease cannabis use, as he felt it had caused him significant financial, interpersonal, psychological and emotional problems. He was not as interested in reducing alcohol use, despite describing a number of potentially problematic situations that had occurred while he was quite intoxicated. After approximately 20 min of rapport building, MI focused primarily on the immediate and long-term issues raised by using cannabis and on the potential difficulties of remaining abstinent. After about 1.75 h of MI, Brendan contracted to attempt abstinence from cannabis for 6 months, after which he would review this decision. Brendan anticipated some difficulty in abstaining from cannabis because of the enjoyment it gave him. On several occasions subsequently, Brendan's motivation to change his cannabis use wavered, as did his insight into its effects on his mental health. At these times, aspects of MI were readministered.

In the remaining 90 min of the intervention, Brendan planned how he would deal with anticipated high-risk situations after discharge (boredom, social situations including his birthday, cravings, and feelings of paranoia). During the sessions, ways of coping with his symptoms and managing lapses in substance use or symptom control were discussed. The therapist explained that Brendan could use the same skills with managing alcohol use. Psychoeducational sessions were conducted by another therapist with Brendan's father, who was encouraged to provide support and structure to assist Brendan to stop his cannabis use.

Brendan remained abstinent for the first 1.5 weeks after discharge (apart from two "cones" on the day of discharge). He then decided to "try just one 'cone'/day to see how he went", and this began a pattern of lapses alternating with periods of abstinence. Overall, he has been abstinent for about 50% of the first 2 months after discharge, and his cannabis intake has been substantially below baseline levels. Mild symptoms of thought disorder and disorganized behaviour persisted. Periods of renewed abstinence followed telephone calls by the therapist in which substance use was assessed and problem solving applied. The initial outcome for this person has therefore been unstable, despite the fact that he was at his first episode when he entered the study.

OUTCOME STUDIES ON THE APPROACH

An initial pilot study examined whether the effects of SOS were superior to those of standard care by the mental health service. It is described more fully in a separate paper (Kavanagh et al, submitted). The participants were 25 inpatients aged 16–40 years who had a consensus diagnosis of any DSM-IV psychosis (including substance-induced psychosis), were in the first 3 years of first diagnosis with psychotic disorder, and were at their first to third episode. They also had to be able to converse in English without an interpreter and not suffer from either developmental disability or amnestic disorder. All of these patients had screened positive for substance-related problems on the DrugCheck (Kavanagh et al, 1999a), and fulfilled criteria for abuse or dependence on one or more substances on the CIDI (World Health Organization, 1997). Exclusion criteria were the receipt of other concurrent treatment for substance misuse and use of heroin more than once a month. The latter criterion was initially an exclusion of people who regularly used any intravenous drug, but was modified part way through the study because of a very high incidence of intravenous amphetamine use. The exclusion of regular heroin use was retained/applied because of the probable need for other intervention within that group. Sampling was undertaken at three Brisbane hospitals, and random allocation to conditions was undertaken separately within each hospital.

In Standard Care (SC), no specific recommendations for treatment were given. The SOS intervention was conducted as described. At 6 weeks, and at 3, 6 and 12 months after discharge, participants were contacted for assessment of their substance use. The final assessment was undertaken by assessors who were blind to treatment group.

Twenty-five participants (13 SOS, 12 SC) participated in the trial, and all but one SC participant were assessed to 6 months. We were able to follow up 11 SOS and 6 SC participants to 12 months, a fact which in itself reflects the greater degree of rapport we were able to retain with SOS. Five participants in SOS (38%) did not proceed beyond initial rapport building. Outcomes of the trial are therefore described in terms of "treated" subjects (including only SOS participants receiving some MI) and "intention to treat" (including all allocated participants). The primary outcome was a blind assessment using all available data, of abstinence or substantial improvement on all substances, versus a lack of improvement on at least one. Improvement required either no problems from ongoing substance use, or at least a 50% reduction of intake in relation to baseline levels, together with a substantial reduction in attendant problems. A negative outcome was substituted for missing data.

There was no significant difference between the groups on substance use at 6 weeks or 3 months. At 6 months, the treated SOS participants had significantly better outcomes than the SC, and this effect was maintained at 12 months. All of the treated SOS participants showed improvement at the 6-month assessment, compared with 58% of those in SC. At 12 months, only one treated SOS participant that we assessed showed a lack of improvement over baseline levels, compared with half of the assessed people in the SC. We were therefore able to demonstrate good maintenance of the results in the treated sample. In this small sample, the outcomes would not reach significance at any stage if an intention to treat analysis were used.

These results were therefore encouraging, especially given the fact that most of the intervention was conducted during an acute psychotic episode. However, they illustrated that the challenge of initial engagement had not been fully solved, given that 38% did not proceed as far as MI.

A second and larger outcome trial is currently under way. In this study, we are comparing the SOS intervention with a nonspecific supportive intervention that effectively stops at the rapport-building stage. We also test whether the impact of the SOS intervention is indeed better in early psychosis, by including anyone with psychosis in the sample. If we continue to obtain positive results from the intervetion, we plan to examine the impact of dissemination into routine mental health care.

CONCLUSION

Brief interventions are known to be effective in the general population in samples with hazardous or harmful alcohol use. There is now some evidence that they might be of some benefit in early psychosis. Our SOS intervention appears promising as a first-line treatment that is compatible with the caseload demands of mental health staff and may be particularly applicable to people with early psychosis. We are confident that a full-scale controlled trial will confirm the utility of SOS, and that it will be readily disseminated throughout mental health services.

REFERENCES

Addington, J. and el Guebaly, N. (1998) Group treatment for substance abuse in schizophrenia. *Canadian Journal of Psychiatry*, **43**: 843–845.

Andreasson, P. and Allebeck, U. (1989) Schizophrenia in users and nonusers of cannabis. *Acta Psychiatrica Scandinavica*, **79**: 505–510.

Arndt, S., Tyrrell, G., Flaum, M. and Andreasen, N.C. (1992) Comorbidity of substance abuse and schizophrenia: the role of premorbid adjustment. *Psychological Medicine*, **22**: 379–388.

Azrin, N.H. (1976) Improvements in the community reinforcement approach to alcoholism. *Behaviour Research and Therapy*, **14**: 339–348.

Bellack, A.S. and DiClemente, C.C. (1999) Treating substance abuse among patients with schizophrenia. *Psychiatric Services*, **50**: 75–80.

Bien, T.H., Miller, W.R. and Tonigan, J.S. (1993) Brief interventions for alcohol problems: a review. *Addiction*, **88**: 315–335.

Birchwood, M. (1992) Early intervention in schizophrenia: theoretical background and clinical strategies. *British Journal of Clinical Psychology*, **31**: 257–278.

Daley, D., Salloum, I., Zuckoff, A., Kirisci, L. and Thase, M. (1998) Increasing treatment adherence among outpatients with depression and cocaine dependence: results of a pilot study. *American Journal of Psychiatry*, **155**: 1611–1613.

Drake, R.E. and Brunette, M.F. (1998) Complications of severe mental illness related to alcohol and other drug use disorders. In M. Galanter (Ed.), *Recent Developments in Alcoholism*, pp. 285–299. New York, Plenum.

Drake, R.E., Mercer-McFadden, C., Mueser, K.T., McHugo, G.J. and Bond, G.R. (1998) Review of integrated mental health and substance abuse treatment for patients with dual disorders. *Schizophrenia Bulletin*, **24**: 589–608.

Drake, R.E. and Wallach, M.A. (1993) Moderate drinking among people with severe mental illness. *Hospital and Community Psychiatry*, **44**: 780–782.

Fleming, M.F., Barry, K.L., Manwell, L.B., Johnson, K. and London, R. (1997) Brief physician advice for problem alcohol drinkers. A randomized controlled trial in community-based primary care practices. *Journal of the American Medical Association*, **277**: 1039–1045.

Green, M. (1996) What are the functional consequences of neurocognitive deficits in schizophrenia? *American Journal of Psychiatry*, **153**: 321–330.

Hellerstein, D.J., Rosenthal, R.N. and Miner, C.R. (1995) A prospective study of integrated outpatient treatment for substance-abusing schizophrenic patients. *American Journal on the Addictions*, **4**: 33–42.

Kaner, E.F., Lock, C.A., McAvoy, B.R., Heather, N. and Gilvarry, E. (1999) ARCT of three training and support strategies to encourage implementation of screening and brief alcohol intervention by general practitioners. *British Journal of General Practice*, **49**: 699–703.

Kavanagh, D.J. (1987) Mood, persistence and success. *Australian Journal of Psychology*, **39**: 307–318.

Kavanagh, D.J. (1992) Self-efficacy and depression. In R. Schwartzer (Ed.), *Self-Efficacy: Thought Control of Action*, pp. 177–193. New York, Hemisphere.

Kavanagh, D.J. (1994) Issues in multidisciplinary training of cognitive-behavioural interventions. *Behaviour Change*, **11**: 38–44.

Kavanagh, D.J. (1995) An intervention for substance abuse in schizophrenia. *Behaviour Change*, **12**: 20–30.

Kavanagh, D.J. and Bower, G.H. (1985) Mood and self-efficacy: impact of joy and sadness on perceived capabilities. *Cognitive Therapy and Research*, **9**: 507–525.

Kavanagh, D.J., Greenaway, L., Jenner, L., Saunders, J., White, A., Sorban, J., Hamilton, G. and the Dual Diagnosis Consortium (2000) Contrasting views and experiences of health professionals on the management of comorbid substance abuse and mental disorders. *Australian and New Zealand Journal of Psychiatry*, **34**: 279–289.

Kavanagh, D.J. and Mueser, K.T. (2001) The future of cognitive and behavioral therapies in early psychosis. *Behavior Therapy*, **32**: 693–724.

Kavanagh, D.J., Piatkowska, O., Clark, D., O'Halloran, P., Manicavasagar, R., Rosen, A. and Tennant, C. (1993) Application of a cognitive-behavioural family intervention for schizophrenia ini multi-disciplinary settings: what can the matter be? *Australian Psychologist*, **28**: 181–188.

Kavanagh, D.J., Saunders, J.B., Young, R., White, A., Jenner, L., Clair, A. and Wallis, J. (1999a) *Evaluation of Screening and Brief Intervention for Substance Abuse in Early Psychosis. A Report to Auseinet.* Adelaide, SA, Flinders University.

Kavanagh, D.J., Young, R., Boyce, L., Clair, A., Sitharthan, T., Clark, D. and Thompson, K. (1998) Substance treatment options in psychosis (STOP): a new intervention for dual diagnosis. *Journal of Mental Health*, **7**: 135–143.

Kavanagh, D.J., Young, R., White, A., Saunders, J., Jenner, L., Clair, A. and Wallis, G. (1999b) *Start Over and Survive (SOS) Treatment Manual.* Brisbane, University of Queensland.

Kavanagh, D.J., Young, R., White, A., Saunders, J.B., Wallis, G., Shockley, N., Jenner, L. and Clair, A. (submitted, 2002) Brief intervention for substance misuse in early psychosis.

Lehman, A.F., Herron, J.D., Schwartz, R.P. and Myers, C.P. (1993) Rehabilitation for young adults with severe mental illness and substance use disorders: a clinical trial. *Journal of Nervous and Mental Disease*, **181**: 86–90.

Lewinsohn, P.M. and Graf, M. (1973) Pleasant activities and depression. *Journal of Consulting and Clinical Psychology*, **41**: 261–268.

Liberman, R.P., Mueser, K.T. and Wallace, C.J. (1986) Social skills training for schizophrenic individuals at risk for relapse. *American Journal of Psychiatry*, **143**: 523–526.

Marlatt, G.A. and Gordon, J.R. (1985) *Relapse Prevention.* New York, Guilford Press.

McGorry, P.D., Edwards, J., Mihalopoulos, C., Harrigan, S.M. and Jackson, H.J. (1996) EPPIC: an evolving system of early detection and optimal management. *Schizophrenia Bulletin*, **22**: 305–326.

Miller, W.R. and Rollnick, S. (1991) *Motivational Interviewing: Preparing People to Change Addictive Behavior.* New York, Guilford.

Minkoff, K. (1989) An integrated treatment model for dual diagnosis of psychosis and addiction. *Hospital and Community Psychiatry*, **40**: 1031–1036.

Monti, P.M., Colby, S.M., Barnett, N.P., Spirito, A., Rohsenow, D.J., Myers, M., Woolard, R., Lewander, W. (1999) Brief intervention for harm reduction with alcohol-positive older adolescents in a hospital emergency department. *Journal of Consulting and Clinical Psychology*, **67**: 989–994.

Mueser, K.T., Drake, R.E. and Wallach, M.A. (1998) Dual diagnosis: a review of etiological theories. *Addictive Behaviors*, **23**: 717–734.

Mueser, K.T., Yarnold, P.R., Levinson, D.F., Singh, H., Bellack, A.S., Kee, K., Morrison, R.L. and Wadalam, K.G. (1990) Prevalence of substance abuse in schizophrenia: demographic and clinical correlates. *Schizophrenia Bulletin*, **16**: 31–56.

Mueser, K.T., Yarnold, P.R., Rosenberg, S.D., Swett, C., Miles, K.M. and Hill, D. (2000) Substance use disorder in hospitalized severely mentally ill psychiatric patients: prevalence, correlates, and subgroups. *Schizophrenia Bulletin*, **26**: 179–192.

Poikolainen, K. (1999) Effectiveness of brief interventions to reduce alcohol intake in primary health care populations: a meta-analysis. *Preventive Medicine*, **28**: 503–509.

Ridgely, M.S., Goldman, H.H. and Willenbring, M. (1990) Barriers to the care of persons with dual diagnoses: organizational and financing issues. *Schizophrenia Bulletin*, **16**: 123–132.

Walitzere, K., Dermen, K. and Connors, G. (1999) Strategies for preparing clients for treatment. *Behavior Modification*, **23**: 129–151.

Wallace, C.J. and Liberman, R.P. (1985) Social skills training for patients with schizophrenia: a controlled clinical trial. *Psychiatry Research*, **15**: 239–247.

Wilk, A.I., Jensen, N.M. and Havighurst, T.C. (1997) Meta-analysis of randomized control trials addressing brief interventions in heavy alcohol drinkers. *Journal of General Internal Medicine*, **12**: 274–283.

World Health Organization (1997) *Composite International Diagnostic Interview: CIDI Auto Version 2.1.* Sydney, WHO.

Chapter 15

PHARMACOLOGICAL MANAGEMENT OF SUBSTANCE MISUSE IN PSYCHOSIS

Ed Day, George Georgiou and Ilana Crome

INTRODUCTION

There is a growing awareness that rates of substance misuse are increasing, and a recognition that use of such substances results in poorer outcomes in patients with co-existing mental health problems. Much recent progress has been made in the development of effective pharmacological treatments, and this chapter will review the evidence for a range of potential medications for treating both psychotic disorders and substance misuse problems. It begins by describing practical treatments for the misuse of opioids, stimulants and alcohol, before moving on to describe the pharmacological therapies available for the underlying causes of psychosis.

One of the challenges facing any service treating patients with co-occurring substance misuse and psychosis is choosing the correct order in which to tackle the various problems. Therefore, three flow diagrams have been incorporated in the chapter in order to aid the clinician in deciding which strategy to adopt at different stages of presentation. Few substances of abuse are without withdrawal symptoms, and pharmacological treatment of these may be an important way of engaging a patient in treatment. Once detoxification has occurred, an assessment of residual symptoms of psychiatric illness can take place, and treatment of these can help prevent relapse and promote attempts at rehabilitation.

Substance Misuse in Psychosis: Approaches to Treatment and Service Delivery.
Edited by Hermine L. Graham, Alex Copello, Max J. Birchwood and Kim T. Mueser.
© 2003 John Wiley & Sons, Ltd.

Finally, it is useful to acknowledge that the combination of substance misuse and psychiatric symptoms leads to additional difficulties in applying treatment strategies developed for either of the problems in isolation. There are several potential reasons why clinicians may be reluctant to prescribe for this group of patients, including the view that drug-misusing patients are unlikely to experience improvement in psychiatric disorders due to the deleterious effects of illicit substance misuse. There is often concern about being "manipulated" by the patient, and even if the doctor does prescribe, concerns remain about unwanted interactions between the drug of abuse and the prescribed medication. Many of these difficulties will be illustrated by a case example at the end of the chapter.

TREATMENT OF SUBSTANCE-USE DISORDERS

There is increasing evidence for the effectiveness of treatment for substance misuse, and it is important to remember that people often demonstrate the capacity for change despite severe problems. The particular components of treatment that yield beneficial results are not readily identifiable, but in some cases engaging patients in a long-term relationship is important in improving outcome. Interventions for drug and alcohol problems have a range of objectives, and treatment may be associated with decreases in substance use, injecting behaviour and improvements in related problems such as forensic or social factors. The spread of the HIV virus in the early to mid-1980s led to the "harm-reduction" model gaining prominence within UK drug treatment services (Department of Health, 1996). However, abstinence should probably be considered the basis or aim of treatment for most people with both substance misuse and psychiatric problems (Goldsmith, 1999). Intensive treatment for severe problems is also associated with improvement, and treatment plans involving both pharmacological and psychological treatments are often the most effective.

Pharmacological interventions for substance misuse problems may include the following:

1. *Maintenance or substitution treatment.* The harm-reduction approach aims to attract people to and retain them in treatment in order to stabilize chaotic lifestyles and reduce criminality, morbidity and mortality. A key feature of this strategy is maintenance or substitute prescribing. Methadone maintenance therapy is the best-known example, although buprenorphine has also recently been licensed.
2. *Detoxification.* There are well-established regimens for most substances producing withdrawal syndromes, and there has been an increasing trend towards undertaking the process as an outpatient with appropriate supervision. Patients with severe psychiatric symptoms in

addition to substance misuse may be an exception to this trend, and an inpatient admission is often useful.

3. *Relapse prevention.* Medications such as disulfiram for alcohol and naltrexone for opioids are most appropriate for people who have decided to abstain but find some extra reassurance useful. However, such drugs have their own complications, and it is suggested that only experienced clinicians should engage patients in this form of treatment.

4. *"Anti-craving" agents.* Craving has been described as an urge to use when not in withdrawal, and is often cited as a reason for lapse after a drug free period. Therefore, pharmacological agents that reduce the problem are highly sought after. Patients with comorbid psychiatric symptoms may describe relapse triggers that are related more to mood swings, boredom and lassitude than pure craving. Even so, "anti-craving" medication, such as naltrexone or acamprosate can have a significant impact on prevention of relapse.

Opioids

Treatment of drug misuse problems tends to be carried out by specialist community-based teams. A spectrum of problems exists, and doctors may provide a range of interventions, the timing of which is highlighted in our first flow chart (Figure 15.1).

Reduction of harm associated with drug misuse

Injecting drug misuse carries a significant risk of infection, particularly when equipment is shared or poorly cleaned. Advice about improved injection technique and cleaning of equipment can be effective in reducing this risk, particularly when combined with the provision of clean needles and syringes via local needle exchange schemes. It is important to remember that this advice is equally applicable to injectors of drugs other than heroin (e.g., amphetamines and cocaine).

Detoxification

A common goal for opioid users is to stop using the drug while avoiding unpleasant withdrawal symptoms. The opioid withdrawal syndrome is not life-threatening, but is unpleasant enough to lead many users to relapse, and so some form of pharmacotherapeutic support is often necessary. This will be particularly so for patients with coexisting mental health problems, as these may be exacerbated during the withdrawal process. The first phase of therapy should include an assessment of the level of dependence as well as any drug-related medical, psychological and social

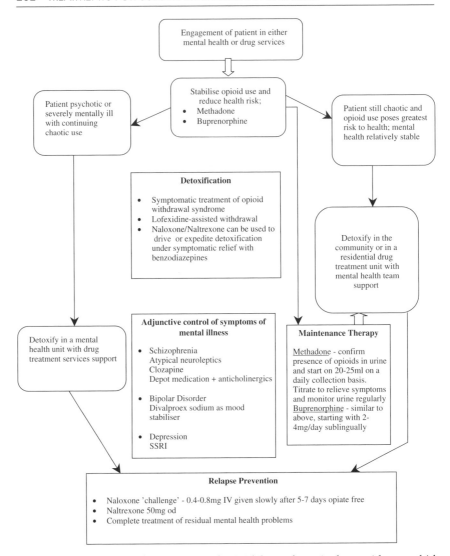

Figure 15.1   Algorithm for treatment of opioid dependence in those with comorbid mental illness

problems, accompanied by an attempt to develop a therapeutic alliance. An explanation of the likely withdrawal side effects and their time course can help to clarify any misunderstandings, and patients using small amounts of heroin may be able to stop abruptly with purely symptomatic support. This may include diazepam to reduce anxiety, muscle cramps and craving, night sedation such as zopiclone, ibuprofen to reduce muscular aches, and loperamide to control diarrhoea.

Those with dependence who are also on higher doses of heroin or with longer histories of drug use may not be able to tolerate such a simple detoxification process, and often require assessment and management by a specialist drug treatment agency. Home detoxification under the supervision of a community drug worker may utilize the above approach in addition to the provision of lofexidine. This is an alpha-2 agonist that reduces the adrenergic surge of the opioid withdrawal syndrome. It was initially developed as an antihypertensive, and so blood pressure must be measured regularly, and it has proven efficacy in both inpatient and out-patient environments (Bearn et al, 1996; Kahn et al, 1997; Carnwath and Hardman, 1998).

Another alternative is an initial period of stabilization on methadone, followed by a slow reduction over a number of weeks. Methadone used in this way has become the mainstay treatment for opioid detoxification in the UK, but the evidence base for its effectiveness as a detoxification treatment is limited. It is also important to recognize the potential for overdose and death if methadone is not initiated at low doses (20–25 mg) and slowly titrated against its effect.

Prescription of substitute medication such as methadone

"Substitute" prescribing implies the use of a legally prescribed drug instead of an illegal drug of unknown purity and quality. Methadone maintenance therapy (MMT) has been used for over 30 years in the management of opioid dependence, and research has demonstrated clear benefits in reducing illicit opioid use, HIV infection and criminal activity (Marsch, 1998). Its effectiveness appears to depend on a range of factors including dose, retention in treatment and psychosocial support (Ball and Ross, 1991), and methadone maintenance programmes vary substantially in their effectiveness. There is evidence to suggest that regimens involving higher daily doses of the substitute drug (approximately 60–80 mg methadone) are the most successful at reducing illicit drug intake (Caplehorn et al, 1993; Ling et al, 1996; Schottenfeld et al, 1997). However, better quality counselling, more medical services, better staff-patient relationships and better management have also been shown to be beneficial, and services in the UK have tended to favour lower methadone doses (Farrell et al, 1994).

Alternatives to methadone such as buprenorphine show considerable potential, but as yet are not widely used in the UK. Buprenorphine is a partial opioid agonist, and so produces less euphoria, sedation or respiratory depression than heroin. It also has a longer half-life, and discontinuation leads to less severe withdrawal symptoms. The evidence base for its effectiveness is beginning to develop, particularly when compared to lower doses (20–35 mg) of methadone (Barnett et al, 2001). Furthermore, it has shown particular promise in treating mixed cocaine and opioid abuse (Schotten-feld et al, 1997).

Psychosis is not a typical feature of the opioid withdrawal syndrome, but it has been reported in some cases after stopping methadone (Levinson et al, 1995). Bloom et al (1976) have proposed that an excess of endogenous opi-oids may have a role in the pathogenesis of schizophrenia. One study even suggests that methadone may be a treatment for schizophrenia (Brizer et al, 1985), and it is sometimes more practical to maintain opioid-dependent schizophrenic patients on a combination of antipsychotic medication and methadone than attempting a detoxification process.

Naltrexone is a long-acting oral opioid antagonist that can be used as a relapse prevention measure in opioid users that have completed a detoxi-fication and are drug-free. The evidence for its effectiveness is limited, but it may have potential on a case by case basis (Report of the National Research Council Committee on Clinical Evaluation of Narcotic Antagonists, 1978; Farren, 1997). Like disulfiram, it is likely to be most effective when con-sumption is supervised (Brewer, 1993a). Polysubstance users may also be particularly suitable candidates, as naltrexone also has potential as a phar-macological agent for the treatment of alcohol dependence, and has been shown to diminish the effects of acute cocaine use in cocaine-dependent patients. It may be given as a daily dose of 50 mg, or else three times per week (100 mg Monday, 100 mg Wednesday and 150 mg Friday). Liver func-tion tests should be performed prior to induction onto naltrexone, and the drug should be avoided if liver transaminases are over three times normal (Farren, 1997).

Stimulant drugs

Most pharmacotherapeutic research into stimulant drug abuse has been conducted in the USA, where cocaine is the major problem. Unfortu-nately, none of the medications tested for treating cocaine dependence has proven to be clearly and unequivocally effective, and many studies are of poor design and involve very few patients. However, cocaine-dependent individuals with psychiatric comorbidity are one group suggested by Kosten (1989) to be particularly likely to benefit from pharmacological treatments, and our second flow chart (Figure 15.2) illustrates the applica-tion of some of the treatments described below.

Chronic use of stimulant drugs causes changes in a number of neuro-transmitter systems in the brain, including serotonin, noradrenaline and dopamine. The reinforcing and rewarding properties of stimulant drugs are probably caused by the inhibition of dopamine reuptake in the mesolimbic and mesocortical reward pathways. Common withdrawal symptoms such

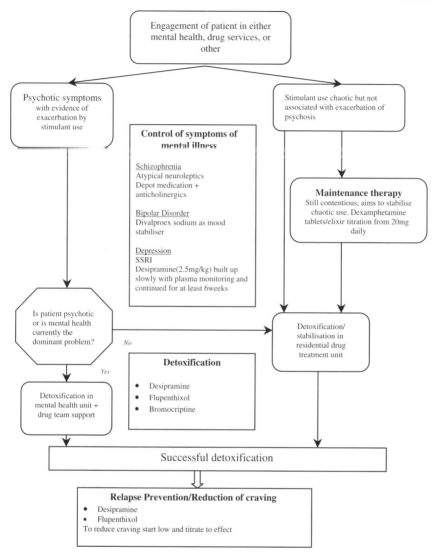

Figure 15.2   Algorithm for treatment of stimulant problems in those with comorbid mental illness

as dysphoria and intense craving may be secondary to underactivity in dopaminergic systems, and chronic use can lead to dopamine depletion and so to supersensitivity of the postsynaptic dopamine receptors. Thus, medications that function as dopamine agonists have been studied as a way to treat the withdrawal syndrome. However, dopamine does not account for all the positive and negative reinforcing properties of cocaine. Other neurotransmitters (serotonin) and mechanisms (brain kindling) have been suggested in the understanding of the neurobiological basis of cocaine addiction.

Pharmacological agents may be useful in two phases of the treatment of stimulant users (Gawin and Kleber, 1986). In the initial withdrawal phase, agents that work as direct or indirect agonists on the dopaminergic system may be most useful, particularly in relieving dysphoria. Both the D2-agonist bromocriptine and the indirect dopamine agonist amantadine have been suggested as potential treatments. However, studies in the treatment of cocaine dependence have tended to yield mixed results, with some evidence of a reduction in drug craving only in the early withdrawal period (Gawin et al, 1989c). L-dopa, methylphenidate and pergolide (a direct dopamine agonist) have also been postulated as potential therapies (Rao et al, 1995), but the most widely tested agents have been the tricyclic antidepressants. The latter have potential value as they may help to reverse some of the cocaine-induced neurochemical changes as well as treating the anhedonia and depression seen during cocaine withdrawal. Desipramine has been the most widely studied, but with equivocal results (Gawin and Kleber, 1984; Gawin et al, 1989b). Not only are adequate doses required (2.5 mg/kg daily), but at least 6 weeks of treatment appears to be necessary, and this may be a problem in a group with poor frustration tolerance. Some patients have experienced symptoms of stimulation, insomnia, and anxiety, ultimately leading to their relapse to cocaine use, and the potential for additive cardiotoxicity should not be forgotten (Lange and Hills, 2001).

Once abstinence has been achieved, pharmacological agents also have a potential role in maintaining it. Craving for stimulant drugs has been much studied, and again tricyclic antidepressants may have a role. Desipramine has been shown to reduce craving for cocaine as well as increasing the length of time that users stay in treatment. However, tricyclic antidepressants appear to take up to 2 weeks to work (Gawin et al, 1989b), and other pharmacotherapies have been sought to bridge the gap. Several studies have shown that dopamine-blocking agents such as haloperidol and chlorpromazine can antagonize some of cocaine's effects in both animal models and human subjects. Flupenthixol has been shown to decrease cocaine craving and use (Gawin et al, 1989a), and this may be a useful option in patients with psychotic symptoms who also abuse stimulant drugs. The use of an acute agent such as a dopamine agonist in combination with a tricyclic antidepressant may improve treatment retention during the first few weeks, but toxicity and the side-effect profile may make this an impractical option. The role of atypical antipsychotic drugs has yet to be evaluated in this area.

Cocaine is a powerful serotonergic reuptake inhibitor, and chronic administration leads to enhanced 5-HT autoregulatory mechanisms, resulting in decreased 5-HT transmission (a mechanism to explain the depressive symptoms of acute withdrawal from cocaine). Animal studies have implicated 5-HT receptors in the mechanisms of stimulant-induced euphoria. Fluoxetine and sertraline have been investigated in small numbers of cases, with both agents showing promise in decreasing cocaine use and improving mood. Phenelzine has shown some efficacy in treating cocaine use and craving (Brewer, 1993b), although potential interactions with stimulant drugs limit its usefulness.

The amount of amphetamine misuse is less widely studied, and the use of substitute prescribing is a controversial area in need of more research. Despite its uncertain status, it seems to be widely practised in the UK, with some evidence that the prescription of dexamphetamine is both safe and effective in bringing about improvements in reduction of illicit drug use (Fleming and Roberts, 1994; White, 2000). A particular concern is substitute prescribing in patients with psychotic phenomena who are also abusing illicit stimulant drugs. Provision of drugs such as dexamphetamine with dopamine agonist activity may be presumed to be inappropriate due to the risk of precipitating or worsening psychotic features. However, each case must be considered on its merits, weighing up the risks and benefits of the treatment. The prescription of a fixed amount of amphetamine of known quality may help reduce illicit and chaotic use, while engaging and retaining the patient in treatment services.

Cannabis

Cannabis is possibly the most commonly abused drug by patients with psychotic disorders. There is some debate about whether there is a clinically important cannabis withdrawal syndrome, but most of the recognized criteria for dependence can be applied, and tolerance is also recognized (Thornicroft, 1990). There are no established pharmacological treatments for cannabis craving, and supportive treatment is recommended for the mild symptoms of nausea and headache experienced by some during withdrawal. Psychological treatments described elsewhere are the treatment of choice.

Benzodiazepines

Dependence on benzodiazepines is seen in a substantial number of people treated by psychiatric services. A useful treatment strategy may be to prescribe an initial maintenance period while other factors are stabilized, followed by a planned slow reduction of the benzodiazepine. The initial aim of such a programme is to convert the total benzodiazepine load to a single drug with a long half-life, such as diazepam. The starting dose and reducing regimen are then negotiated between doctor and patient, in order to minimize withdrawal symptoms. Clear criteria for review and goals of progress are also established before starting, and the frequency of reduction and stringency of required adherence to the regimen vary with levels of motivation and co-occurring medical or psychosocial problems. Complicated cases with extensive comorbidity may require a period of inpatient treatment.

Alcohol

Individuals that meet the criteria for alcohol dependence are likely to require pharmacological help in order to provide an effective intervention. There has been considerable expansion in the development of new pharmacological agents in the treatment of alcohol problems in the past few years. Analysis of the research data on novel psychotropic drugs has engendered some scepticism (Schuckit, 1996; Moncrieff and Drummond, 1997), but there is no dispute that this is a developing area.

Detoxification

Most patients do not experience serious complications during alcohol withdrawal, and detoxification can usually be done safely, successfully and cost-effectively at home. The general practitioner may have a role in prescribing for these patients, usually in conjunction with a community alcohol team. However, patients with severe medical or psychiatric problems, a history of withdrawal fits or delirium tremens, or few social supports are likely to require inpatient admission. Detoxification is best seen as the start of the therapeutic process rather than a treatment in its own right (see our third flow chart; Figure 15.3), but, in the case of severe alcohol dependence, the process can also be seen as a harm-reduction measure as it may prevent other potentially life-threatening complications such as delirium tremens.

In "medicated" detoxification, the severity of withdrawal symptoms is minimized (or completely suppressed) by the administration of a drug, with gradual reduction of the substitute medication after the peak of the withdrawal syndrome has passed. Benzodiazepines are the mainstay of treatment for the acute effects of withdrawal, as they are cross-tolerant with alcohol and also have anticonvulsant and anxiolytic properties. Longer-acting drugs such as diazepam and chlordiazepoxide are the favoured option, although short-acting benzodiazepines, such as lorazepam and oxazepam, are preferred when liver dysfunction is a problem. A meta-analysis on the pharmacological management of alcohol withdrawal

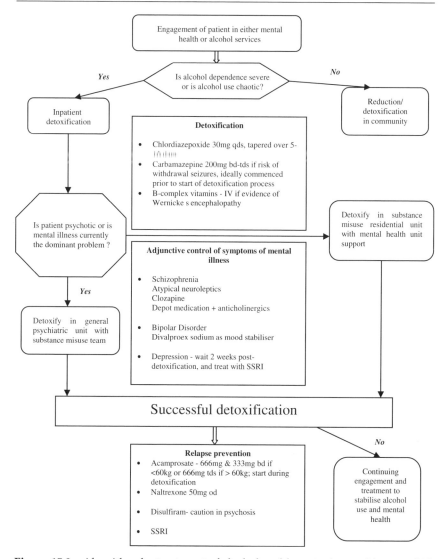

Figure 15.3   Algorithm for treatment of alcohol problems in those with comorbid mental illness

has demonstrated that benzodiazepines reduce withdrawal severity, the incidence of delirium, and the risk of seizures (Mayo-Smith, 1997). Beta-blockers, clonidine, carbamazepine and phenothiazines also affect withdrawal severity, but have less proven effect on delirium and convulsions, and so should be regarded as adjunctive therapy only. Chlormethiazole should not be administered as a first-line drug due to abuse potential and respiratory depression. Caution must be exercised when prescribing benzodiazepines to polysubstance users, and there is a risk that dependence on alcohol may be substituted for benzodiazepine dependence if treatment is not carefully supervised. Close attention should also be paid to the possibility of nutritional deficits. B-complex vitamins should be administered intravenously or intramuscularly to patients with confusion, ataxia, ophthalmoplegia, hypotension or other signs of malnutrition (Cook and Thomson, 1997).

Relapse prevention

Although psychosocial methods are the most commonly used treatment modalities for alcohol problems, there is a growing body of evidence for new forms of medication to reduce drinking in the rehabilitation phase of management. However, decisions to use such medications depend on the history and severity of dependence, personality profile, psychiatric symptomatology and available support network. Pharmacotherapy is likely to be enhanced in combination with psychosocial interventions, and should not be viewed as a simple answer to a complicated problem.

The search for a pharmacological therapy to help the patient through the post-detoxification period has led to the evaluation of a variety of agents, including disulfiram, bromocriptine, tiapride, ritanserin, buspirone and desipramine. Selective serotonin reuptake inhibitors (SSRIs) have been shown to produce a small but definite decrease in drinking (Naranjo et al, 1992), but it is not certain that serotonergic drugs can reduce craving and the risk of relapse in detoxified dependent drinkers.

Naltrexone has been shown to reduce alcohol craving and the number of days in which any alcohol was consumed (Volpicelli et al, 1997). Acamprosate is reported as a useful adjunct for maintaining abstinence in detoxified alcohol-dependent patients (Pelc et al, 1997). The mechanism of action is thought to involve stimulation of inhibitory GABA transmission and antagonism of excitatory amino acids such as glutamate (Littleton, 1995). Little is known about the use of these drugs in patients with coexisting mental health problems, and there has been some suggestion of poor toleration of naltrexone in patients with bipolar disorder (Sonne and Brady, 2000).

A review of 38 studies using either oral or implanted disulfiram concluded that there was no justification for the use of the implanted form, and that oral disulfiram reduced alcohol consumption without evidence that abstinence was maintained (Hughes and Cook, 1997). The key features that improved efficacy were supervision and social stability in the context of a total treatment package. The use of disulfiram in younger or older age groups should be implemented with extreme caution, as psychotic episodes have been reported in a small number of patients treated with disulfiram.

Anxiolytic agents may be administered to patients who experience anxiety disorders separately from any problems related to substances. Buspirone may also have a useful role in this group, but if benzodiazepines are used, it is vital to prescribe short courses and monitor symptoms closely. Longer-acting benzodiazepines are preferred because of their lower abuse liability, although daytime drowsiness and cumulative toxicity is a problem. Psychological treatments are the preferred option.

TREATMENT OF PSYCHIATRIC DISORDERS

Schizophrenia

The consequences of substance misuse in schizophrenia are substantial, as misuse of alcohol, cannabis and stimulants is associated with exacerbation of psychotic symptoms, more frequent hospitalization, poor social functioning, homelessness, increased suicide rate and poor treatment response. However, when substance-free and treated, this group may have a milder symptom profile than other hospitalized schizophrenics. The "self-medication hypothesis" suggests that such patients use substances as an attempt to reduce a variety of symptoms (Siris, 1990), and that these symptoms may provide the basis of a therapeutic strategy (Krystal et al, 1999). Relatively little research has been done on the pharmacological treatment of patients with coexisting schizophrenia and substance-use disorders, with many studies focusing on psychosocial treatment and providing patients with standard pharmacotherapy.

Alcohol and cannabis use often precede the onset of positive symptoms, and delusions or hallucinations may promote substance abuse as an attempt to self-medicate (Krystal et al, 1999). Patients with schizophrenia report using substances for pleasure and to relieve boredom, but also to relieve feelings of anxiety, sadness or distress (Mueser et al, 1995). However, vigorous attempts to optimize the pharmacological management of such symptoms with typical antipsychotics may lead to further problems. There is evidence that substance-using patients respond differently to conventional antipsychotics from non-substance-users, one study showing a poorer therapeutic response to fixed doses of haloperidol and perphenazine (Bowers et al, 1990). Several studies have suggested a higher incidence of neuroleptic-induced movement disorders and tardive dyskinesia in alcohol-abusing schizophrenic patients taking neuroleptic drugs than in schizophrenic patients that do not use alcohol (Olivera et al, 1990). Schizophrenic patients who abuse stimulants tend to receive larger typical neuroleptic doses during hospitalization than patients that do not, thus leading to an increased risk of extrapyramidal and dysphoric side effects. Nicotine, cannabis and cocaine may reduce extrapyramidal effects by stimulating dopamine release, and alcohol may do so through GABA-A receptor potentiation and NDMA receptor antagonism (Krystal et al, 1999). Therefore, attempts to reduce unwanted side effects by adjusting neuroleptic dose, adding anticholinergic medications, or switching to novel antipsychotics with more favourable efficacy or side-effect profiles may be useful.

There is much interest in the use of atypical antipsychotics in this group, but again there is little good research evidence. The serotonergic system has been implicated in the control of alcohol consumption (Amit et al, 1991); thus, antipsychotic agents with serotinergic action may have the added benefit of decreasing alcohol consumption while exerting their antipsychotic effect. Several reports have suggested that clozapine may be effective in this population. Moderate substance abuse has been found not to alter the response to clozapine (Buckley et al, 1994), and many authors report a reduction in substance use in patients treated with clozapine for psychotic symptoms (Buckley et al, 1994; Marcus and Snyder, 1995; Tsuang et al, 1999). Drake et al (2000) report significant reductions in severity of alcohol abuse and days of alcohol use in patients with either schizophrenia or schizoaffective disorder while on clozapine. A retrospective study by Zimmet et al (2000) found that more than 85% of patients actively using substances at the initiation of the administration of clozapine actively decreased their substance use over the treatment period. Other atypical antipsychotics are also likely to be useful in schizophrenic patients that misuse substances, particularly as they have fewer extrapyramidal side effects and may have antidepressant effects. However, there is little good evidence for their effectiveness in this group as yet (Conley et al, 1998).

Low mood may be a motivator for substance use in schizophrenic patients (Brunette et al, 1997), and there is evidence that antidepressant treatment is helpful in some cases (Ziedonis et al, 1992). The link between negative symptoms and substance use is far from clear; indeed, negative symptoms may be less severe in substance-using patients with schizophrenia than in other schizophrenic patients. Non-compliance with medication is common among substance users; therefore, patients with schizophrenia may benefit from motivational enhancement work to improve adherence to pharmacological treatment. Depot neuroleptics are useful for some patients, but produce an increased rate of extrapyramidal side effects. Patients may refuse medications that they feel cause low mood or are ineffective.

Bipolar disorder

There is a strong link between bipolar disorder and substance misuse; the ECA study showed that more than 60% of people with a diagnosis of bipolar I disorder had a lifetime diagnosis of substance-use disorder (Regier et al, 1990). Furthermore, a combination of the two problems may present a serious diagnostic challenge as it can be difficult to tell which of the two problems is primary, and intoxication and withdrawal effects may be hard to distinguish from hypomania. There is some evidence that individuals with concurrent substance-use problems and bipolar disorder are more likely to have more mixed or dysphoric manic episodes (Sonne et al, 1994) or rapid cycling. This is significant, as evidence is accumulating that subtypes of bipolar disorder have varying responses to different mood stabilizers, and the mixed or rapid cycling types are less responsive to lithium than the classic euphoric mania (Goldberg, 2000; Sachs et al, 2000). Use of drugs or alcohol has been associated with poor outcome with lithium treatment (O'Connell et al, 1991), and an open trial of lithium showed little efficacy for cocaine abusers with bipolar spectrum disorders (Nunes et al, 1990).

Substance-misusing bipolar patients may respond well to anticonvulsant medications, and divalproex sodium has been suggested to be safe and effective (Hertzman, 2000; Sachs et al, 2000). This may also have the advantage of treating both alcohol withdrawal and mania at the same time in the acutely ill patient (Hammer and Brady, 1996), and divalproex appears to produce fewer side effects and have better rates of compliance than lithium. However, it does have the potential to cause liver toxicity, and so liver enzymes must be carefully monitored in substance-misusing patients, who may have compromised their liver function in other ways. Carbamazepine, lamotrigine and gabapentin may also be useful in patients with bipolar disorder that misuse substances (Nemeroff, 2000), as are traditional agents such as neuroleptics and benzodiazepines. However, when one uses benzodiazepines, it is important to ensure that prescriptions are time-limited and targetted at particular symptoms, and the potential for abuse should not be forgotten (Sonne and Brady, 1999).

Depression

Symptoms of depression are common in people that misuse drugs and alcohol, although depressive symptoms observed in substance-dependent individuals often resolve with abstinence, and are probably substance-induced mood disorders. Tricyclic antidepressants have been the most widely studied in populations with depression and coexisting alcohol abuse. Studies using imipramine have demonstrated favourable results (Nunes et al, 1993; McGrath et al, 1996), although the optimum dose of imipramine is not clear, as heavy alcohol consumption alters the drug's clearance, and plasma level monitoring is usually necessary for effective treatment. Another practical concern is the risk of the potentiation of the side effects of tricyclic drugs by alcohol. Imipramine has been shown to enhance the sedative-hypnotic effects of alcohol for psychomotor performance, memory assessments and some subjective ratings in normal subjects (Frewer and Lader, 1993).

More recently, the SSRIs have been investigated, and studies evaluating cerebrospinal fluid (CSF) levels of the main metabolite of serotonin (5-hydroxyindolacetic acid) have suggested that low serotonergic functioning is associated with depression, suicidality and alcohol abuse (Cornelius et al, 1997). A double-blind, placebo-controlled study involving a detoxified inpatient population found a significantly greater improvement in the fluoxetine group than in the placebo group, as well as a lower total alcohol consumption during the trial (Cornelius et al, 1997). As SSRIs have also been shown to decrease alcohol ingestion in animal studies, studies have been conducted to determine whether fluoxetine decreases the alcohol consumption of problem drinkers who do not have comorbid major depression, with modest positive results. Higher doses of SSRI may be needed due to alcohol's inducing effect on hepatic microsomal activity. Overall, depression that persists for 2 weeks of abstinence is generally thought to merit consideration for pharmacotherapy. SSRIs are probably the first-choice antidepressant, but are only clearly effective in patients with a depressive disorder after detoxification from alcohol.

In contrast, opioid-dependent individuals with depressive symptoms often benefit from a period of stabilization with substitute prescribing rather than detoxification. Tricyclic antidepressants have also been used in such patients, but a variety of studies have given inconclusive results. In one study, 57% of 84 adequately treated patients receiving imipramine were rated as responders compared with 7% of 42 receiving placebo, and imipramine also appeared to reduce substance abuse among patients whose mood improved (Nunes et al, 1998). Doxepin has also been shown to relieve symptoms of depression, anxiety and drug craving in studies of methadone-maintained patients. Plasma-level monitoring is again important, as methadone-maintained patients often have plasma levels of tricyclic drugs twice as high as prior to methadone administration. The use of antidepressants in the treatment of cocaine-dependent patients has tended to focus on the treatment of cocaine dependence rather than the treatment of depression (see above). There is a risk of cardiotoxicity with the co-administration of tricyclic antidepressants and cocaine or other stimulant drugs.

CASE EXAMPLE

The following case example illustrates some of the issues raised by the pharmacological management of this client group.

Martin is a 30-year-old man who presented to substance-misuse treatment services 5 years ago with a 15-year history of drug and alcohol use. His pattern of use was chaotic and included large doses of benzodiazepines (up to 120 mg of temazepam and 80 mg of diazepam per day), amphetamines, cocaine and heavy use of alcohol (up to 12 pints of beer per day). He would also occasionally use opioids in the form of heroin or methadone, with varying degrees of dependence. He was inconsistent in his preferred route of drug use and would often inject a selection of substances including amphetamines, cocaine, heroin and temazepam. His lifestyle was similarly chaotic; he found it difficult to reside in furnished flats for any length of time, and often chose to live on the streets and wander from city to city.

At initial presentation, Martin also described a wide variety of psychotic phenomena including clear third-person hallucinations and delusional paranoid beliefs. He talked of hearing voices talking about him in a derogatory way that were so distressing that he became depressed and suicidal. On one occasion, he had deliberately walked onto the carriageway of a motorway. He had discovered that listening to music on a Walkman helped him cope with the content of the voices, and he was observed to have the volume turned up very high during his initial contact with the addiction treatment service. On occasions, he also worried that he was being poisoned, and he once hit a girlfriend when he suspected that she was part of a plot to kill him. Martin described using a variety of substances to help relieve his symptoms. He felt that using large doses of benzodiazepines was the only way to reduce his anxiety and induce sleep. However, he was able to acknowledge that he quickly became tolerant to them and then suffered withdrawal symptoms if he could not obtain a regular supply. By contrast, amphetamines helped lift his mood and motivated him to get up each day, and cocaine and heroin were used at different times to help him escape from his various problems.

Like many other patients, Martin initially came to the attention of the health services when his unusual behaviour began to attract the attention of the police. A psychiatrist was called to assess him after an overnight detention in a police cell, but he was discharged because it was felt that his mental health symptoms were "drug-induced". Soon afterwards, Martin felt that he had reached a low and approached the addiction treatment services for the first time. At the time of first presentation, he felt that he needed replacement prescribing for his various dependencies. In particular, he asked for large doses of temazepam or diazepam, methadone, and dexamphetamine. His experiences with other psychotropic medication was very negative, and he was unwilling to consider antipsychotic medicines. The initial treatment goal was to stabilize his chaotic injecting behaviour and to engage him in a longer-term therapeutic relationship. A plan was formulated, and he was started on moderate doses of diazepam (30 mg daily in divided doses) and oral methadone mixture 1 mg/ml (40 ml daily), which he collected from the pharmacy on a daily basis. Regular monitoring of his drug consumption and mental state was carried out, and initially the doses of prescribed medication were gradually increased to try to cut down his need for street drugs.

Over a number of weeks and months, Martin became accustomed to visits to the treatment centre and began to confide in members of staff about his true level of substance use and his high levels of distress. At various times, it was clear that his mental health symptoms had deteriorated, and he would appear extremely pre-occupied by auditory hallucinations, and was both tearful and agitated. Twice in the first year, a decision was made to admit him on an informal basis to the addiction service inpatient unit for a period of evaluation and treatment of both his mental health and drug misuse problems. These episodes lasted between 2 and 4 weeks, and, in retrospect, proved to be of critical importance in Martin's long-term management. An evaluation of his mood while drug-free led to the prescription of an SSRI, and, subsequently, his use of stimulant medication reduced dramatically. During a third such admission, he reduced his methadone dose by 50%, using a steady linear reduction, and was also able to rationalize his use of benzodiazepines. As his illicit drug use came under control, he also began to understand more about his mental health symptoms, and was eventually persuaded to undertake a trial of antipsychotic medication.

Martin had previously been prescribed haloperidol and chlorpromazine, and talked bitterly about the side-effects that he had experienced. An atypical neuroleptic was therefore commenced, but again his compliance was poor, and he initially attributed any physical discomfort that he experienced to the medication. With much reassurance, he began to replace self-medication with illicit drugs with longer periods of antipsychotic medication, and as he did so, he began to acknowledge that it did have some beneficial effect on his psychotic symptoms. Periodically, crises would develop that led to a further period of use of street drugs, but each time he would eventually return to the addiction treatment services and reinstate his treatment plan. Five years after entering treatment, he had reached a better level of symptom control by taking a combination of an atypical antipsychotic, an SSRI and a small dose of methadone (25 ml per day). His injecting behaviour had completely stopped, as had his binges on cocaine and amphetamines. This change led to his being taken on by a local assertive outreach mental health team, with a consequent improvement in his housing situation.

CONCLUSIONS

People that have psychiatric disorders and also misuse substances are difficult to treat, and the best results appear to be obtained by combining medications with psychosocial interventions. Each case must be treated on its merits, and the treatment strategy developed will depend on the psychiatric diagnosis and the types of substances abused. Pharmacological management of this patient group has been underresearched, and further double-blind, placebo-controlled clinical trials are required with larger samples and longer follow-up periods.

REFERENCES

Amit, Z., Smith, B.R. and Gill, K. (1991) Serotonin uptake inhibitors: effects on motivated consummatory behaviours. *Journal of Clinical Psychiatry*, **55**: 55–60.

Ball, J.C. and Ross, A. (1991) *The Effectiveness of Methadone Maintenance Treatment: Patients, Progress, Services and Outcomes*. New York, Springer-Verlag.

Barnett, P.G., Rodgers, H.H. and Bloch, D.A. (2001) A meta-analysis comparing buprenorphine to methadone for treatment of opiate dependence. *Addiction*, **96**: 683–690.

Bearn, J., Gossop, M. and Strang, J. (1996) Randomised double-blind comparison of lofexidine and methadone in the in-patient treatment of opiate withdrawal. *Drug and Alcohol Dependence*, **43**: 87–91.

Bowers, M.B., Mazure, C.M., Nelson, J.C. and Jatlow, P.I. (1990) Psychotogenic drug use and neuroleptic response. *Schizophrenia Bulletin*, **16**: 81–85.

Brewer, C. (1993a) Naltrexone in the prevention of relapse and opiate detoxification. In C. Brewer (Ed.), *Treatment Options in Addiction*. London, Gaskell.

Brewer, C. (1993b) Treatment of cocaine abuse with monoamine oxidase inhibitors. *British Journal of Psychiatry*, **163**: 815–816.

Brizer, D.A., Hartman, N., Sweeney, J. and Millman, R.B. (1985) Effect of methadone plus neuroleptics on treatment-resistant chronic paranoid schizophrenia. *American Journal of Psychiatry*, **142**: 1106–1107.

Brunette, M.F., Mueser, K.T., Xie, H. and Drake, R.E. (1997) Relationships between symptoms of schizophrenia and substance abuse. *Journal of Nervous and Mental Disease*, **185**: 13–20.

Buckley, P., Thompson, P., Way, L. and Meltzer, H.Y. (1994) Substance abuse among patients with treatment-resistant schizophrenia: characteristics and implications for clozapine therapy. *American Journal of Psychiatry*, **151**: 385–389.

Caplehorn, J.R.M., Bell, J., Kleinbaum, D.G. and Gebski, V.J. (1993) Methadone dose and heroin use during maintenance treatment. *Addiction*, **88**: 119–124.

Carnwath, T. and Hardman, J. (1998) Randomised double-blind comparison of lofexidine and clonidine in outpatient treatment of opiate withdrawal. *Drug and Alcohol Dependence*, **50**: 251–254.

Conley, R.R., Kelly, D.L. and Gale, E.A. (1998) Olanzapine response in treatment-refractory schizophrenic patients with a history of substance abuse. *Schizophrenia Research*, **33**: 95–101.

Cook, C.C.H. and Thomson, A.D. (1997) B-complex vitamins in the prophylaxis and treatment of Wernicke-Korsakoff syndrome. *British Journal of Hospital Medicine*, **57**: 461–465.

Cornelius, J.R., Salloum, I.M., Ehler, J.G., Jarrett, P.J., Cornelius, M.D., Perel, J.M., Thase, M.E. and Black, A. (1997) Fluoxetine in depressed alcoholics. *Archives of General Psychiatry*, **54**: 700–705.

Department of Health (1996) *Task Force to Review Services for Drug Misusers: Report of an Independent Review of Drug Treatment Services in England*. London, Department of Health.

Drake, R.E., Xie, H., McHugo, G.J. and Green, A.I. (2000) The effects of clozapine on alcohol and drug use disorders among patients with schizophrenia. *Schizophrenia Bulletin*, **26**: 441–449.

Farrell, M., Ward, J., Mattick, R., Hall, W., Stimson, G.V., des Jarlais, D., Gossop, M. and Strang, J. (1994) Fortnightly Review: Methadone maintenance treatment in opiate dependence: a review. *British Medical Journal*, **309**(6960): 997–1001.

Farren, C.K. (1997) The use of naltrexone, an opiate antagonist, in the treatment of opiate addiction. *Irish Journal of Psychological Medicine*, **14**: 31–34.

Fleming, P.M. and Roberts, D. (1994) Is prescription of amphetamine justified as a harm reduction measure? *Journal of the Royal Society of Health*, **114**: 127–131.

Frewer, L.J. and Lader, M. (1993) The effects of nefazadone, imipramine and placebo, alone and combined with alcohol, in normal subjects. *International Clinical Psychopharmacology*, **8**: 13–20.

Gawin, F.H., Allen, D. and Humbelstone, B. (1989a) Outpatient treatment of crack cocaine smoking with flupenthixol decanoate. *Archives of General Psychiatry*, **46**: 322–325.

Gawin, F.H. and Kleber, H.D. (1984) Cocaine abuse treatment. Open pilot trial with desipramine and lithium carbonate. *Archives of General Psychiatry*, **41**: 903–909.

Gawin, F.H. and Kleber, H.D. (1986) Abstinence symptomatology and psychiatric diagnosis in chronic cocaine abusers. *Archives of General Psychiatry*, **43**: 322–325.

Gawin, F.H., Kleber, H.D., Byck, R., Rounsaville, B.J., Kosten, T.R., Jatlow, P.I. and Morgan, C. (1989b) Desipramine facilitation of initial cocaine dependence. *Archives of General Psychiatry*, **46**: 117–121.

Gawin, F.H., Morgan, C., Kosten, T.R. and Kleber, H.D. (1989c). Double-blind evaluation of the effect of acute amantadine on cocaine craving. *Psychopharmacology*, **97**: 402–403.

Goldberg, J.F. (2000) Treatment guidelines: current and future management of bipolar disorder. *Journal of Clinical Psychiatry*, **61** (Suppl 13): 12–18.

Goldsmith, R.J. (1999) Overview of psychiatric comorbidity. *Psychiatric Clinics of North America*, **22**: 331–349.

Hammer, B.A. and Brady, K.T. (1996) Valproate treatment of alcohol withdrawal and mania. *American Journal of Psychiatry*, **153**: 1232.

Hertzman, M. (2000) Divalproex sodium to treat concomitant substance abuse and mood disorders. *Journal of Substance Abuse Treatment*, **18**: 371–372.

Hughes, J.C. and Cook, C.C.H. (1997) The efficacy of disulfiram: a review of outcome studies. *Addiction*, **92**: 381–395.

Kahn, A., Mumford, J.P., Rogers, G.A. and Beckford, H. (1997) Double-blind study of lofexidine and clonidine in the detoxification of opiate addicts in hospital. *Drug and Alcohol Dependence*, **44**: 57–61.

Kosten, T.R. (1989) Pharmacotherapeutic interventions for cocaine abuse: matching patients to treatments. *Journal of Nervous and Mental Disease*, **177**: 379–389.

Krystal, J.H., D'Souza, D.C., Madonick, S. and Petrakis, I.L. (1999) Toward a rational pharmacotherapy of comorbid substance abuse in schizophrenic patients. *Schizophrenia Research*, **35**: S35–S49.

Lange, R.A. and Hills, L.D. (2001) Cardiovascular complications of cocaine use. *New England Journal of Medicine*, **345**: 351–358.

Levinson, I., Galynker, I.I. and Rosenthal, R.N. (1995). Methadone withdrawal psychosis. *Journal of Clinical Psychiatry*, **56**: 73–76.

Ling, W., Wesson, D.R. and Charuvastra, C. (1996) A controlled trial comparing buprenorphine and methadone maintenance in opioid dependence. *Archives of General Psychiatry*, **53**: 401–407.

Littleton, J. (1995) Acamprosate in alcohol dependence: how does it work? *Addiction*, **90**: 1179–1188.

Marcus, P. and Snyder, R. (1995) Reduction of comorbid substance abuse with clozapine. *American Journal of Psychiatry*, **152**: 959.

Marsch, L.A. (1998) The efficacy of methadone maintenance interventions in re-
ꓳꓳꓳ ꓳꓳ ꓳꓳꓳꓳꓳ ꓳꓳꓳꓳꓳꓳ ꓳꓳꓳ, ꓲꓲꓲ ꓳꓳꓳꓳ ꓳꓳꓳꓳꓳꓳꓳꓳꓳꓳ ꓳꓳꓳꓳꓳꓳꓳꓳ: ꓳ ꓳꓳꓳꓳꓳꓳꓳꓳꓳꓳꓳ. *Addiction*, **93**: 515–532.

Mayo-Smith, M.F. (1997) Pharmacological treatment of alcohol withdrawal: a meta-analysis and evidence-based practice guideline. American Society of Addiction Medicine Working Group on Pharmacological Management of Alcohol Withdrawal. *Journal of the American Medical Association*, **278**: 144–151.

McGrath, P.J., Nunes, E.V., Stewart, J.W., Goldman, D., Agosti, V., Ocepek-Welikson, K. and Quitkin, F.M. (1996) Imipramine treatment of alcoholics with primary depression. A placebo-controlled clinical trial. *Archives of General Psychiatry*, **53**: 232–240.

Moncrieff, J. and Drummond, D.C. (1997) New drug treatments for alcohol problems: a critical appraisal. *Addiction*, **92**: 939–947.

Mueser, K.T., Nishith, P., Tracy, J.I., DeGirolamo, J. and Molinaro, M. (1995) Expectations and motives for substance use in schizophrenia. *Psychiatric Clinics of North America*, **21**: 367–378.

Naranjo, C.A., Poulos, C.X., Bremner, K.E. and Lanctot, K.L. (1992) Citalopram decreases desirability, liking, and consumption of alcohol in alcohol-dependent drinkers. *Clinical Pharmacology and Therapeutics*, **51**: 729–739.

Nemeroff, C.B. (2000) An ever-increasing pharmacopeia for the management of patients with bipolar disorder. *Journal of Clinical Psychiatry*, **61** (Suppl 13): 19–25.

Nunes, E.V., McGrath, P.J., Quitkin, F.M., Stewart, J.P., Harrison, W., Tricamo, E. and Ocepek-Welikson, K. (1993) Imipramine treatment of alcoholism with comorbid depression. *American Journal of Psychiatry*, **150**: 963–965.

Nunes, E.V., McGrath, P.J., Wager, S. and Quitkin, F.M. (1990) Lithium treatment for cocaine abusers with bipolar spectrum disorder. *American Journal of Psychiatry*, **147**: 655–657.

Nunes, E.V., Quitkin, F.M., Donovan, S.J., Deliyannides, D., Ocepek-Welikson, K., Koenig, T., Brady, R., McGrath, P.J. and Woody, G. (1998) Imipramine treatment of opiate-dependent patients with depressive disorders. *Archives of General Psychiatry*, **55**: 153–160.

O'Connell, R.A., Mayo, J.A., Flatlow, L., Cuthbertson, B. and O'Brien, B.E. (1991) Outcome of bipolar disorder on long-term treatment with lithium. *British Journal of Psychiatry*, **159**: 123–129.

Olivera, A.A., Kiefer, M.W. and Manley, N.K. (1990) Tardive dyskinesia in psychiatric patients with substance use disorders. *American Journal of Drug and Alcohol Abuse*, **16**: 57–66.

Pelc, I., Verbanck, P., Bon, O.L., Gavrilovic, M., Lion, K. and Lehert, P. (1997) Efficacy and safety of acamprosate in the treatment of detoxified alcohol-dependent patients. *British Journal of Psychiatry*, **171**: 73–77.

Rao, S., Ziedonis, D. and Kosten, T. (1995) The pharmacotherapy of cocaine dependence. *Psychiatric Annals*, **25**: 363–368.

Regier, C.A., Farmer, M.E. and Rae, D.S. (1990) Comorbidity of mental disorders with alcohol and other drug abuse results from the epidemiologic catchment area (ECA) study. *Journal of the American Medical Association*, **264**: 2511–2518.

Report of the National Research Council Committee on Clinical Evaluation of Narcotic Antagonists (1978) Clinical evaluation of naltrexone treatment of opiate-dependent individuals. *Archives of General Psychiatry*, **35**: 335–340.

Sachs, G.S., Printz, D.J., Kahn, D.A., Carpenter, D. and Docherty, J.P. (2000) The Expert Consensus Guideline Series: "Medication Treatment of Bipolar Disorder 2000". *Postgraduate Medicine, Special Issue* (April): 1–104.

Schottenfeld, R.S., Pakes, J.R., Oliveto, A., Ziedonis, D. and Kosten, T.R. (1997) Buprenorphine vs methadone maintenance treatment for concurrent opioid dependence and cocaine abuse. *Archives of General Psychiatry*, **54**: 713–720.

Schuckit, M.A. (1996) Recent developments in the pharmacotherapy of alcohol dependence. *Journal of Consulting and Clinical Psychology*, **64**: 669–676.

Siris, S.G. (1990) Pharmacological treatment of substance-abusing schizophrenic patients. *Schizophrenia Bulletin*, **16**: 111–122.

Sonne, S.C. and Brady, K.T. (1999) Substance abuse and bipolar comorbidity. *Psychiatric Clinics of North America*, **22**: 609–627.

Sonne, S.C. and Brady, K.T. (2000) Naltrexone for individuals with comorbid bipolar disorder and alcohol dependence. *Journal of Clinical Psychopharmacology*, **20**: 114–115.

Sonne, S.C., Brady, K.T. and Morton, W.A. (1994) Substance abuse and bipolar affective disorder. *Journal of Nervous and Mental Disease*, **182**: 349–352.

Thornicroft, G. (1990). Cannabis and psychosis. Is there epidemiological evidence for an association? *British Journal of Psychiatry*, **157**: 25–33.

Tsuang, J.W., Eckman, T.E., Shaner, A. and Marder, S.R. (1999) Clozapine for substance-abusing schizophrenic patients. *American Journal of Psychiatry*, **156**: 1119–1120.

Volpicelli, J.R., Rhines, K.C., Rhines, J.S., Volpicelli, L.A., Alterman, A.I. and O'Brien, C.P. (1997) Naltrexone and alcohol dependence. *Archives of General Psychiatry*, **54**: 737–742.

White, R. (2000) Dexamphetamine substitution in the treatment of amphetamine abuse: an initial investigation. *Addiction*, **95**: 229–238.

Ziedonis, D., Richardson, T., Lee, E., Petrakis, I. and Kosten, T.(1992) Adjunctive desipramine in the treatment of cocaine abusing schizophrenics. *Psychopharmacology Bulletin*, **28**: 309–314.

Zimmet, S.V., Strous, R.D., Burgess, E.S., Kohnstamm, S. and Green, A.I. (2000) Effects of clozapine on substance use in patients with schizophrenia and schizoaffective disorder: a retrospective survey. *Journal of Clinical Psychopharmacology*, **20**: 94–98.

Part IV

SPECIAL POPULATIONS

INTRODUCTION

Hermine L. Graham

A number of assumptions regarding homogeneity are often made when we think about appropriate interventions for people with SMP. However, this section will provide an opportunity for service providers and clinicians to take a more in-depth look at the issues specific to a number of subgroups within the SMP population. These will include young people experiencing their first episode of psychosis, forensic populations, the homeless, and people with HIV/AIDS, all of whom present special challenges to effective treatment provision.

In Chapter 16, Edwards and colleagues focus on cannabis and first-episode psychosis. Consideration is given to the difficulties encountered in attempting to implement early intervention strategies with young people in light of the liberal attitudes today regarding recreational cannabis use. The psychosocial intervention outlined seeks to integrate the treatment of cannabis use into the treatment of psychosis, by educating clients about the critical links between the two and building motivation to change to enhance the recovery process.

In Chapter 17, Beck and colleagues explore the relationship between violent behaviour and SMP. It is suggested that there is an increased likelihood of violent behaviour among those with severe mental health problems, particularly after admission for the first psychotic episode and problematic polysubstance use. A number of significant challenges to the development of integrated treatment for this population are considered. The integrated relapse-prevention model and the forensic behaviour treatment unit described point a possible way forward for clinicians and service providers.

In Chapter 18, Pickett-Schenk and colleagues go on to highlight the marked negative outcomes, particularly social and housing, associated with those with SMP and the vicious cycle that ensues. An integrated demonstration project specifically tailored to the needs of this subgroup and its impact are described.

The final chapter in this section continues the theme of focusing on improving negative outcomes for the SMP population. Razzano draws attention to the issue of the prevalence of HIV among those with SMP and the significant risk factors inherent in substance-using behaviours, the associated lifestyle and experiencing mental health problems. Integrating a health education model into treatment is demonstrated, highlighting the need to consider increased sensitivity to psychotropic medication and drugs/alcohol and their interactions.

Chapter 16

CANNABIS AND FIRST-EPISODE PSYCHOSIS: THE CAP PROJECT

Jane Edwards, Mark Hinton, Kathryn Elkins and Olympia Athanasopoulos

Hi, my name is Hugh, I go to an inner-city high school, I am 17 years of age, and in 1998 I had psychosis. Today, I'm going to talk to you about having a psychosis and smoking dope. These are the pamphlets I used to help me [*displays two booklets and a pamphlet about cannabis and a fact sheet on cannabis and psychosis*]. These pamphlets are available out there.... There is help out there for you. I started smoking when I was 14. I was young and one of my mates asked if I wanted a bong. He had a gram on him and he mulled up and we hit-one-out in a coke bong. It was the first time I ever smoked and I started coughing my lungs out. Even the smell made me high. I started sort of hallucinating—when I closed my eyes I could imagine a box with pictures in it. That was really trippy. After that, I thought I'd never smoke again but a week later me and my friend decided that we'd have another smoke. This time it didn't hit me as hard but I was still knocked off my arse. After that I continued smoking weekly, then it went to daily, then all the time—by that I mean sessions every few hours. I was 16 by this time. The smoke made me feel relaxed and it gave me new friends who I still have today. I also tried some other drugs. When I was 14 I started dealing heroin and eventually ended up smoking it. Also tried cocaine, acid, ecstasy and speed. I liked ecstasy and used it quite regularly at raves. When I was 17 I was smoking a few grams a day—this eventually led on to me getting psychosis. Psychosis is really really really trippy. You don't actually know what you are thinking isn't true. Even when people tell you sense you make it out to be wrong. My psychosis involved me thinking I was the Son of God and that people were always talking about me and stuff and that my room was bugged. I used to catch a train twice a day to get from home to school. I used to sit on the train and think all the business people were talking about me. Friends told me I was just tripping and paranoid but I thought I couldn't be. I was *really* scared and anxious and I just wanted

Substance Misuse in Psychosis: Approaches to Treatment and Service Delivery.
Edited by Hermine L. Graham, Alex Copello, Max J. Birchwood and Kim T. Mueser.
© 2003 John Wiley & Sons, Ltd.

to get off the train. Things got worse from there and I went to hospital for a little while. After going to EPPIC, the people there really helped me get back on my feet and after about a month I almost felt back to my old self. I realized the stuff wasn't true and I felt relieved. I took medication for a while and am still taking it now. It makes sleeping and concentrating hard sometimes, which makes school harder, but on the brighter side it keeps the psychosis away. I had to make some other changes too. I stopped smoking dope and dropping ecstasy. I still really miss dope and ecstasy, not all the time, but sometimes it is hard. But I'd rather be sane than on drugs. My friends are really supportive in me not smoking dope. They don't offer me bongs, and if I ask for one, they just say "No way, man." They know I've had a psychosis and don't want me to have it again. I even worked at practising how to say "No, no thanks—I don't smoke dope any more." I am confident that I can say no and stay off dope. So today I want to tell you, but most importantly, I want to tell myself why I am not going to smoke dope again. I *never* want to have a psychosis again. It's scary and embarrassing. I don't like the person it made me. It is such a price to pay for a few minutes of pleasure, to have a relapse because I smoked dope. My friends and family would kill me if I smoked dope again, and I don't want to disappoint them.

[Transcript of video made by client and CAP therapist]

The literature regarding the coexistence of severe mental illness and substance use indicates that there is a substantial overlap of problems, particularly in adolescents and young adults (Linszen and Lenior, 1999). However, there are few data available, and treatment has been retarded (Selzer and Lieberman, 1993). The limited literature on cannabis and psychosis supports anecdotal evidence, and it suggests that cannabis use is associated with worse outcome in schizophrenia and related disorders (Hall and Degenhardt, 2000). Linszen et al (1994) argue that "treatment strategies have to be developed to discourage cannabis abuse by schizophrenic patients" and that "further studies should include cannabis abuse intervention programs" (p. 278).

The Early Psychosis Prevention and Intervention Centre (EPPIC) is a comprehensive community mental health service for individuals 15–29 years of age with first-episode psychosis (FEP) (Edwards and McGorry, 1998; McGorry and Edwards, 1997; McGorry et al, 1996). Between 1998 and 2001, the Victorian Government Department of Human Services (Australia) funded EPPIC to develop and evaluate a brief treatment intervention for individuals experiencing FEP and cannabis use, the Cannabis and Psychosis (CAP) project. Considerable experience had been gained with EPPIC clients who were continuing to use cannabis, and basic intervention strategies had been formulated. Additional advice was sought from relevant experts.[*]

---

[*]Expert consultants to the CAP project were Jon Evans, Geoff Munro, Stephen Allsop, Wayne Hall, David Kavanagh, Jean Addington, Kim Mueser and Roger Roffman. Allan Kellehear, Donald Linszen and Martin Hambrecht provided initial project support.

EPPIC aims to reduce the level of both primary and secondary morbidity in individuals with early psychosis through the dual strategy of identification of patients at the earliest stage from onset of psychosis and provision of intensive phase-specific treatment up to 18 months. Its philosophy and practice (McGorry and Edwards, 1997) adhere to the Australian Clinical Guidelines for Early Psychosis (National Early Psychosis Project Clinical Guidelines Working Party, 1998). The EPPIC catchment area covers the western metropolitan region of Melbourne, which is serviced by two public psychiatric hospitals and four adult mental health services. Important features of the region include large proportions of people born overseas or with at least one parent born overseas, low fluency in English, low-income households, high unemployment, a low proportion of people with university qualifications, and few private psychiatrists.

This chapter introduces the CAP intervention, which was developed over the past 3 years, and is further detailed in a treatment manual (http://www.eppic.org.au). The background and key influences of the CAP project are described, followed by FEP considerations. Comment is made on the need to integrate drug and alcohol with mental health treatment practices. The content of the CAP intervention is then summarized. The randomized, controlled trial is outlined and an illustrative CAP case provided.

It should be noted that the CAP intervention was developed to support early psychosis case managers (Edwards et al, 1999). CAP therapists are expected to have

1. experience in assessment and treatment of serious mental illness
2. familiarity with the early psychosis literature (e.g., Birchwood et al, 2000; McGorry, 1998; McGorry and Jackson, 1999)
3. an understanding of the principles and techniques of cognitive-behavioural therapy.

These three bodies of literature are not reviewed here.

BACKGROUND TO CAP

Substance misuse (abuse or dependence) has been reported to be a common comorbid problem in FEP (Curry et al, 1999; Hambrecht and Häfner 1996; Rabinowitz et al, 1998; Strakowski et al, 1995, 1996). EPPIC data suggest that approximately 70% of all FEP patients have used illicit substances, predominantly cannabis, within 12 months prior to initial presentation for treatment (Power et al, 1998), and that about 50% have used cannabis in the month prior to initial assessment (Rolfe et al, 1999). While it can be argued that the relationship between the amounts of cannabis consumed and the effects on mental state varies, there is little doubt that daily cannabis use increases the risk of relapse and continuing/increased symptoms in schizophrenia and related disorders, even in the early phase of illness (Gleeson et al, 2001; Kovasznay et al, 1997; Linszen et al, 1994).

Young people presenting with FEP who are daily cannabis users often do not receive the basic elements of treatment. There are many reasons for "missing out", including non-attendance, poor engagement, medication non-compliance, and the resultant failure to achieve stabilization of psychotic and mood symptoms. The heavy cannabis user is frequently in crisis, and the case manager must undertake numerous tasks related to financial, accommodation, legal, general health, family and/or other interpersonal problems. These clients require active intervention geared for assertive outreach, with a focus on education about psychosis, cannabis, and the relationship between the two.

There is an extensive literature on the dual diagnosis of substance misuse and mental illness (e.g., Addington and el-Guebaly, 1998; Bellack and DiClemente, 1999; Levin et al, 1998; Maisto et al, 1999). Samples have comprised, for the most part, multiple substance users from the USA with long-standing psychotic conditions. The majority of studies have focused on polysubstances or "serious" drugs such as heroin or cocaine.

However, there is a dearth of published randomized, controlled trials for substance misuse. Lehman et al (1993) randomized 54 dually diagnosed individuals to intensive case management and an innovative group programme. The subjects were aged 18–40 years, and most had severe disorders. This trial failed to show any significant benefit, a result which was mostly attributed to a large drop-out rate and lack of readiness to engage in treatment. The only interventions for cannabis specifically are those targetted at the general school-age population (e.g., Klepp et al, 1995). Such studies have been undertaken in an educational environment and have not led to a sustained reduction in alcohol and cannabis use.

TREATMENT INFLUENCES

In developing the CAP intervention, we drew on current trends in the treatment of substance misuse and results from an EPPIC study undertaken by Rolfe et al (1999).

Brief interventions

Research interest has been growing in brief interventions, particularly in the alcohol field, targetting those who use alcohol excessively and who show few, if any, signs of dependence. These individuals often present for assistance in general health facilities for reasons not identified as associated with alcohol use (Rollnick et al, 1992), and health workers are presented with a brief opportunity to intervene. In a review of brief-intervention studies in the alcohol field, Bien et al (1993) concluded: "Brief interventions are more effective than no counselling, and often as effective as more extensive treatment" (p. 315).

Harm minimization

The focus of CAP is "problematic" cannabis use among young people with a psychotic illness in a "harm minimization" framework. Labelling cannabis use in negative terms and insisting that individuals reduce or totally abstain from cannabis use is largely unsuccessful. Rather, cannabis is considered with a view to exploring harm to the individual. Harm to self and others includes exacerbation of psychosis, failure to respond to treatment, persistent illness, and ongoing problems such as poor finances, poor nutrition, poor clothing, isolation, homelessness, and health and forensic consequences. The harm minimization framework is a non-judgemental and non-confrontational approach that promotes open discussion of cannabis use. Discussion of the quantity and quality of cannabis use is relevant only with regard to assessing potential harm.

Stages of change

Prochaska and DiClemente (1986) developed the "Transtheoretical model of behaviour change" to account for the process of achieving successful, permanent change in problematic substance use. They suggest that individuals cycle through six stages: precontemplation, contemplation, determination, action, maintenance, and relapse. They reinforce the need to match treatment to an individual's position in the model. Clinicians often assume that patients are at the "action stage"; however, most substance users are ambivalent about change and are, at best, contemplating change. Motivational interviewing techniques are used in the CAP intervention to enhance and develop commitment to change substance use.

Cannabis and psychosis link

It is our experience that a first psychotic episode can serve as powerful motivator to change substance use habits, since patients are frequently traumatized by the psychotic experience and its implications. There is a group of individuals for whom cannabis use has an immediate, aversive impact upon their psychosis, producing or exacerbating noxious symptoms. Rolfe et al (1999) suggest that approximately 50% of those who are using cannabis in the month prior to initial presentation cease use in the 6–8 weeks thereafter (within a context of receiving routine clinical care at EPPIC) for this reason. For others who are slower to draw a link between cannabis use and their illness course, or who do not experience negative consequences immediately after use, education about the potential impact of cannabis upon psychosis can serve as a powerful motivator of behaviour change. The latter is often witnessed via some experimentation with the drug, at varying times and in differing quantities, as the individual monitors the effects upon symptoms.

FIRST-EPISODE CONSIDERATIONS

There are a number of considerations for the FEP population that suggest modification to substance-use interventions.

Age of clients

Young people do not respond well to lecturing and confrontation. This can be even more pronounced in individuals with a psychotic illness, who often present with tentative engagement, loss of confidence, paranoia, fragile self esteem, and mood disturbance. The destructive influence of a confrontational intervention style has been discussed at length by Miller (1983), who suggests that the clinician must not adopt an authoritarian parental role.

Treatment entry

The circumstances that bring individuals to treatment demand sensitivity with regard to establishing rapport and raising the issue of cannabis use. As a result of the potential risk of harm to self others associated with a psychotic illness, many patients who enter mental health services are coerced into treatment. Frequently, individuals with FEP present as unconcerned about cannabis use. Such circumstances are very different from those of clients who attend drug and alcohol services either wanting to or "having to" examine their substance use. In early CAP sessions, the focus is on engagement and establishing rapport as priorities in treatment.

Variability

FEP clients present with comorbid DSM IV Axes I and II (American Psychiatric Association, 1994) disorders, varying patterns of substance use, and at different phases of recovery from the psychotic illnesses. There is a need for sound clinical judgement about individual needs, reviewed on a session-to-session basis, and considerable flexibility in treatment.

Impact of psychosis

The following factors potentially compromise the ability of an individual with a psychotic illness to respond to treatment: confusion and thought disorder; cognitive function deficits, particularly in relation to mental control; concentration, attention, and memory problems; paranoia; distraction associated with enduring positive symptoms; poor motivation; and asociality associated with enduring negative symptoms. While EPPIC adopts a "start low, go slow" medication policy (National Early Psychosis Project Clinical Guidelines Working Party, 1998), side effects can also have a marked physical and psychological impact, and can compromise active engagement in treatment. The introduction of strategies to assist with understanding and retention of information may be required.

Negative effects of cannabis

Use of cannabis frequently destabilizes the mental state and leads to poor motivation. Considerable stress can be caused by the financial demands of the drug. Cannabis can exacerbate respiratory problems such as asthma and bronchitis. Family disapproval and legal issues are also potentially problematic. These factors can prolong recovery and/or increase the risk of relapse. The result is that the individual neither achieves a stable mental state nor develops the supportive environment necessary to achieve behaviour change with regard to cannabis use. Thus, on occasions, the first step may be to secure a safe, "cannabis-free" environment in which the patient can achieve a stable mental state prior to attempts to influence motivation for behaviour change.

Social network

The social network for an individual experiencing FEP and abusing substances often presents a major challenge to intervention. Many individuals with FEP have drifted toward or further immersed themselves in drug-using social circles in recent times. Most patients have numerous friends or family members who use more cannabis than they do without having developed psychotic disorders. The early phases of CAP involve much psychoeducation—the issue of individual differences and vulnerabilities is raised with regard to impact of cannabis on mental health. Moreover, "belonging" to a cannabis-using network is often viewed favourably by the client. Strategies for lifestyle modifications and surviving in a cannabis-permissive social group are approached in the later CAP sessions.

INTEGRATING THERAPEUTIC APPROACHES

The delivery of effective interventions has been complicated by the split between drug and alcohol services and mental health services in many countries, including Australia. The differences in therapeutic approaches between clinicians from "drug and alcohol" and "mental health" professional backgrounds are quite marked. Within the drug and alcohol context, clients are expected to make appointments and attend at the time arranged, and to present in a manner that suggests interest in examining current substance use. FEP clients presenting to mental health services are typically viewed as more fragile, with their mental state potentially in flux, relapse an ongoing possibility, and the need constantly to review risk assessment. Additionally, their insight and motivation may be poor. As such, the mental health clinicians tend to demonstrate greater flexibility in terms of boundaries and expectations, and at times are required to take responsibility for treatment decisions on the client's behalf.

The question is how to align the two approaches to produce a consistent response to the individual presenting with the dual problem of FEP and problematic cannabis use. By way of resolution, it is important that the clinician adopts a position that reflects the dual philosophies. The patient has responsibility for management of substance use, as is generally the case with psychotic illness; however, the necessary support is provided to promote goal-directed activity when deficits associated with psychosis prove a handicap. The clinician must repeatedly question whether the patient's difficulties are associated with psychotic illness or an avoidance of responsibility for, and poor commitment to, cannabis-use goals.

The CAP intervention takes the following approach to the obstacles encountered:

Non-attendance

The client is contacted within 24 h of missing an appointment. Clinicians inquire about the barriers preventing the participant from attending the previous appointment and strategies which might be used to assist in overcoming these barriers in the future. A further appointment is then offered.

Intoxication

The issue of intoxication is discussed in the introductory sessions. Clinicians contract with clients to attend sessions with sensorium uncompromised by substances. The rationale is that the participant's memory, concentration and attention can be affected by substances. Clinicians demonstrate some flexibility by negotiating appointment times at which participants are more likely to manage to abstain from using (e.g., morning appointments). When participants attend appointments intoxicated, sessions are terminated and a further appointment is made.

Crisis

Clinicians approach crises with some flexibility. All crises are acknowledged by the clinician and briefly discussed at the commencement of the session. Thereafter, a course of action is agreed between the clinician and the participant. If the client's anxieties can be allayed, the session proceeds. Alternatively, if the crisis warrants immediate attention, the session is terminated and an appointment is made for a later date. Routine crisis procedures used by the mental health service are adopted.

Confidentiality

Establishing the obligations and boundaries of confidentiality in the introductory sessions is critical in developing rapport. Suspicious or paranoid individuals experience difficulty with engagement, and this can be exacerbated when discussing use of a prohibited substance such as cannabis. Frank discussion of the role of the clinician with regard to other professionals (e.g., the referrer, treatment team, and the supervisor), and the nature of case documentation and access to the same, can be helpful. A full explanation of the circumstances in which confidentiality may be breached, such as risk to the safety of clients or others, should be provided.

CAP INTERVENTION

When assessment indicates ongoing cannabis use at 4–6 weeks after initiation of treatment for FEP, a "cannabis-focused" approach is recommended. It is assumed that, prior to a cannabis-focused intervention, clients will have been assigned a case manager and attempts made to provide psychoeducation. Ideally, psychoeducation involves provision of information about the nature and course of psychosis, medication and other treatment approaches, the nature of recovery, relapse prevention, and service system details (see McGorry and Edwards, 1997: Module 9). Clearly, use of other substances will also be a focus of treatment if indicated—see approaches to other substances outlined in this book.

The CAP approach involves six phases of treatment. The goals and strategies of each phase of treatment are outlined in Table 16.1 and should be examined alongside the summaries outlined below. The clinician needs to be sensitive to the selection of the appropriate phase of treatment and timing of the progression from phase to phase. The client is seen individually with the aim of personalizing treatment (Jarvis et al, 1995). Individual treatment is preferred to a group intervention, as the latter is difficult with regard to varying stages of change among participants. Sessions are highly structured, last 20–60 min and occur on a weekly basis. As clients achieve the goals of each phase, and their cannabis use stabilizes, sessions become less frequent, and the time period between interviews can be increased. Clinicians are encouraged to identify and reinforce successful solutions already within the client's repertoire (DeShazer, 1985; Walter and Peller, 1992). Positive reinforcement of clients' belief that they can achieve their goals is supported at every opportunity.

Phase one—entry

The goal of phase 1 is to engage clients and raise the issue of their cannabis use. The focus is on assessment, particularly history taking (see Table 16.2) and gaining an understanding of the clients' explanatory model. Feedback, including comment on cannabis use, should be linked with psychoeducation. Emphasis is placed on the interaction of cannabis use and psychosis, and differentiation of problematic and non-problematic cannabis use. Information regarding readiness to change cannabis use should be apparent from assessment data. A cannabis use diary can be introduced to

Table 16.1   Aims and strategies of the six phases of the CAP intervention

Phase	Aims	Strategies
1. Entry	Engagement Commitment to treatment Raise the issue of problematic cannabis use	Case formulation Feedback of findings from assessment Exploring explanatory model of psychosis Exploring views on interaction of cannabis and psychosis Assess readiness to change Psychoeducation Explore and problem solve barriers to attendance
2. Commitment	Building commitment to a goal of non-problematic cannabis use	Motivational interviewing Harm minimization Psychoeducation about Cannabis Psychosis Cannabis and psychosis
3. Goal setting	Reinforcing commitment to change Setting a non-problematic cannabis goal Development of goal achievement strategies	Motivational interviewing revisited Goal setting Psychoeducation
4. Challenges	Adopting a sound approach to potential challenges to cannabis reduction goals	Withdrawal counselling Problem solving Relapse prevention Psychoeducation Personalized feedback
5. Lifestyle	Examination of factors that are "threats" to the short-term achievement and long-term maintenance of non-problematic cannabis use Consider positive lifestyle change to support cannabis goals	Relapse prevention Cannabis refusal skills Time management Motivational interviewing revisited Psychoeducation
6. Maintenance	Maintenance of motivation to a commitment to non-problematic cannabis use Ongoing consideration of positive lifestyle change to support cannabis goals	Relapse prevention Coping skills Time management Motivational interviewing revisited Psychoeducation Reinforcement of psychoeducation

Table 16.2   Questions to ask the CAP client

Psychosis
Why are you attending this service?
What is your understanding of the word "psychosis"?
What does your treating team say the diagnosis is?
Do you know anyone who has a psychotic illness?
What do your family and friends think has happened?
Why has this happened now?

Cannabis
What do you know about cannabis?
What do you think of your cannabis use?
What does cannabis do for you? (i.e., what function does it serve?)
What about you and cannabis in the future?
Does your cannabis use differ from that of others?

Cannabis and psychosis
Do you think cannabis has an effect on psychosis, or vice versa?
What has been the effect upon your psychosis when you use cannabis?
What do you know about cannabis and psychosis? Have you met anyone
    who uses cannabis and has experienced psychosis?
What would you advise others who are thinking of using cannabis for the
    first time?
What would you say to others who have a psychotic illness and use cannabis?

---

acquire baseline information when the client agrees to participate in future
sessions.

Phase 2—commitment

The goal of phase 2 is to persuade clients that their cannabis use is potentially problematic and, therefore, to consider a goal of non-problematic
cannabis use. Motivational interviewing (Miller and Rollnick, 1991) is
applied, after discussion of "current thinking" about the impact of
cannabis use on psychosis. Educational resources are introduced, such as
the *Cannabis and Psychosis Fact Sheet* (<http://www.dhs.vic.gov.au/phd/
hdev/cannabis/booklet/contents.htm>), a cannabis video titled *What's
Your Poison?* (Bell, 1997), the booklets *A Guide to Quitting Marijuana*
(Grenyer et al, 2001) and *Mulling It Over* (Bleeker and Malcolm, 1998),
and relevant websites (e.g., <http://www.abc.net.au/quantum/poison/
marijuan/marijuan.htm>).[*]

---

[*]The cannabis booklets and video can be purchased through the Australian Drug Foundation
(ADF) (http://www.adf.org.au). It should be noted that the ADF has also produced *How
Drugs Affect You: Cannabis* (pamphlet) and *Dealing with Cannabis Use: A Guide for Parents*
(booklet).

Phase 3—goal setting

In phase 3, the clinician revisits the client's "statement of intent" with the aim of formulating clear goals for cannabis reduction in the immediate, short-term, and long-term future. The strategy for goal achievement includes securing support from significant others where possible. If the goal involves continuing to use cannabis (e.g., gradual reduction), then strategies to reduce the harm associated with obtaining, using, being intoxicated with, or coming off cannabis are considered. For example, clients may be encouraged to limit use to safe or familiar environments, or to use cannabis in food to reduce the harmful effects of smoking. Suggestions to use weaker cannabis or to switch to low-tar cigarettes may also be helpful.

Phase 4—challenges

The focus in phase 4 is the identification of immediate challenges to cannabis reduction goals and the introduction of a general approach to problem solving (D'Zurilla and Goldfried, 1971). Withdrawal counselling is usually indicated. This involves education about cannabis withdrawal and the development of strategies to assist coping with distressing withdrawal symptoms. Construction of a risk hierarchy (i.e., hierarchy of threats to the client's cannabis reduction goals) is undertaken, and strategies to manage risk situations are developed. Clients are first encouraged to approach a situation that is minimally challenging to test coping strategies before attempting more difficult situations (e.g., going to the movies "straight" with parents before driving with friends).

Phase 5—lifestyle

Maintenance of a commitment to change cannabis use rests on providing a positive lifestyle change that reinforces initial decisions to modify past cannabis habits. The focus of phase 5 is to assist the client to identify lifestyle issues that could contribute to relapse, including skill deficits, socializing with cannabis-using friends, and boredom. Relapse triggers such as negative emotional states (e.g., loneliness, anxiety, anger, and depression) and interpersonal conflict should be identified and addressed.

Phase 6—maintenance

In phase 6 treatment, clinicians contact clients, after a predetermined period of time (i.e., 6–12 weeks), with the objective of reinforcing strategies and "boosting" motivation to maintain goals. Given evidence of the unhelpful cognitive distortions that emerge with the passage of time after an initial decision to modify substance use (e.g., fond recall of "the good times" and a blank on "the bad times" associated with cannabis use), booster sessions are a reminder of the initial reasons that change in cannabis use was indicated. Furthermore, clients report that having to provide feedback on progress with regard to cannabis reduction goals serves as an incentive to maintain goals, particularly when they are feeling vulnerable to lapse.

CAP RANDOMIZED CONTROLLED TRIAL (RCT)

The purpose of the CAP project is to examine the relationship between cannabis use and FEP, and to evaluate a brief intervention for "problematic" cannabis use. The design of the RCT involves EPPIC patients who have used cannabis in the previous month, as assessed at the second of four assessment time points (i.e., 6–8 weeks after initiation of treatment), being randomized into CAP therapy or the control condition—in this case, psychoeducation (see McGorry and Edwards, 1997: Module 9). All patients continue to receive routine EPPIC case-management services. The assessment instruments used in the study are listed in Table 16.3.

The participants comprised 193 individuals assessed at entry (T1) to EPPIC; 57% used cannabis in the previous month (first use: mean [M] age = 14.8, SD = 3.2; regular use: M age = 17.0, SD = 3.2), and 30% used daily. Reassessment of 130 individuals (M age: 21.7, SD = 3.6) was done 6–8 weeks subsequently (T2). We defined "non-problem" as no cannabis use in the previous month, and "problem users" as using cannabis in the previous month, regardless of the amount. There was a trend for a greater percentage of the T2 drop-outs to be problem users (60.3%) than of the T2 completers (49% problem users), although this was not significant. Of the 64 problem users at T1, 48% reported not using cannabis in the month preceding T2. At T2, problem users scored significantly higher than the non-problem group on the BPRS (total score, psychotic subscale, and depression item) and BDI; there were no significant differences between groups on the BPRS anxiety and suicidality items and the SANS (see Table 16.3 for full names of these assessment instruments). The pattern of other substance use was similar across non-problem and problem users, with alcohol being the most frequently reported substance used. The results on psychopathology measures for non-problem and problem users were covaried for alcohol use, and the results remained similar. A number of problem users refused the intervention trial, and the remainder were randomized to one of the two treatment conditions—23 CAP and 23 psychoeducation. All post-intervention follow-ups (T3) are complete, and the final 6-month post-intervention assessments

Table 16.3 CAP assessment instruments

Illness
- SCID-DSM-IV (First et al, 1996)
- Brief Psychiatric Rating Scale—Expanded (BPRS-E) (Lukoff et al, 1986)
- Scale for the Assessment of Negative Symptoms (SANS) (Andreasen, 1984)
- Beck Depression Inventory—Short Form (BDI-SF) (Beck and Beck, 1972), Liverpool
- University Neuroleptic Side-Effect Rating Scale (LUNSERS) (Day et al, 1995)
- Knowledge Questionnaire (KQ) (Birchwood et al, 1992)—a modified version

Substance
- Cannabis and Substance Use Assessment Schedule (CASUAS), adapted from the Schedule for Clinical Assessment in Neuropsychiatry (SCAN) (Wing et al, 1990)
- Addiction Severity Index (ASI) (McLellan et al, 1985)
- Readiness to Change Questionnaire—Cannabis (RCQ-C) (Rollnick et al, 1992)

Cognitive and General
- Social and Occupational Functioning Scale (SOFAS) (American Psychiatric Association, 1994)
- Health of the Nation Outcome Scale (HoNOS) (Wing et al, 1996)
- National Adult Reading Test (NART) (Nelson and Willison, 1991)
- WAIS-R—4 sub-tests (Kaufman, 1990)
- Premorbid Functioning Assessment Scale (PAS) (Cannon-Spoor et al, 1982)
- Quality of Life Scale (QLS) (Lehman, 1988)

(T4) are in progress. Treatment results have not yet been examined for fear of biasing the therapists.

"STEVE": CAP CASE NOTES

The following case of Steve illustrates CAP as provided within the 10-session (maximum) framework of a RCT. The phase approach previously described is undertaken within the time constraints. Obviously, many clients will not proceed through all the stages consecutively (certainly not in 10 sessions), and there may be more flexibility outside the research situation.

Steve, a 22-year-old, single man of Greek origin, lived with his parents in the western suburbs of Melbourne, and was employed in computer sales. He was referred to the EPPIC by his mother, who reported significant behaviour change and increasing cannabis use over the past 12 months. He was described as argumentative and irritable, believing that others were out to "get him", and that people on the radio and television were talking about him. Steve first used cannabis at age 18 and had since experimented with speed, heroin, and ecstasy. After completion of high school, he attempted a university computer course, but this was interrupted by his deteriorating mental state.

Steve disputed his mother's concerns and refused involvement with the EPPIC. He was eventually admitted to the EPPIC inpatient unit and discharged 3 days later on a community treatment order (i.e., legal requirement to continue medication). At the second CAP assessment, 6 weeks post-entry to the EPPIC, he admitted to using cannabis in the previous month. He had returned to full-time work and reluctantly agreed to see a CAP therapist after work. His psychotic symptoms had partially remitted.

Sessions 1 and 2

The therapist empathized with Steve's distress at the EPPIC follow-up, but asked why his mother had been concerned. He spoke about his cannabis use, giving the therapist the opportunity to explore current and past substance use. A detailed history was gathered and his substance use was neither condoned nor supported by the therapist. Asked about his explanatory model of psychosis and the interaction between cannabis and psychosis, Steve said he did not have a psychosis but had heard that drugs can make you "trip out". The therapist tried to stimulate curiosity about cannabis and psychosis, and requested his comments on the information from the "experts" contained in the *Cannabis and Psychosis Fact Sheet*. The therapist expressed interest in Steve's views on a video about cannabis titled *What's Your Poison?* and suggested they view it together at the next session. Didactic discussion about the nature of psychosis ensued. Steve agreed to attend the following week.

Session 3

The therapist further investigated Steve's comments about cannabis "making you trip out". They watched the video. Steve was given the remote control and encouraged to pause if he wished to comment on key points. He became more relaxed and admitted knowing little about the negative effects of cannabis. He said that he was waiting to see if "it was going to start up again", and that he had tripped out the last time he smoked. The therapist enquired about the impact of cannabis on his thoughts, behaviour, motivation, and relationships. Steve asked questions about the video. He used personal information in the discussion about cannabis and psychosis that ensued.

Session 4

Steve began to think that he may have had psychosis and that cannabis could have contributed to his condition. The therapist explored his experience of

Table 16.4 Steve's Decisional Balance Grid

	Making up your mind exercise	
	Using	Changing
Benefits	Relax Fit in with mates, "what we do" Passes time Helps me sleep	Keeps me sane Prevents the psychosis from coming back Makes me feel better Get along with family Less paranoid More money to spend on other stuff Not dependent on it No cravings when you are over it

Costs	Makes you "trip out"
	Financial costs
	Makes me paranoid
	I have arguments over it with
	  my family
	Involved with the wrong crowd
	Have got into theft
	Bad for your health
	Don't want to do it for ever
	Don't want my brother to
	  smoke
	Can't imagine smoking in
	  a relationship
		Lost some friends
		Don't go to the same places I used to

psychosis and acknowledged difficulty in coming to grips with what had happened. Current and future cannabis use was examined. The therapist suggested that he could take an active part in his recovery by controlling cannabis use. The Decisional Balance Grid, summarized in Table 16.4, was used to weigh up the costs and benefits before setting a goal for future cannabis use. Steve said he wanted to work towards abstinence because he did not want to risk a relapse or exacerbation of symptoms. He agreed to keep a cannabis use diary.

Sessions 5 and 6

Steve reported 2 weeks of not using cannabis. Withdrawal symptoms were outlined, and the therapist encouraged him to take "one day at a time", emphasizing the temporary nature of withdrawal symptoms. Boredom after work, difficulties in sleeping and peer influence were determined to be risk factors for relapse. Activities after work were planned, good sleeping habits were outlined, and scenarios of being offered cannabis were role-played with the aim of being assertive and practising saying "no".

Session 7

Steve reported that he had had two "bongs" on the previous Saturday night to see what would happen. He said he had felt no ill effects and queried whether cannabis would affect him again. The costs and benefits of continuing cannabis use were re-examined via reference to the Decisional Balance Grid. Steve renewed his commitment to work on his goal despite the lapse. The therapist elicited other high-risk situations and focused on developing problem-solving skills. Steve and the therapist reviewed the factors initially contributing to cannabis use, and the therapist reinforced the need to consider future lifestyle changes.

Sessions 8 and 9

Steve reported being "back on track". Since the last session, he had been confronted with a further situation where he was tempted to use cannabis, but this time he was able to say "no". The therapist commenced planning for termination. Steve was asked what would remind him about his negative experience with cannabis and motivate him to pursue his commitment to abstinence. He suggested that a written statement of his goal and rationale for the same would be helpful. Steve and therapist wrote such as statement together during the last session.

The first three sessions with Steve were devoted to *phase 1* tasks and involved engagement, history taking and assessment of cannabis use, and exploration of an explanatory model. The "facts" seemed to help Steve understand how cannabis had affected his thinking. As the psychotic symptoms further improved, he began to make the link between psychosis and cannabis, facilitated by psychoeducation. *Phases 2* and *3* followed in tandem—*phase 2* focused on commitment to change, and *phase 3* concerned goal setting. With developing insight, Steve become fearful of relapse and decided that he was going to do something about "the bit" he could control, i.e., cannabis. *Phases 4, 5 and 6* concerned both the immediate challenges and the lifestyle changes required to maintain Steve's goal in the future.

> After two years with psychosis it was difficult for anyone to make me understand that I had it after I got out of hospital. I was overwhelmed with joy that my life was given back to me. It took me more than six months to work out what reality was inside me. Slowly I've been remembering more detail about what I went through which keeps me in line my behaviour towards certain substances. My life has been great ever since and I never want to look at drugs again.
>   [Steve's faxed response to reading the above case notes, 14/12/2000]

SUMMARY

"Do you think purple butterflies can fly?"
"What the fuck is that supposed to mean? It's that kind of shit I'm talking about. You can't go around saying shit like that. Nobody knows what the hell you're talking about. You need to see someone. You're completely fucked. You haven't slept or eaten in days, and you're acting really weird. Do you want to end up like your uncle?"
"Hmm, maybe they can fly, but I doubt it. Can you pass the bong?"
[Extract from essay shown to EPPIC case manager]

Cannabis use in young people with FEP often plays a major role in inhibiting recovery. The crisis of initiation of treatment for FEP provides an opportunity to encourage these individuals to rethink old habits in the context of new health risks. The early psychosis mental health worker is in an ideal position to influence the choices made at this phase of illness. The aim of CAP is to package a "do-it-yourself", user-friendly intervention strategy that, ideally, the busy case manager can apply in such situations. A randomized, controlled trial is under way, and results will be analysed during 2002.

ACKNOWLEDGEMENTS

CAP is funded by the Victorian Government Department of Human Services. Kerri Donovan, Michelle Downing, and Christina Curry collected the CAP assessments. Susy Harrigan completed data analyses. We are most grateful to the three individuals who gave permission to include the video transcript, case notes/fax, and essay extract ("Have a Nice Trip" by Jayne Cossar).

REFERENCES

Addington, J. and el-Guebaly, N. (1998) Group treatment for substance abuse in schizophrenia. *Canadian Journal of Psychiatry*, **43**: 843–845.

American Psychiatric Association (1994) *Diagnostic and Statistical Manual of Mental Disorders* (4th edn, Rev.). Washington, DC, APA.

Andreason, N.C. (1984) *Scale for the Assessment of Negative Symptoms (SANS)*. Iowa, University of Iowa.

Beck, A.T. and Beck, R.W. (1972) Screening for depressed patients in family practice: a rapid technique. *Postgraduate Medicine*, **52**: 81–85.

Bell, J. (Producer) (1997) *What's Your Poison? Part 3. Marijuana*. Australia, ABC Science Unit.

Bellack, A.S. and DiClemente, C.C. (1999) Treating substance abuse among patients with schizophrenia. *Psychiatric Services*, **50**: 75–80.

Bien, T.H., Miller, W.R. and Tonigan, J.S. (1993) Brief interventions for alcohol problems: a review. *Addiction*, **88**: 315–333.

Birchwood, M., Fowler, D. and Jackson, C. (Eds.) (2000) *Early Intervention in Psychosis: A Guide to Concepts, Evidence and Interventions*. Chichester, Wiley.

Birchwood, M., Smith, J. and Cochrane, R. (1992) Specific and non-specific effects of educational intervention for families with schizophrenia: a comparison of three methods. *British Journal of Psychiatry*, **160**: 806–814.

Bleeker, A. and Malcolm, A. (1998) *Mulling It Over: Health Information for People Who Use Cannabis* [Booklet]. Manly, NSW: Manly Drug Education and Counselling Centre.

Cannon-Spoor, E., Potkin, S. and Wyatt, R.J. (1982) Measurement of pre-morbid adjustment in chronic schizophrenia. *Schizophrenia Bulletin*, **8**: 470–484.

Curry, C., Smith, D. and McGorry, P.D. (1999) The intensity, prevalence, and client characteristics of cannabis use in first onset psychosis. Paper presented at the Inaugural International Cannabis and Psychosis Conference, Melbourne, Australia.

Day, J.C., Wood, G., Dewey, M. and Bentall, R.P. (1995) A self-rating scale for measuring neuroleptic side effects: validation in a group of schizophrenic patients. *British Journal of Psychiatry*, **166**: 650–653.

DeShazer, S. (1985) *Keys to Solution in Brief Therapy*. New York, Norton.

D'Zurilla, T.J. and Goldfried, M. (1971) Problem solving and behavior modification. *Journal of Abnormal Psychology*, **78**: 107–126.

Edwards, J., Cocks, J. and Bott, J. (1999) Preventive case management in first-episode psychosis. In P.D. McGorry and H.J. Jackson (Eds.), *Recognition and Management of Early Psychosis: A Preventive Approach*, pp. 308–337. New York, Cambridge University Press.

Edwards, J. and McGorry, P.D. (1998) Early intervention in psychotic disorders: a critical step in the prevention of psychological morbidity. In C. Perris and P.D. McGorry (Eds.), *Cognitive Psychotherapy of Psychotic and Personality Disorders*, pp. 167–195. Chichester, Wiley.

First, M.B., Spitzer, R.L., Gibbon, M. and Williams, J.B.W. (1996) *Structured Clinical Interview for DSM-IV Axis I Disorders*. New York, Biometrics Research Department, New York State Psychiatric Institute.

Gleeson, J.F., McGorry, P.D., Rawlings, D. and Jackson, H.J. (2001) Predictors of first episode psychotic relapse following remission in first-episode psychosis: a 12-month prospective follow-up. *Schizophrenia Research*, **49** (Suppl): Special Issue: Abstracts VIIIth International Conference on Schizophrenia Research, pp. 13–14.

Grenyer, B., Solowij, N. and Peters, R. (2001) *What's the Deal on Quitting* [Booklet]. New South Wales, National Drug and Alcohol Research Centre, University of New South Wales.

Hall, W. and Degenhardt, L. (2000) Cannabis use and psychosis: a review of clinical and epidemiological evidence. *Australian and New Zealand Journal of Psychiatry*, **34**: 26–34.

Hambrecht, M. and Häfner, H. (1996) Substance abuse and the onset of schizophrenia. *Biological Psychiatry*, **40**: 1155–1163.

Jackson, H.J., Edwards, J., McGorry, P.D. and Hulbert, C. (1999) Recovery from psychosis: psychological interventions. In P.D. McGorry and H.J. Jackson (Eds.), *Recognition and Management of Early Psychosis: A Preventive Approach*, pp. 265–307. New York, Cambridge University Press.

Jarvis, J.T., Tebbutt, J. and Mattick, R. (1995) *Treatment Approaches for Alcohol and Drug Dependence: An Introductory Guide*. New York, Wiley.

Kaufman, A.S. (1990) *Assessing Adolescent and Adult Intelligence*. Boston, Allyn & Bacon.

Klepp, K.I., Kelder, S.H. and Perry, C.L. (1995) Alcohol and marijuana use among adolescents: long-term outcome of the class of 1989 study. *Annals of Behavioral Medicine*, **17**: 19–24.

Kovasznay, B., Fleischer, J., Tanenberg-Karant, M., Jandorf, L., Miller, A.D. and Bromet, E. (1997) Substance use disorder and the early course of illness in schizophrenia and affective psychosis. *Schizophrenia Bulletin*, **23**: 195–201.

Lehman, A.F. (1988) A quality of life interview for the chronically mentally ill. *Evaluation and Programme Planning*, **11**: 51–62.

Lehman, A.F., Herron, J.D., Schwartz R.P. and Myers C.P. (1993) Rehabilitation for adults with severe mental illness and substance abuse disorders. *Journal of Nervous and Mental Disease*, **181**: 86–90.

Levin, F.R., Evans, S.M., Coomaraswammy, S., Collins, E.D., Regent, N. and Kleber, H.D. (1998) Flupenthixol treatment for cocaine abusers with schizophrenia: a pilot study. *American Journal of Drug and Alcohol Abuse*, **24**: 343–360.

Linszen, D.H., Dingemans, P.M. and Lenior, M.E. (1994) Cannabis abuse and the course of recent-onset schizophrenic disorders. *Archives of General Psychiatry*, **51**: 273–279.

Linszen, D.H. and Lenior, M.E. (1999) Early psychosis and substance abuse. In P.D. McGorry and H.J. Jackson (Eds.), *Recognition and Management of Early Psychosis: A Preventive Approach*, pp. 363–375. New York, Cambridge University Press.

Lukoff, D., Neuchterlein, K.H. and Ventura, J. (1986) Manual for the Expanded Brief Psychiatric Rating Scale. *Schizophrenia Bulletin*, **12**: 594–602.

Maisto, S.A., Carey, K.B., Carey, M.P., Purnine, D.M. and Barnes, K.L. (1999) Methods of changing patterns of substance use among individuals with co-occurring schizophrenia and substance use disorder. *Journal of Substance Abuse Treatment*, **17**: 221–227.

McGorry, P.D. (Ed.) (1998) Verging on reality. *British Journal of Psychiatry*, **173** (Suppl 33).

McGorry, P.D. and Edwards, J. (1997) *Early Psychosis Training Pack*. Cheshire, Gardiner-Caldwell Communications. [online] Available: http://www.eppic.org.au/~resources

McGorry, P.D., Edwards, J., Mihalopoulos, C., Harrigan, S. and Jackson, H.J. (1996) Early psychosis prevention and intervention centre: an evolving system for early detection and intervention. *Schizophrenia Bulletin*, **22**: 305–326.

McGorry, P.D. and Jackson, H.J. (Eds.) (1999) *Recognition and Management of Early Psychosis: A Preventive Approach*. New York, Cambridge University Press.

McLellan, A.T., Luborsky, L., Cacciola, J., Griffith, J., Evans, F., Barr, H.L. and O'Brien, C.P. (1985) New data from the Addiction Severity Index. Reliability and validity in three centers. *Journal of Nervous and Mental Disease*, **173**: 412–423.

Miller, W.R. (1983) Motivational interviewing with problem drinkers. *Behavioural Psychotherapy*, **11**: 147–172.

Miller, W.R. and Rollnick, S. (1991) *Motivational Interviewing: Preparing People To Change Addictive Behavior*. New York, Guilford.

National Early Psychosis Project Clinical Guidelines Working Party (1998) *Australian Clinical Guidelines for Early Psychosis*. Melbourne, National Early Psychosis Project, University of Melbourne.

Nelson, H.E. and Willison, J. (1991) *National Adult Reading Test (NART, 2nd edn): Test Manual*. Windsor, NFER Nelson.

Power, P., Elkins, K., Adlard, S., Curry, C.M., McGorry, P.D. and Harrigan, S. (1998) Analysis of the initial treatment phase in first-episode psychosis. *British Journal of Psychiatry*, **172** (Suppl 33): 71–77.

Prochaska, J.O. and DiClemente, C.C. (1986) Toward a comprehensive model of change. In W.R. Miller and N. Heather (Eds)., *Treating Addictive Behaviours: Processes of Change*, pp. 3–27. New York, Plenum.

Rabinowitz, J., Bromet, E.J., Lavelle, G., Carlson, B., Kovasznay, B. and Schwartz, J.E. (1998) Prevalence and severity of substance use disorder and onset of psychosis in first-admission psychotic patients. *Psychological Medicine*, **28**: 1411–1419.

Rolfe, T., McGorry, P.D., Longley, T. and Plowright, D. (1999) Cannabis use in first-episode psychosis: incidence and short-term outcome [Abstract]. *Schizophrenia Research*, **36**: 313–314.

Rollnick, S., Heather, N., Gold, R. and Hall, W. (1992) Development of a short "readiness to change" questionnaire for use in brief, opportunistic interventions among excessive drinkers. *British Journal of Addiction*, **87**: 743–754.

Selzer, J.A. and Lieberman J.A. (1993) Schizophrenia and substance abuse. *Psychiatric Clinics of North America*, **16**: 401–412.

Strakowski, S.M., Keck, P.E., McElroy, S.L., Lonczak H.S. and West, S.A. (1995) Chronology of comorbid and principal syndromes in first-episode psychosis. *Comprehensive Psychiatry*, **36**: 106–112.

Strakowski, S.M., McElroy, S.L., Keck, P.E., Jr. and West, S.A. (1996) The effects of antecedent substance abuse on the development of first-episode psychotic mania. *Journal of Psychiatric Research*, **30**: 59–68.

Walter, J.L. and Peller, J.E. (1992) *Becoming Solution-Focused in Brief Therapy*. New York, Brunner/Mazel.

Wing, J.K., Babor, T., Brugha, T., Burke, J., Cooper, J.E., Giel, R., Jablensky, A., Regier, D. and Sartorius, N. (1990) SCAN. Schedules for Clinical Assessment in Neuropsychiatry. *Archives of General Psychiatry*, **47**: 589–593.

Wing, J.K., Curtis, R.H. and Beevor, A.S. (1996) *HoNOS: Health of the Nation Outcome Scales: Report on Research and Development July 1993–December 1995*. London, Royal College of Psychiatrists Research Unit.

Chapter 17

COMORBID SEVERE MENTAL HEALTH PROBLEMS AND SUBSTANCE ABUSE IN FORENSIC POPULATIONS

Alison Beck, Tom Burns and Tim Hunt

SUBSTANCE ABUSE AND SEVERE MENTAL HEALTH PROBLEMS

Evidence from well-designed North American studies (e.g., Regier et al, 1990) appears to indicate higher rates of alcohol and substance abuse in people with severe mental health problems than in the general population. This is particularly true of young, male, chronically mentally ill patients. European research into comorbid substance abuse and severe mental health problems has been more limited (Smith and Hucker, 1993). However, the findings are similar, with the highest prevalence rates of substance abuse being found in young, chronically mentally ill, males. This group has consistently been found to display the highest prevalence rates of substance abuse (Mueser et al, 1990; Cuffel et al, 1993; Soyka et al, 1993; Smith and Hucker, 1994). Young males are also overrepresented among the "mentally disordered offenders" who make up forensic populations. Furthermore, those severe mental health problems that are associated with a higher risk of comorbid substance abuse, such as schizophrenia and affective disorder, are disproportionately over-represented (as a proportion of all diagnosable disorders) in forensic populations.

Substance Misuse in Psychosis: Approaches to Treatment and Service Delivery.
Edited by Hermine L. Graham, Alex Copello, Max J. Birchwood and Kim T. Mueser.
© 2003 John Wiley & Sons, Ltd.

Within psychotic populations, all substances have not been found to be equally popular. For example, among individuals with schizophrenic illnesses, alcohol has been found to be the most popular substance (although not consistently so; see, for example, Cantwell et al, 1999), followed by cannabis, stimulants and hallucinogens (Mueser et al, 1990; Soyka et al, 1993; Menezes et al, 1996). There is evidence to suggest (Beck and Hunt, in press) that patterns of abuse in forensic populations may differ from those in non-forensic populations. The authors found a fourfold odds of poly-substance abuse and a nearly 13-fold odds of abusing solvents in their high-security hospital population compared to their non-forensic psychiatric population. It is possible that forensic populations may abuse greater numbers of substances and that their pattern of abuse may be more chaotic.

COMORBIDITY AND VIOLENCE

Mental disorders have been found to increase the risk of criminal behaviour in general (Modestin and Ammann, 1996; Belfrage, 1998; Wallace et al, 1998) and of violent behaviour in particular (Steadman et al, 1998; Hodgins et al, 1996; Monahan, 1992; Swanson et al, 1990). The relative risks associated with mental illness compared to characteristics such as socio-economic status or history of violence, are unclear (Mulvey, 1994). However, the factors that have been found to predict dangerous behaviour in the non-mentally ill population, such as history of violence, age (young) or gender (male), have also been found to predict such behaviour in the mentally ill population (Krakowski et al, 1986). On the basis of limited evidence, some authors suggest that a history of violence in response to psychotic symptoms may be a risk factor for future violence in response to psychotic symptoms (McNiel, 1994). Nevertheless, only a small proportion of mentally ill individuals are at risk of committing serious violence (Crichton, 1995). Furthermore, this small subgroup probably account for a disproportionately large amount of the violence perpetrated by mentally ill individuals (Mulvey, 1994). The overlap between this small subgroup and the forensic population, namely, individuals detained in secure hospital conditions or as outpatients of forensic services, is probably high.

Swanson et al (1996) found that after controlling for socio-demographic covariants, schizophrenia and the major affective disorders were associated with about a fourfold increase in the odds of violence in 1 year compared to the general population. This relationship is correlational. A connection could not be made between the timing of violent episodes and the occurrence of psychotic states because psychotic symptoms were measured over the lifetime since age 18, whereas violence was measured in the last year. Many other studies have reported on correlations between mental illness and violence. For example, Krakowski et al (1986) reported that the severity of psychotic symptomatology is correlated with violence.

From a review of the literature, Krakowski et al (1986) found evidence to suggest that violent incidents are more likely to occur shortly after admission, and particularly after admission for a first psychotic episode, than later in the course of the illness. The authors also reported that violence is inversely correlated with compliance with medication where the latter significantly affects psychotic symptomatology.

Several studies have begun to explore the complex causal pathways linking mental illness and violent behaviour. A common feature of many of these studies is the focus on the meaning of the psychotic experience for the individual. For example, Link and Stueve (1994) found an association between certain types of active psychotic symptoms, which they termed "threat/control override" symptoms (TCO), and violence.

Although the meaning individuals give to their experiences may be important in terms of understanding causal pathways, this should not distract from the context in which the individual operates. Estroff et al (1994) argued that people with severe mental health problems who behave violently often do so in the context of constricted social networks, financial dependency and otherwise threatening environments. These factors are also important in terms of understanding their behaviour. Support for this contextual emphasis is widespread in the literature. For example, several studies of inpatient violence have found that violence is more common when there is little structured activity (for a review, see Crichton, 1995).

COMMUNITY STUDIES

Several studies have confirmed the association between Substance misuse with psychosis (SMP) and increased risk of violence in community populations. Cuffel et al (1994) undertook a longitudinal study of 103 individuals with schizophrenia or schizoaffective disorder who were seen in an outpatient clinic for treatment. After controlling for age, sex and ethnicity, they found that those who abused multiple substances were 12 times more likely to behave violently in the next 3 months than those who did not abuse substances. Odds of violence were particularly elevated for those individuals who had a pattern of polysubstance abuse. However, individuals who used only alcohol or marijuana did not have a higher risk of violence than individuals with these mental disorders who did not abuse substances.

Using ECA data, Swanson (1994) reported on the relative risks of lifetime violence associated with mental disorders and substance abuse. He concluded that while having a major mental disorder alone elevated the risk of violence over lifetime from 15% in the non-disordered population to 33%, a much greater relative risk of violence was associated with substance abuse. Substance abuse increased the lifetime risk of violence from 15% to 55%. SMP increased the lifetime risk of violence to 64%.

One methodological challenge common to all studies of SMP and violence is how to define the terms. Different studies use different definitions of violence, making comparison between them difficult. Definitions of violence had a marked effect on the results reported by Swanson (1994). He noted that the addition of an item about "drinking and fighting" brought about a substantial increase in the estimated prevalence of violence. The data were collected by self-report, and the author concluded that respondents perceived fighting while drinking as distinct from the other violent behaviours about which they had been asked to report. Apparently small differences in methodology can account for substantially different results between studies.

By comparison with the fourfold increase in the odds of violence in 1 year associated with schizophrenia and major affective disorders, Swanson et al (1996) reported that, after controlling for socio-demographic covariants, SMP increased the odds ratio for violent behaviour to 16.8. In other words, comorbid individuals were found to be 16.8 times more likely than the general population to have behaved violently in the past year.

Scott et al (1998) compared offending among SMP individuals and individuals with psychosis only, who were in contact with an inner London adult mental health team. They found that 25.7% of the "dually diagnosed" group and 10.9% of the "psychosis only" group reported a lifetime history of having committed a violent offence. SMP increased the odds of violent offending by 2.6.

STUDIES OF SECURE HOSPITAL PATIENTS

In a Swedish study, Lindqvist and Allebeck (1989) examined the case records of 644 people with schizophrenia hospitalized in Stockholm County over a 14-year period from 1971 to 1985. They found that 38 patients had convictions for violent offences, of whom 55% were recorded as having substance abuse problems.

In the UK Smith and Hucker (1994) examined 33 consecutive admissions to a regional secure unit. They found that 73% of the people with schizophrenia fulfilled DSM-III-R criteria for drug or alcohol abuse. However, only 20% of these individuals were intoxicated at the time of their index offence.

In another British study of schizophrenic patients in a regional secure facility, Wheatley (1998) found that 64% of the substance abusers had a forensic history compared with only 29% of the patients who did not abuse substances.

In a survey of males discharged from a maximum-security hospital in the second half of the 1970s, Norris (1984) found that one in five had an alcohol problem in addition to severe mental health problems. Furthermore, this group was much more likely to reoffend than their non-abusing counterparts. Quayle and Clarke (1992) found that 7% of the patients in one Special Hospital had severe alcohol dependence, and 15–17% were in the high-dependency category; 33% of the patients were found to have been drinking at the time of the offence that led to their admission. All the patients in these samples had severe comorbid mental health problems.

In a study of 61 mentally disordered patients detained in another high-security hospital, Thomas and McMurran (1993) identified 18% as having "alcohol-related problems". The alcohol abusers showed more serious criminality than the non-abusers, having significantly more previous convictions, and being responsible for 29% of the total number of murder and manslaughter offences in the sample.

Quayle et al (1998) examined reported weekly levels of alcohol abuse in a typical week prior to admission in a sample of patients from two English Special Hospitals, and a secure hospital for Scotland and Northern Ireland. They found that 49.3% of the men in their sample reported weekly levels of alcohol consumption above the health-risk limit of 50 units per week. Furthermore, 67.9% of the female patients in their sample reported weekly rates of alcohol consumption above their health-risk limit of 35 units per week. These findings might be broadly compared with general population base rates. For example, Hedges (1996) found that 6% of males and 2% of females in the general population consume above these respective health-risk limit quantities. Quayle et al (1998) also found, at interview, that 42% of their sample reported drinking at the time of their index offence.

The literature suggests, therefore, that the prevalence of SMP in secure hospital populations is very high, but how does this compare with non-forensic populations?

COMPARING SMP IN FORENSIC AND NON-FORENSIC POPULATIONS

Two of the authors undertook a study (Beck and Hunt, in press) comparing mentally ill patients (that is, individuals diagnosed with a psychotic illness according to DSM-IV) with and without SMP across levels of hospital security. The sample consisted of 80 patients detained in a medium-security unit and 139 detained in a maximum-security hospital. In addition, 209 community outpatients (from community mental health teams) were also included as a "non-secure" comparison group. Information on any history of substance abuse was obtained from a thorough review of patients' medical records. We found that the prevalence of substance abuse (at any time across the lifetime) was significantly higher in the high-security sample than the non-secure sample for the following substances: solvents (OR 12.47, CI 2.39–64.9), hallucinogens (OR 2.2, CI 1.1–4.5) and cocaine (OR 6.15, CI 2.2–17.2). These results persisted even after controlling for age, ethnicity, sex, having committed a violent crime and number of hospitalizations. Furthermore, polysubstance abuse was found to increase with increasing level of hospital security.

We were surprised by a "reverse finding" for alcohol abuse whereby non-forensic community patients were significantly more likely to have abused alcohol at some time in their lives than those detained in a high-security hospital. While this finding may be a result of methodological weaknesses in the study (such as a reliance on medical records), it might also be the case that patients at higher levels of hospital security have higher tolerance for deviancy. For these individuals, belonging to a social group that abuses illegal or "unacceptable" substances may help them to gain a sense of identity. In other words, patients with a propensity to abuse substances who are contained at higher levels of hospital security may be more likely to select more socially unacceptable substances.

Across the whole sample of forensic and non-forensic patients, we found, after controlling for socio-demographic covariants, an increased risk of having been convicted of a violent crime among those mentally ill individuals with a lifetime prevalence of abuse of cannabis (OR 1.97, CI 1.2–3.3), solvents (OR 4.54, CI 1.2–17.8), hallucinogens (OR 2.37, CI 1.2–4.5) and polysubstances (OR 2.59, CI 1.3–5.1) by comparison with non-abusers with a mental illness.

Even after controlling for whether or not the patients had committed a violent crime, we found that the odds of lifetime substance abuse increased with increasing level of hospital security. This finding requires further elucidation with a more sensitive measure of crime severity. However, it suggests that irrespective of whether or not the individuals concerned had committed a violent crime, those with SMP problems were more likely to be detained at higher levels of security than those with a mental disorder alone. The most likely explanation for this is that the patients with SMP in this sample were more likely than the patients with a single diagnosis to have other problems that warranted their detention at higher levels of

security. For example, they may have displayed more challenging behaviours or have been more likely to abscond. All this suggests that forensic
patients with comorbid problems may differ in many ways from non-
forensic patients with SMP, and not simply in terms of their increased
propensity for violent offending.

INTERACTION EFFECT

How do severe mental health problems and substance abuse interact to
increase the risk of violence? What other factors influence the interaction
so as to increase the risk of a violent outcome in a comorbid forensic
population?

Johns (1997) proposed that substance abuse may predispose individuals
to violence in a number of ways. This section considers some examples in
the context of active psychosis. Assuming that the meaning of a psychotic
experience for individuals is crucial in determining their subsequent behaviour, it stands to reason that concomitant substance abuse may well
alter that meaning. Johns (1997) suggested that the desired effects of a substance may increase the likelihood of violence. For example, among the
immediate effects of crack cocaine are feelings of intense energy, increased
libido, euphoria and self-confidence. In the context of active psychosis,
the meaning of psychotic symptoms is likely to be altered by these effects.
For example, one of the authors (A.B.) worked with a patient detained
in a medium-security unit suffering from a disorder involving erotoman-
ical delusions. When this man was well, he was considered sexually in-
hibited. However, when ill, he was likely to overvalue the inadvertent
glance of a woman, conclude that she had propositioned him and recipro-
cate with a sexual advance towards her. Certain personality features and
pro-offending patterns of thought, prevalent in forensic populations and
present in this individual, increase the likelihood that individuals such as
this man might, especially under the influence of a substance such as crack
cocaine, behave in a sexually aggressive manner.

Intoxication may be accompanied by irritability, autonomic arousal and
cognitive impairment, which individuals may experience as aversive. Co-
occurring psychotic symptoms may exacerbate these problems. For example, a patient diagnosed with paranoid schizophrenia was seen by A.B.
Despite being detained in a medium-security hospital, he was known to
abuse cannabis regularly. He reported feeling less in control and more
threatened (two TCO symptoms) when intoxicated. The behavioural expression of this experience may be influenced by a variety of factors
including cultural (MacAndrew and Edgerton, 1969) and peer-group effects (Lang et al, 1979). This individual, like many paranoid personalities

prevalent among forensic populations, was particularly vulnerable to respond aggressively in the context of experiencing TCO symptoms.

TREATMENT CHALLENGES AND SANCTIONS

Providing treatment for people with SMP presents many challenges, not least because the emphasis is on management rather than "cure". However, the management of SMP forensic patients differs radically from the management of non-forensic patients. Non-forensic patients may be encouraged to steer their own care programme, whereas forensic patients are usually managed and actively monitored by mental health professionals. Forensic patients may be subject to long periods of detention in hospital, and even when discharged they may remain subject to various legal requirements aimed at directing their behaviour. These differences set the parameters for the differences in service provision for forensic and non-forensic comorbid patients and for the different treatment philosophies adopted by these services.

INPATIENT TREATMENT CHALLENGES

Patients in medium-or high-security hospitals are nearly always detained on an involuntary basis. This contrasts with the eligibility criteria of many non-forensic addiction services that require voluntary commitment to treatment.

Forensic patients detained under treatment orders of the Mental Health Act 1983 (MHA 1983) must be suffering from a mental disorder within the meaning of the Act. As a result, the mental disorder is considered primary in many hospitals. The MHA 1983 expressly states that behaviour due solely to "promiscuity or other immoral conduct, sexual deviancy or dependence on alcohol or drugs" is excluded from the definition of mental disorder (MHA 1983 s.1(3)). Many forensic services have, at least traditionally, operated primarily as single disorder services. Furthermore, it is often assumed that it is the mental disorder that has the biggest impact on the risk of violence posed by the patient. This is somewhat at odds with the literature pertaining to the relative importance of substance abuse and mental disorder on subsequent violent behaviour. However, it must be remembered that forensic patients are a small subgroup of the mentally disordered population, and the relative risks associated with their violent behaviour are complex and multifaceted. Forensic patients with comorbid problems often demonstrate a variety of factors that increase their risk of violence beyond both their mental disorder and their abuse of substances.

Another reason why mental disorder is usually the primary target of treatment in forensic services may be that the mental health professionals who staff these services are primarily trained in the treatment of mental disorders. The end result is often that substance abuse difficulties are treated only when they are clearly associated with a mental disorder. For example, one symptom of a borderline personality disorder might be "impulsive substance abuse". In this case, treating the substance abuse might be considered an integral part of the treatment of the core mental disorder. In practice, however, treatment of forensic patients is rarely so circumscribed. Treatment of one disorder may be fused with treatment of the other. For example, a relapsing psychotic illness cannot be managed long-term unless comorbid substance abuse, which unfettered might precipitate a psychotic relapse, is also treated. Treatment of both might involve the patient in learning about the relapse-prevention (RP) model (Marlatt and Gordon, 1985).

The first author of this chapter (A.B.) has developed an RP model suitable for use with people with psychosis (Beck-Sander, 1999). This model is described in detail elsewhere; however, an outline is provided in Figure 17.1. Comparisons with other RP models used in the treatment of substance abuse and offending behaviour are easily made. It may be useful, when working with individuals with comorbid problems, to consider these parallels and to explore the possibilities for integrated treatments. For example, with reference to Figure 17.1, individuals might abuse a substance at stage 2, as a habitual way of coping (probably negatively) with difficulties in their life. This abuse might led them to a high-risk situation (stage 3), such as stopping maintenance medication, which in turn might place them at greater risk of developing early signs of psychotic relapse (defined here as lapse stage 4). In some individuals, psychotic relapse (stage 5) may be associated with an increased likelihood of offending behaviour. The model described in Figure 17.1 emphasizes the possibilities of using one model to coordinate treatments for psychosis, substance abuse and offending behaviour. It highlights the multiple points, or stages, in the relapse process at which interventions aimed at reducing the likelihood of relapse might be directed. For example, reducing face-to-face contact with a high expressed emotion (EE) relative (to less than 35 h per week) has been shown to reduce the risk of psychotic relapse, particularly in the first 9 months following psychotic decompensation (stage 1). Other interventions might aim to maintain non-offending or control over substance abuse. A high-risk situation (stage 3) is a concurrence of factors which markedly increase the risk of a relapse. Prolonged imbalance between stressors and effective coping resources, a preponderance of negative coping strategies or severe one-off stressful events may all give rise to a high-risk situation. Intervention at this stage might focus on reducing the stressors (e.g., by providing

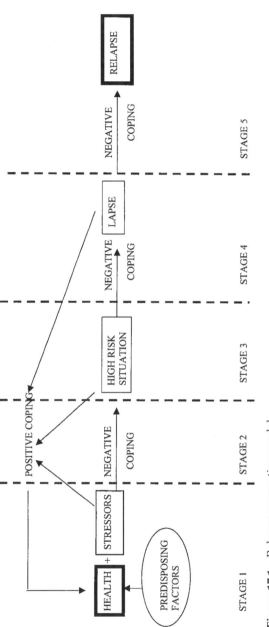

Figure 17.1 Relapse prevention model

financial assistance) or bolstering the positive coping strategies (e.g., by offering psychosocial support). These interventions may be useful in the management of psychosis, substance abuse and offending behaviour.

OUTPATIENT TREATMENT CHALLENGES

Forensic outpatients may be subject to statutory legislation which directs their behaviour. Therefore, the treatment challenges, which have been dealt with in one way in the provision of services to people with severe mental health problems who abuse substances, may be dealt with differently in a forensic setting. For example, patients with comorbid problems typically have poorer outpatient attendance records and higher drop-out rates than those who do not abuse substances (Hall et al, 1977). Similarly, they are more likely to be non-compliant with prescribed medication than patients who do not abuse substances (Alterman et al, 1980; Kofoed et al, 1986; Drake et al, 1989). Several pieces of statutory legislation may be employed to direct the behaviour of forensic patients:

Part III of the MHA 1983 makes provision for the admission of patients to hospital on the order of a court or from a prison. Restriction orders can be made by a Crown Court where necessary to protect the public from serious harm. These orders restrict the discharge of patients from hospital, usually for an open-ended period at the discretion of the Home Secretary. The clinical team managing the patient's care may make recommendations to the Home Secretary that restrictions be imposed and become conditions of discharge. For example, conditions may stipulate where patients reside, that they regularly attend outpatient appointments, that they abstain from drugs or alcohol, or that they comply with regular drug screening. Failure to comply with these restrictions may (although not necessarily) result in the Home Secretary recalling the patient to hospital.

A Supervised Discharge Order (SDO) may be made under section 25(a) of MHA 1983. However, these orders are essentially "toothless" in that there may be little that can be done if a patient consistently fails to comply. SDOs may require a patient who is being considered for discharge from a treatment order to reside at a specific address and/or to attend for treatment. They may also require patients to be conveyed to their residences and/or treatment appointments. However, patients cannot be compelled to take their medication, and if they persistently leave their residence or treatment appointments, there may be little point in returning them. No other sanctions follow.

Other orders may be pertinent in a forensic setting, such as a guardianship order (Section 7, MHA 1983). In addition, NHS Trusts often hold local supervision registers of difficult patients. These operate within the framework of the Care Programme Approach to guide good practice by ensuring that care plans are drawn up and monitored. However, these orders cannot compel patients who persistently choose not to. More potent are the drug treatment orders available under the Crime and Disorder Act 1998 and supervised by a probation officer.

SERVICES FOR COMORBID FORENSIC PATIENTS

Treating comorbid substance abuse problems in forensic patients is fraught with difficulties. Differences between the treatment philosophies of forensic and addiction services often make it difficult for the two services to coordinate their practice. For example, the use of neuroleptic medication in forensic services may conflict with the emphasis in some addiction services on drug-free treatment programmes. As a result, particularly forensic outpatients are in danger of being passed from one service to the next. This undermines the consistency of the care they receive. Furthermore, forensic patients are often difficult to manage, flouting the boundaries set by services. They may find themselves either refused admission to (Smith and Hucker, 1993) or prematurely discharged from addiction services (Galanter and Castaneda, 1988).

Current research suggests that integrated treatment is superior to sequential or parallel treatment (Mueser et al, 1992; Zimberg, 1993; Minkoff, 1989; Carey, 1995). Single programmes, which combine diverse elements of both addiction and mental health services, are better at providing integrated treatment because they are more cost-effective and easier for patients to navigate than sequencing separate treatments (Mueser et al, 1992). All treatment is provided by one clinician or team of clinicians, reducing conflicts between providers, reducing the patients' burden of attending two clinics and the potential for hearing conflicting messages, and reducing financial or other barriers to access and retention (Minkoff, 1989).

Enthusiasm for integrated services is not universal. For example, Johnson (1997) argues that specialist programmes run counter to the established practice in Britain and Europe of multidisciplinary teams (MDTs). A specialist service would disrupt the continuity of care provided by MDT-based services. She suggests that one strategy for Britain might be, instead of creating specialist teams, to develop means of delivering integrated care within the existing mental health teams. McKeown et al (1996a; b) and Quayle et al (1996) describe the shift made in one maximum-security hospital from MDT management of the "main" mental disorder (with add-on extra interventions for addictive behaviours such as alcohol education packages, Alcoholics Anonymous groups, and relapse prevention provided on an ad hoc basis) to the establishment of a Forensic Addictive Behaviours Unit.

The aim of the Forensic Addictive Behaviours Unit is to treat an SMP population, which is potentially very dangerous, with a view to reducing the likelihood of relapse of their substance abuse, their offending behaviour, other addictive behaviours or a combination. The unit provides a service solely to inpatients. Within the MDT structure of the hospital patients may be "referred" to the unit. Dependent on the outcome of a thorough assessment, the unit provides treatment on either an "in" or "out" patient basis; in other words, patients are either admitted to reside on the ward, or come on to the unit from other wards on a daily basis. The unit is run, as far as security permits, along the lines of a therapeutic community (TC). Psychodynamic and general groups run parallel with the rest of the programme, and there is provision for individual work as well. Patients are expected to work through the programme over a 2–3-year period. The unit also provides support for clinical teams on other wards in order for them to respond appropriately to the needs of the comorbid patients in their care.

CONCLUSIONS

There are a number of ways in which forensic patients with SMP are similar to non-forensic patients with SMP. There are also a number of ways in which the two populations differ radically. In both populations, the risk of violence associated with SMP is higher than with either disorder alone. Likewise, in both populations, certain demographic groups (young, chronically ill males) are at increased risk of violence. Furthermore, the likelihood of violent behaviour may be described in both forensic and non-forensic populations by a model which considers the meaning of the psychotic experience in the context of substance abuse for the individual concerned.

However, forensic and non-forensic populations differ in that a much higher prevalence of violent offending is associated with the former group. Individuals classified as "forensic" are often at increased risk of violence by virtue of a variety of factors other than their SMP difficulties (such as personality or social circumstances). These are generally not so pertinent in non-forensic populations. Furthermore, differences are to be found in the types of substances SMP forensic patients abuse and in the patterns of their substance abuse. The possibility that these differences affect their propensity to violence cannot be ruled out.

The increased risks associated with forensic populations are widely recognized, and they are reflected in mental health legislation. It follows that the contexts in which SMP forensic patients are treated often differ radically from the contexts in which non-forensic SMP patients are treated. Forensic patients are typically hospitalized for longer periods. Integrated inpatient treatments are still in their infancy. However, pioneering work, such as the Forensic Addiction Unit at Broadmoor Hospital, has begun. In an outpatient context, forensic patients may be subject to a number of legal sanctions which may guide the management of their substance abuse and mental disorder. Outpatient services for comorbid forensic patients often continue to operate in parallel, with all the pitfalls associated with such provision. Integrated service provision remains exceptional for this client group.

REFERENCES

Alterman, A.I., Erdlen, F.R., McLellan, A.T. and Mann, S.C. (1980) Problem drinking in hospitalized schizophrenic patients. *Addictive Behaviours*, **5**: 273–276.

Beck, A. and Hunt, T. (2002, in press) Co-morbidity across levels of hospital security. *Addiction Research*.

Beck-Sander, A. (1999) Relapse prevention: a model for psychosis? *Behaviour Change*, **16**: 191–202.

Belfrage, H. (1998) Making risk predictions without an instrument. Three years' experience of the new Swedish law on mentally disordered offenders. *International Journal of Law and Psychiatry*, **21**: 59–64.

Cantwell, R., Brewin, J., Glazebook, C., Dalkin, T., Fox, R., Medley, I. and Harrison, G. (1999) Prevalence of substance misuse in first-episode psychosis. *British Journal of Psychiatry*, **174**: 150–153.

Carey, K.B. (1995) Treatment of substance use disorders and schizophrenia. In: A.F. Lehman and L.B. and Dixon (Eds), *Double Jeopardy: Chronic Mental Illness and Substance Use Disorders*, pp. 85–108. Switzerland, Harwood Academic Publishers.

Crichton, J. (1995) A review of psychiatric in-patient violence. In: Crichton, J. (Ed), *Psychiatric Patient Violence: Risk and Response*. London, Duckworth.

Cuffel, B.J., Heithoff, K.A. and Lawson, W. (1993) Correlates of patterns of substance abuse among patiens with schizophrenia. *Hospital and Community Psychiatry*, **44**: 247–251.

Cuffel, B.J., Shumway, M., Chouljian, T.L. and McDonald, T. (1994) A longitudinal study of substance use and community violence in schizophrenia. *Journal of Nervous and Mental Disorders*, **182**: 704–708.

Drake, R.E., Osher, F.C. and Wallach, M.A. (1989) Alcohol use and abuse in schizophrenia: a prospective study. *Journal of Nervous and Mental Disease*, **177**: 408–414.

Estroff, S.E., Zimmer, C. and Lachicotte, W.S. (1994) The influence of social networks and social support on violence by persons with serious mental illness. *Hospital and Community Psychiatry*, **45**: 669–679.

Galanter, M. and Castaneda, R. (1988) Substance abuse among general psychiatric patients: place of presentation, diagnosis and treatment. *American Journal of Alcohol and Drug Abuse*, **14**: 211–235.

Hall, R.C.W., Popkin, M.K., De Vaul, R. and Stickney, S.K. (1977) The effect of unrecognized drug abuse on diagnosis and theraputic outcome. *American journal of Drug and Alcohol Abuse*, **4**: 455–465.

Hedges, B. (1996) Alcohol consumption. In H. Colhoun and P. Prescott-Clarke (Eds), *Health Survey for England 1994*. Department of Epidemiology and Public Health. London, HMSO.

Hodgins, S., Mednick, S.A., Brennan, P.A., Sculsinger, F. and Engburg, M. (1996) Mental disorder and crime: evidence form a Danish cohort. *Archives of General Psychiatry*, **53**: 489–496.

Johns, A. (1997) Substance misuse: a primary risk and a major problem of comorbidity. *International Review of Psychiatry*, **9**: 233–241.

Johnson, S. (1997) Dual diagnosis of severe mental illness and substance misuse: a case for specialist services? *British Journal of Psychiatry*, **171**: 205–208.

Kofoed, L.L., Konio, J. Walsh, T. and Atkinson, R. (1986) Outpatient treatment of patients with substance abuse and coexisting psychiatric disorders. *American Journal of Psychiatry*, **143**: 867–872.

Krakowski, M., Volavka, J. and Brizer, D. (1986) Psychopathology and violence: a review of the literature. *Comprehensive Psychiatry*, **27**: 131–148.

Lang, A.R., Goeckner, D.J. Adesson, V.J. and Marlatt, G.A. (1979) Effects of alcohol on aggression in male social drinkers. *Journal of Abnormal Psychology*, **84**: 508–518.

Link, B.G. and Stueve, A. (1994) Psychotic symptoms and the violent/illegal behaviour of mental patients compared to community controls. In J. Monahan and H.J. Steadman (Eds), *Violence and mental Disorder: Developments in Risk Assessment*, pp. 137–159. Chicago: University of Chicago Press.

Lindqvist, P. and Allebeck, P. (1989) Schizophrenia and assaultive behaviour: the role of alcohol and drug abuse. *Acta Psychiatrica* Scandinavica, **82**: 191–195.

MacAndrew, C. and Edgerton, R.B. (1969) *Drunken Comportment: A Social Explanation*. London, Nelson.

Marlatt, G.A. and Gordon, J.R. (Eds) (1985) *Relapse Prevention*. London, Guilford Press.

Mckeown, O., Forshaw, D.M., McGauley, G., Fitzpatrick, J. and Roscoe, J. (1996a) Forensic addictive behaviours unit: a case study (part I). *Journal of Substance Misuse*, **1**: 27–31.

Mckeown, O., McGauley, G., Forshaw, D.M., Carlyle, J. and Fitzpatrick, J. (1996b) Forensic addictive behaviours unit: a case study (part II). *Journal of Substance Misuse*, **1**: 97–103.

McNiel, D. (1994) Hallucinations and violence. In J. Monahan and H.J. Steadman (Eds), *Violence and Mental Disorder: Developments in Risk Assessment*, pp. 183–203. Chicago, University of Chicago Press.

Menezes, P.R., Johnson, S., Thorncroft, G., Marshall, J., Prosser, D., Bebbington, P. and Kuipers, E. (1996) Drug and alcohol problems among individuals with severe mental illness in south London. *British Journal of Psychiatry*, **168**: 612–619.

Minkoff, K. (1989) An integrated treatment model for dual diagnosis of psychosis and addiction. *Hospital and Community Psychiatry*, **40**: 1031–1036.

Modestin, J. and Ammann, R. (1996) Mental disorder and criminality: male schizophrenia. *Schizophrenia Bulletin*, **22**: 69–82.

Monahan, J. (1992) Mental disorder and violent behaviour: perceptions and evidence. *American Psychologist*, **47**: 511–521.

Mueser, K.T., Yarnold, P.R., Levinson, D.F, Singh, H., Bellack, A.S., Kee, K., Morrison, R.L. and Yadalam, K.G. (1990) Prevalence of substance abuse in schizophrenia: demographic and clinical correlates. *Schizophrenia Bulletin*, **16**: 31–57.

Mueser, K.T., Bellack, A.S. and Blanchard, J.J. (1992) Comorbidity of schizophrenia and substance abuse: implications for treatment. *Journal of Consulting and Clinical Psychology*, **60**: 845–856.

Mulvey, E.P. (1994) Assessing the evidence of a link between mental illness and violence. *Hospital and Community Psychiatry*, **45**: 663–668.

Norris, N. (1984) *Intergration of Special Hospital Patients into the Community*. Aldershot, Gower.

Quayle, M., Clark, F., Renwick, S.J., Hodge, J. and Spencer, T. (1998) Alcohol and secure hospital patients. I. An examination of the nature and prevalence of alcohol problems in secure hospital patients. *Psychology, Crime and Law*, **4**: 27–41.

Quayle, M. and Clarke, F. (1992) The role of alcohol in the offences of special hospital patients. *An Internal Broadmoor Hospital Report, UK*.

Quayle, M., Darling, P., Perkins, D., Lumsden, J., Forshaw, D.M. and Mckeown, O. (1996) Forensic addictive behaviours unit: a case study (part III). *Journal of Substance Misuse*, **1**: 160–164.

Regier, D., Farmer, M.E., Rae, D.S., Locke, B.Z., Keith, S.J., Judd, L.L. and Goodwin, F.K. (1990) Comorbidity of mental disroders with alcohol and other drug abuse: result from the epidemiological catchment area (ECA) study. *Journal of the American Medical Association*, **264**: 2511–2518.

Scott, H., Johnson, S., Menezes, P., Thornicroft, G. Marshall, J., Bindman, J. Bebbington, P. and Kuipers, E. (1998) Substance misuse and risk of aggression and offending among the severely mentally ill. *British Journal of Psychiatry*, **172**: 325–350.

Smith, J. and Hucker, S. (1993) Dual diagnosis patients: substance abuse by the severely mentally ill. *British Journal of Hospital Medicine*, **50**: 651–654.

Smith, J. and Hucker, S. (1994) Schizophrenia and substance abuse. *British Journal of Psychiatry*, **165**: 13–21.

Soyka, M., Albus, M., Kathmann, N., Finelli, A., Hoftstetter, S., Immler, B. and Sand, P. (1993) Prevalence of alcohol and drug abuse in schizophrenic inpatients. *European Archives of Psychiatry and Clinical Neuroscience*, **242**: 362–372.

Steadman, H.J., Mulvey, E.P., Monahan, J., Robbins, P.C., Appelbaum, P.S., Grisso, T., Roth, L.H. and Silver, E. (1998) Violence by people discharged from acute psychiatric inpatient facilities and by others in the same neighbourhoods. *Archives of General Psychiatry*, **55**: 393–401.

Swanson, J., Holzer, C., Ganju, V. and Jono, R. (1990) Violence and psychiatric disorder in the community: evidence from the Epidemiologic Catchment Area Surveys. *Hospital and Community Psychiatry*, **41**: 761–770.

Swanson, J. (1994) Mental disorder, substance abuse, and community violence: an epidemiological approach. In J. Monahan and H. Steadman (Eds), *Violence and Mental Disorder: Developments in Risk Assessment*, pp. 101–136. Chicago, University of Chicago Press.

Swanson, J., Borum, R., Swartz, M.S. and Monahan, J. (1996) Psychotic symptoms and disorders and the risk of violent behaviour in the community. *Criminal Behaviour and Mental Health*, **6**: 309–329.

Thomas, G. and Mcmurran, M. (1993) Alcohol related offending in male special hospital patients. *Medicine, Science and the Law*, **33**: 29–33.

Wallace, C., Mullen, P. and Burgess, P. (1998) Serious criminal offending and mental disorder. *British Journal of Psychiatry*, **172**: 477–484.

Wheatley, M. (1988) The prevalence and relevance of substance use in detained schizophrenic patients. *Journal of Forensic Psychiatry*, **9**: 114–129.

Zimberg, S. (1993) Introduction and general concepts of dual diagnosis. In J. Solomon, S. Zimberg and E. Sholler (Eds), *Dual Diagnosis: Evaluation, Treatment, Training and Program Development*. New York, Plenum.

Chapter 18

INTEGRATED TREATMENT OUTCOMES FOR HOMELESS PERSONS WITH SEVERE MENTAL ILLNESS AND CO-OCCURRING SUBSTANCE USE DISORDERS

Susan A. Pickett-Schenk, Michael Banghart and Judith A. Cook

INTRODUCTION

This chapter describes the problems faced by homeless persons with severe mental illness (HSMI) who have substance abuse problems. We briefly review the research on treatment models and outcomes for this population, and then shift our focus to site-specific findings from a federal research demonstration programme which provided integrated treatment services to HSMI clients, many of whom had a co-occurring substance use disorder. A case example is used to illustrate the problems these individuals faced, the services offered to them, and their treatment outcomes.

HOMELESSNESS, MENTAL ILLNESS, AND SUBSTANCE ABUSE

Persons with substance misuse and psychosis (SMP) who abuse drugs and alcohol suffer numerous negative outcomes (Drake et al, 1998). Substance abuse has been found to be associated with high rates of psychiatric

Substance Misuse in Psychosis: Approaches to Treatment and Service Delivery.
Edited by Hermine L. Graham, Alex Copello, Max J. Birchwood and Kim T. Mueser.
© 2003 John Wiley & Sons, Ltd.

symptom relapse and hospitalization, medication and treatment non-compliance, aggressive and violent behaviour, criminal activity, poor money management, and loss of social support (Abram and Teplin, 1991; Cuffel et al, 1994; Owen et al, 1996; Shaner et al, 1995; Swofford et al, 1996). Perhaps most noteworthy, however, is that substance abuse also leads to greater housing instability and homelessness among persons with mental illness (Drake et al, 1991; Drake and Wallach, 1989). This increased vulnerability to homelessness among persons with SMP may be perceived as part of a vicious cycle involving the negative outcomes listed above. Many of these individuals initially lose their homes as a result of psychiatric hospitalization and/or incarceration. Once homeless, these outcomes become obstacles to finding and maintaining housing (Fischer, 1990). Rent money is spent on drugs and alcohol. Ties with families and friends are broken. Shelters will not tolerate substance use or violent behaviour.

TREATMENT PROGRAMMES AND OUTCOMES

Given their multifarious needs, HSMI individuals who abuse drugs and alcohol may be one of the most difficult-to-serve populations (Bebout, 1997; Drake et al, 1997). Indeed, traditional mental health and substance use treatment programmes have failed to meet the needs of this group by treating problems separately rather than conjointly (Drake et al, 1996). In recent years, service providers and researchers have focused their attention on treatment programmes which deliver integrated services to HSMI individuals with co-occurring substance use problems. As Drake et al (1998) note, these programmes use multidisciplinary teams consisting of case managers, addictions counsellors, and residential staff to deliver mental health, substance abuse treatment, and housing services. Many of these programmes use a harm-reduction philosophy in which substance use and relapse are tolerated and expected, but are not considered grounds for terminating treatment (Mueser et al, 1992).

Recent research suggests that integrated treatment programmes may improve outcomes for HSMI individuals who abuse drugs and alcohol. Drake et al (1997) compared outcomes for 217 HSMI subjects with co-occurring substance use disorders; 158 subjects received integrated treatment services and 59 subjects received standard treatment services. Subjects in the first group received integrated mental health treatment, substance abuse counselling, and housing services from a single agency. These services were delivered by a multidisciplinary team which included case managers, substance abuse counsellors, and housing support staff. Subjects in the second group received services through multiple mental health, substance abuse, and housing agencies. Little coordination existed among these agencies. At 18 months, subjects who received integrated services had spent a greater number of days in stable housing situations (defined as own or other person's apartment, boarding house, or group home) than did subjects who received standard treatment services. Subjects who received integrated treatment services also showed greater progress in recovery from their substance use disorders (e.g., moving from severe dependence to use without impairment), and reported decreased psychiatric symptoms and increased social support, as compared to subjects who received standard treatment services.

Other positive outcomes associated with integrated treatment services ̶h̶a̶v̶e̶ ̶b̶e̶e̶n̶ ̶r̶e̶p̶o̶r̶t̶e̶d̶.̶ ̶H̶o̶s̶p̶i̶t̶a̶l̶i̶z̶a̶t̶i̶o̶n̶,̶ ̶d̶e̶t̶o̶x̶i̶f̶i̶c̶a̶t̶i̶o̶n̶,̶ ̶a̶n̶d̶ ̶a̶r̶r̶e̶s̶t̶ ̶r̶a̶t̶e̶s̶ ̶w̶e̶r̶e̶ significantly reduced among subjects who received services from an integrated treatment team (Detrick and Stiepock, 1992). Blankertz and Cnaan (1992) found that HSMI subjects with substance use problems who received integrated mental health, substance abuse treatment, and residential services had better rates of abstinence than individuals who did not received integrated care. Increased community tenure and decreased treatment drop-out rates also have been reported among integrated service recipients (Meisler et al, 1997). Overall, these findings suggest that integrated treatment services may be beneficial to HSMI individuals with co-occurring substance use disorders by increasing housing stability, reducing psychiatric recidivism, and improving recovery from addiction.

THE ACCESS PROGRAMME

The Access to Community Care and Effective Supports and Services (ACCESS) programme was a federally funded research demonstration project conducted from 1994 to 1999. The ACCESS programme examined the effect of service system integration on improving HSMI individuals' service use, housing and health status, and quality of life (Lam and Rosenheck, 1999). Funds were awarded in the USA to nine states: Connecticut, Illinois, Kansas, Missouri, North Carolina, Pennsylvania, Texas, Virginia, and Washington. Two sites in each state provided intensive outreach and case management services to 100 clients per project year, with a total of 400 clients served by each site (800 clients served per state). Outreach services involved making initial contact with potential clients on the street, in shelters, and at soup kitchens, drop-in centres, and community health-care facilities. Case management services, which began upon enrolment in the ACCESS programme, included a wide array of ongoing services (e.g., medication evaluation and management, housing assistance, counselling, medical and dental care, substance abuse treatment, and entitlement and employment assistance) designed to stabilize symptoms and prevent relapse, and improve community functioning and quality of life (Johnsen et al, 1999). These services were provided in the community to clients via either an assertive community treatment (ACT) (Stein and Test, 1980), a continuous treatment team (Torrey, 1986), or a strengths model of case management (Rapp and Chamberlin, 1985). ACCESS programme components and service delivery models have been described in detail elsewhere (Johnsen et al, 1999; Lam and Rosenheck, 1999; Randolph et al, 1997; Rosenheck et al, 1998).

HSMI individuals were required to be untreated—that is, they could not be receiving ongoing community treatment—and meet psychiatric illness and homelessness criteria in order to enroll in the ACCESS programme (Rosenheck and Lam, 1997). These eligibility criteria were assessed by ACCESS staff during the outreach and engagement process. Presence of psychiatric illness was measured by a 30-item screening instrument (Shern et al, 1994), which measured the presence of depressive, psychotic, and manic symptoms. Homelessness was measured as the subject's having spent at least 7 of the 14 days prior to initial contact with ACCESS outreach workers on the streets, or in a shelter, car, or abandoned building. HSMI individuals who met eligibility criteria were invited to receive ACCESS case-management services.

Upon enrolment, all ACCESS clients were asked to take part in the evaluation component, which consisted of three face-to-face interviews. These interviews were administered at the time of enrolment in the ACCESS programme (also referred to as baseline), 3 months post-enrolment, and 12 months post-enrolment. The interviews assessed several areas of the clients' lives, including their history of homelessness and current housing status, psychiatric history and treatment, substance use and treatment, service needs and use, and demographic characteristics. All interviews were conducted by trained researchers who were not a part of the ACCESS outreach and case management teams.

Given that the authors supervised and conducted the evaluation component at the ACCESS Illinois site—and thus are most familiar with this site's outcomes—this chapter describes the substance use treatment services provided by the ACCESS Illinois case-management teams and the outcomes of the ACCESS Illinois clients who received these integrated services.

THE ACCESS ILLINOIS PROGRAMME

Each of the ACCESS Illinois sites was located in Chicago. One site served the downtown business section of the city, where HSMI individuals could be found congregating in the parks, alleys, and subway trains. The other site served a highly multicultural, economically depressed neighbourhood whose numerous halfway houses and single occupancy hotels were frequented by recently discharged psychiatric patients. Both sites used the ACT model to deliver integrated mental health, substance use, and housing services to clients. These services were delivered by a multidisciplinary staff which included case managers, nurses, psychiatrists, and certified alcohol and drug treatment counsellors (CADCs).

Characteristics of the ACCESS Illinois clients

Of the 800 HSMI individuals who participated in the ACCESS Illinois programme, 60% were male and 40% were female. The majority of clients were African-American (58%); 31% were Caucasian; 5% were of mixed race; 4% were Hispanic; 2% were Native American; and 1% were Asian-American. ACCESS Illinois clients had an average age of 40 years, and experienced their first episode of homelessness at age 31. At the time of enrolment in ACCESS services, they had experienced, on average, five episodes of homelessness, and had a lifetime duration of homelessness of 42 months, or 3.5 years. ACCESS Illinois clients had an average number of nine psychiatric inpatient admissions. Most of the clients (61%) had diagnoses of schizophrenia.

Clients with substance misuse and psychosis (SMP)

The Clinical Rating Scale of Alcohol Use Scale and Drug Use Scales (Mueser et al, 1995) were used to assess ACCESS clients' substance use. These 5-point scales range from 1 (abstinent) to 5 (severe dependence). Ratings for each client were made by ACCESS case-management staff at enrolment and at each of the follow-up interviews. Clients with SMP were those individuals who had ratings from 3 to 5 (abuse, dependence, or severe dependence). A total of 324 (41%) of ACCESS Illinois participants were SMP clients.

T-test and chi-square analyses of baseline interview data show that, compared to non-SMP clients, SMP clients were more likely to be male, African-American, younger, and less educated, and to have been convicted of a crime. SMP clients spent fewer days in stable housing situations (e.g., staying at a single room occupancy facility [SRO], hotel, or boarding home, or their own or someone else's apartment) in the 60 days prior to enrolment in the ACCESS programme than did non-SMP clients. A greater proportion of SMP clients than non-SMP clients were on parole and awaiting trial. SMP clients also reported less contact with their families.

Substance use treatment services

Both of the ACCESS Illinois sites provided similar substance use treatment services. The CADCs conducted individual assessments of clients' drug and alcohol use, provided individual counselling with SMP clients, and led groups which focused on substance abuse issues. Individual counselling and group sessions employed a harm-reduction philosophy and sought to help SMP clients understand how their mental health and substance use problems interacted and affected their quality of life. The sites also offered housing programmes designed specifically for SMP clients. These programmes provided the safety, structure, and services SMP clients needed to help them reduce their drug and alcohol use without fear of being sent back to the streets. ACCESS Illinois teams referred—and at times accompanied—SMP clients to Alcoholics Anonymous (AA), Narcotics Anonymous (NA), and other self-help groups. Staff also helped SMP clients access detoxification services and inpatient residential treatment programmes. In all work with SMP clients, ACCESS Illinois staff used a harm-reduction philosophy in which relapse was expected and not used as a reason to end treatment.

Assessment of 12-month outcomes

Given the prior results of integrated treatment services previously described, we posed two questions about the clients with SMP who participated in the ACCESS Illinois programme. First, do SMP and non-SMP clients have similar outcomes? Second, does receipt of integrated treatment services improve outcomes for SMP clients? To answer these questions, we examined the following 12-month follow-up outcomes: housing status, mental health status, substance use status, criminal activity, and family contact. Housing status was assessed as the number of days clients reported that they had spent homeless (living on the streets, outdoors, in a car, and/or in an abandoned building) and the number of days they spent in stable housing situations (in a SRO, own apartment, and/or someone else's apartment) in the 60 days prior to the interview. Mental health status was assessed as the number of days clients were hospitalized for psychiatric treatment in the 60 days prior to the interview, and whether they were taking prescribed medication for psychiatric problems. Substance use status included the number of days SMP clients drank alcohol and used drugs in the month before the interview, and case managers' ratings of SMP clients' drug and alcohol abuse. Criminal activity was assessed as the number of days clients spent in jail in the 60 days before the interview. Family contact was measured as the amount of face-to-face contact clients had with any member of their family during the past year.

SMP and non-SMP client outcomes

In order to answer our first question, we conducted a series of *t*-tests, and we conducted chi-square analyses to determine whether significant differences occurred between SMP and non-SMP ACCESS Illinois clients on each of the above outcomes (with the exception of substance use) at the time of their 12-month follow-up interview. SMP clients spent a greater number of days homeless and a fewer number of days in stable housing situations in the 60 days prior to their 12-month follow-up interview than non-SMP clients. Specifically, SMP clients spent 2 days homeless and 50 days housed; non-SMP clients spent 1 day homeless and 54 days housed. There were no significant differences between SMP and non-SMP clients on mental health status, criminal activity, or family contact at the time of the 12-month follow-up interview.

Outcomes among SMP clients

To answer our second question, we conducted a series of paired t-tests and chi-square analyses examining differences between SMP clients' baseline and 12-month follow-up interviews on housing, substance use, mental health, criminal activity, and family contact outcomes. SMP clients experienced a significant decrease in the number of days spent homeless (from 9 to 2 days). They also reported a significant increase in the number days spent in stable housing situations from baseline to 12-month follow-up (from 15 to 39 days). Regarding substance use outcomes, SMP clients reported significant decreases in the number of days that they had used drugs in the month prior to the interview (1 day to 0.29 day); the number of days that they used alcohol also decreased (4.5 to 4 days), but this decrease was not significant. Changes in case managers' assessment of SMP clients' substance use from baseline to 12 months also were significant. Ratings improved, moving from the "abuse" category for both drugs and alcohol to the "use without impairment" category. There were no significant changes between baseline and 12-month follow-up in the number of days SMP clients had spent in a psychiatric hospital. A significantly greater proportion of SMP clients reported that they were taking prescribed medication for psychiatric problems at the time of the 12-month follow-up interview (78%) compared to those who reported taking psychotropic medication at baseline (48%). SMP clients experienced a slight, but significant increase in the number of days spent in jail from baseline to 12-month follow-up (1 to 3 days). Changes in family contact were not significant.

SMP clients' experiences: the case of Mr Y

The following case example illustrates the problems faced by the SMP clients who participated in the ACCESS Illinois programme, the integrated services they received, and the ways in which these integrated services may have helped them achieve positive outcomes.

Mr Y, a 39-year-old African-American with schizophrenia, was referred to ACCESS Illinois case-management services by staff at a local homeless shelter where he had been staying for the past 6 months. Mr Y had experienced three lifetime episodes of homelessness. He had been incarcerated six times over the past 21 years for drug-related charges. After his most recent release from prison, Mr Y returned to using crack cocaine, and, as a result, had no money for rent. The shelter staff reported that his angry outbursts were jeopardizing his ability to continue stay at the shelter. Although he reported experiencing auditory and visual hallucinations, he had never been hospitalized, probably as a result of his lengthy incarceration history. Mr Y denied having any drug or alcohol problems, but reported that he had used crack for over 12 years and marijuana for over 27 years. He suffered from both bronchitis and epilepsy.

Mr Y was resistant to the mental health services offered by the ACCESS team. He did not believe that he had psychiatric problems and therefore saw no need to take medications. In addition, he was highly suspicious of the service providers. In order to establish a therapeutic relationship with Mr Y, the ACCESS team first sought to meet his immediate needs for housing and medical care. This involved working with shelter staff to prolong his stay until long-term housing became available, and taking Mr Y to a local health clinic to treat his bronchitis and epilepsy. Slowly, over the next few months, Mr Y agreed to see the team psychiatrist and to take psychotropic medication. With the encouragement and support of ACCESS staff, he began attending NA meetings and agreed to receive inpatient treatment for his substance abuse problem.

After completing the inpatient treatment programme, ACCESS staff secured an apartment for Mr Y in a residential substance abuse treatment programme. This programme, developed specifically for SMP clients, provided individuals with their own apartments, on-site substance abuse treatment, and mental health-care services. ACCESS team members coordinated their efforts with housing programme staff in order to provide Mr Y with the integrated case-management services he needed to help him maintain his sobriety and live successfully in the community. After 8 months of sobriety, Mr Y decided to stop taking his medication and began using drugs. He became extremely psychotic and was hospitalized. However, rather than refusing treatment as he had in the past, Mr Y agreed to the inpatient stay and, after his symptoms subsided, he asked to return to the SMP housing programme. The ACCESS team worked with housing staff to allow Mr Y to return to the programme after his hospital stay. At the time of his 12-month follow-up interview, Mr Y was living in the SMP housing programme, taking his medication, regularly attending NA meetings and SMP group meetings sponsored by ACCESS and his housing programme, and seeking employment. He had experienced no additional drug relapses or psychiatric hospitalizations.

CONCLUSIONS

SMP clients demonstrated significant changes from the time they entered the ACCESS Illinois programme to 1-year follow-up on several important outcomes. First, the time spent homeless decreased and the time spent housed significantly increased during their year in the ACCESS programme. Second, as suggested by the changes in substance use, they made significant strides in their recovery process. Third, they increased their compliance with taking prescribed psychotropic medication. Similar to other studies (Drake et al, 1997; 1998), these findings suggest that integrated treatment may help HSMI clients with co-occurring substance use disorders find and keep housing, as well as positively influence their ability to reduce drug and alcohol use, and take prescribed psychotropic medication.

The coordination between service providers also may have helped SMP clients achieve positive outcomes. As the case example suggests, ACCESS Illinois team members were able to work successfully with shelter and housing staff to ensure that Mr Y did not become homeless. The ACCESS Illinois team also declined to terminate Mr Y's treatment when he relapsed. Instead, they continued to work with him and help him regain his ability to function in the community. By not "bouncing" between systems and not being expelled from services, Mr Y was better able to achieve his goals.

Criminal activity was the one outcome area in which improvement did not occur among the SMP clients. Indeed, they spent more days in jail at the time of the 12-month follow-up interview than at baseline. This may be due in part to the buildings in which the SMP clients were living. Many of these facilities were located in high-crime neighbourhood where drugs were readily available. It is possible that some SMP clients, particularly those who were actively using drugs and alcohol, may have committed crimes in order to support their substance use. These SMP clients also may have been arrested for public intoxication and vagrancy.

Although our results are cursory, they do suggest that integrated services may be an effective treatment programme for HSMI individuals with co-occurring substance use disorders. Additional analyses examining how specific components of these integrated services influence outcomes are needed. Future studies examining long-term outcomes of this population also are needed in order to understand how receipt of integrated services affects these individuals' community functioning after treatment has ended.

REFERENCES

Abram, K.M. and Teplin, L.A. (1991) Co-occurring disorders among mentally ill jail detainees: implications for public policy. *American Psychologist*, **46**: 1036–1045.

Bebout, R.R., Drake, R.E., Xie, H., McHugo, G. and Harris, M. (1997) Housing status among formerly homeless dually diagnosed adults. *Psychiatric Services*, **48**: 936–941.

Blankertz, L. and Cnaan, R. (1992) Principles of care for dually diagnosed homeless persons: findings from a demonstration project. *Research on Social Work Practice*, **2**: 448–464.

Cuffel, B.J., Shumway, M., Chouljian, T.L. and MacDonald, T. (1994) A longitudinal study of substance use and community violence in schizophrenia. *Journal of Nervous and Mental Disease*, **182**: 704–708.

Detrick, A. and Stiepock, V. (1992) Treating persons with mental illness, substance abuse, and legal problems: the Rhode Island experience. In L.I. Stein (Ed.), *Innovative Community Mental Health Programs. New Directions in Mental Health Services, Vol. 56*. San Francisco, Jossey-Bass.

Drake, R.E., McHugo, G.J., Clark, R.E., Teague, G.B., Xie, H., Miles, K. and Ackerson, T.H. (1998) Assertive community treatment for patients with co-occurring severe mental illness and substance use disorder: a clinical trial. *American Journal of Orthopsychiatry*, **68**: 201–215.

Drake, R.E., Mueser, K.T., Clark, R.E. and Wallach, M.A. (1996) The course, treatment, and outcome of substance disorder in persons with severe mental illness. *American Journal of Orthopsychiatry*, **66**: 42–51.

Drake, R.E., Osher, F.C. and Wallach, M.A. (1991) Homelessness and dual diagnosis. *American Psychologist*, **46**: 1149–1158.

Drake, R.E. and Wallach, M.A. (1989) Substance abuse among the chronic mentally ill. *Hospital and Community Psychology*, **40**: 1041–1046.

Drake, R.E., Yovetich, N.A., Bebout, R.R., Harris, M. and McHugo, G.J. (1997) Integrated treatment for dually diagnosed homeless adults. *Journal of Nervous and Mental Disease*, **185**: 298–305.

Fischer, P.J. (1990) *Alcohol and Drug Abuse and Mental Health Problems Among Homeless Persons: A Review of the Literature, 1980–1990*. Rockville, MD, National Institute on Alcohol Abuse and Alcoholism.

Gonzalez, G. and Rosenheck, R. (2002, in press). Outcome and service use among seriously mentally ill persons who are homeless and have substance abuse diagnoses. *Psychiatric Services*.

Johnsen, M., Samberg, L., Calsyn, R., Blasinksy, M., Landow, W. and Goldman, H. (1999) Case management models for persons who are homeless and mentally ill: the ACCESS demonstration project. *Community Mental Health Journal*, **35**: 325–346.

Lam, J.A. and Rosenheck, R. (1999) Street outreach for homeless persons with serious mental illness: is it effective? *Medical Care*, **37**: 894–907.

Meisler, N., Blankertz, L., Santos, A.B. and McKay, C. (1997) Impact of assertive community treatment on homeless persons with co-occurring severe psychiatric and substance use disorders. *Community Mental Health Journal*, **33**: 113–122.

Mueser, K.T., Bellack, A.S. and Blanchard, J.J. (1992) Comorbidity of schizophrenia and substance abuse: implications for treatment. *Journal of Consulting and Clinical Psychology*, **60**: 845–856.

Mueser, K.T., Drake, R.E., Clark, R.E., McHugo, G.M., Mercer-McFadden, C. and Anderson, T. (1995) *Evaluating Substance Abuse in Persons with Severe Mental Illness*. Cambridge, MA, Human Services Research Institute.

Owen, R.R., Fischer, E.P., Booth, B.M. and Cuffel, B.J. (1996) Medication Noncompliance and Substance Abuse Among Patients with Schizophrenia. *Psychiatric Services*, **47**: 853–858.

Randolph, F., Blaskinsky M., Leginski, W., Parker L.B. and Goldman H. (1997) Creating integrated service systems for homeless persons with mental illness: the ACCESS program. *Psychiatric Services*, **48**: 369–373.

Rapp, C.A. and Chamberlain, R. (1985) Case management for the chronically mentally ill. *Case Management Services*, Sept–Oct: 417–422.

Rosenheck, R. and Lam, J.A. (1997) Homeless mentally ill clients' and providers' perceptions of service needs and clients' use of services. *Psychiatric Services*, **48**: 381–386.

Rosenheck, R., Morrissey, J., Lam, J., Calloway, M., Johnsen, M., Goldman, H., Randolph, F., Blaskinsky, M., Fontana, A., Calysn, R. and Teague, G. (1998) Service system integration, access to services, and housing outcomes in a program for homeless persons with severe mental illness. *American Journal of Public Health*, **88**: 1610–1615.

Shaner, A., Eckman, T.A., Wilkins, J.N., Tucker, D.E., Tsuang, J.W. and Mintz, J. (1995) Disability income, cocaine use, and repeated hospitalization among schizophrenic cocain abusers. *New England Journal of Medicine*, **333**: 777–783.

Shern, D.L., Lovell, A.M., Tsembris, S., Anthony, W., LaComb, C.A., Richmond, L., Winarski, J. and Cohen, M. (1994) The New York City outreach project: serving a hard-to-reach population. In Center for Mental Health Services (Ed.), *Making a Difference: Interim Status Report of the McKinney Demonstration Program for Homeless Adults with Mental Illness*. Rockville, MD, Center for Mental Health Services.

Stein, L.I. and Test, M.A. (1980) An alternative to mental hospital treatment. I. Conceptual model, treatment program, and clinical evaluation. *Archives of General Psychiatry*, **37**: 392–397.

Swofford, C.D., Cask, J.W., Schuller-Gulch, G. and Inderbitzen, L.B. (1996) Substance abuse: a powerful predictor of relapse in schizophrenia. *Schizophrenia Research*, **20**: 145–151.

Torrey, E.F. (1986) Continuous treatment teams in the care of the chronically mentally ill. *Hospital and Community Psychiatry*, **37**: 1243–1247.

Chapter 19

ISSUES IN COMORBIDITY AND HIV/AIDS

Lisa Razzano

INTRODUCTION: HIV/AIDS AMONG MENTAL HEALTH CONSUMERS

Reports from the Centers for Disease Control and Prevention estimate that, as of June 2000, more than 750 000 AIDS cases have been documented in the USA. Currently, more than an estimated 120 000 people are living with HIV, with another 311 000 living with AIDS (Centers for Disease Control, 2000). Many groups within the general population, however, have been shown to be disproportionately affected by the HIV epidemic, such as injection drug users (IVDUs), youth, women, and people of colour. In addition to these groups, studies have demonstrated the vulnerability of people with mental illnesses to HIV infection (Cournos and McKinnon, 1997; McKinnon and Rosner, 2000). In one review of the literature examining studies estimating the seroprevalence of HIV/AIDS among mental health consumers, Cournos and McKinnon (1997) report an overall infection rate of approximately 7.8%. Although many of these investigations were conducted among psychiatric inpatients, other studies examining seroprevalence among community-based samples with laboratory blood tests, as well as those with self-reports of HIV infection, also indicate that HIV infection rates among mental health clientele are substantially higher (i.e., ≈3%) (Cook et al, 1994; Rosenberg et al, 2001). With the rate of HIV infection among the population at-large estimated at 0.4–0.9%, infection rates among mental health consumers are nearly eight times higher than in the general population.

Substance Misuse in Psychosis: Approaches to Treatment and Service Delivery.
Edited by Hermine L. Graham, Alex Copello, Max J. Birchwood and Kim T. Mueser.
© 2003 John Wiley & Sons, Ltd.

Clients diagnosed with substance misuse and psychosis (SMP) may be the most vulnerable to HIV infection, compared to other consumers without this comorbid factor. In fact, documented HIV infection rates are highest among SMP clients (i.e., 18%) (McKinnon and Rosner, 2000). Rates of HIV infection among SMP clients, however, vary with regard to drugs of choice. While intravenous (IV) drug use is a direct route of transmission and the second most common HIV risk factor (Ferrando and Bataki, 2000; Centers for Disease Control, 1999), other recreational drugs and alcohol have been shown to affect HIV infection rates among the SMP clientele. In particular, more than 33% of SMP clients using IV drugs presented with HIV infection compared to 15% among SMP clients who used non-IV recreational drugs, 10% among alcohol users, and slightly over 2% for clients who did not meet the diagnostic criteria for SMP (Cournos and McKinnon, 1997).

Numerous studies have established the connection between HIV infection and unprotected sex, and use of alcohol, recreational drugs, and IV drugs (Carey et al, 1991; McKinnon and Rosner, 2000; Rosenberg et al, 2001). Among the findings included in these reports, data consistently support the assumption that mental health consumers are more likely to have multiple sex partners, engage in sexual encounters without using condoms, and have sex while under the influence of alcohol and/or other recreational drugs (including IVDUs). In fact, the rates in published accounts indicate that as many as 45% of the consumers reported unsafe sexual activity while under the influence, while as many as 69% of the respondents indicated that they had exchanged sex for drugs or money to buy drugs in the past year.

While it is unlikely that simply having a diagnosis of mental illness directly increases consumers' chances of becoming HIV+, it is more likely that specific symptoms of mental illness affect the risk behaviours in which mental health consumers engage. There is conflicting evidence regarding the specific nature of the relationship between mental illness and HIV risks, but the majority of major psychiatric disabilities present with symptoms such as impaired concentration, disruptions in judgement, difficulties with impulse control, libidinal changes, and deficits in problem-solving skills. These symptoms disrupt "normal" activities and relationships, often resulting in problems in developing and maintaining stable social and sexual relationships, as well as the use of IV drugs, other recreational drugs, and alcohol. For example, McDermott et al (1994) report a significantly higher incidence of IV drug use based on diagnosis, such that clients diagnosed with major depression reported the highest rates of use, followed by those diagnosed with schizophrenia; the lowest rates were reported among clients diagnosed with bipolar disorder. Another study indicated that, when standardized diagnostic interview schedules are used, no relationships are revealed among IV drug use and psychiatric symptomatology, level of function or impairment, or specific diagnostic categories (Horwath et al, 1996).

Studies have examined the relationship between psychiatric diagnoses, symptoms, and other HIV risk behaviours, such as unsafe sexual activities. Similar to the published findings regarding symptoms, alcohol and drug use, and HIV risk, there is conflicting evidence regarding the connection between symptoms and HIV risks related to sexual activities. While no relationship between different mental health diagnoses and being sexually active was found in one investigation, findings from the same study demonstrated relationships between sexual behaviour and particular diagnoses (i.e., schizophrenia and depression), but not others (i.e., bipolar disorder) (Cournos et al, 1993). However, another study (McDermott et al, 1994) explored aspects of sexual behaviour among psychiatric clientele in the 3 months prior to their most recent psychiatric hospitalization, and found that rates of intercourse among people with psychiatric disabilities were significantly lower than those reported by the non-psychiatric comparison group, suggesting that during the recurrence of symptoms, many mental health consumers actually reported being less sexually active. Similarly, findings regarding the impact of specific psychiatric symptoms, rather than broad diagnostic categories, on risk of HIV infection for consumers also were mixed. For example, mental health consumers with more severe positive symptoms of psychosis were more than three times more likely to engage in unsafe behaviours with multiple sex partners than those with less severe positive symptoms (McKinnon et al, 1996). Findings also indicated that many mental health consumers reported engaging in unsafe sexual activities in response to auditory hallucinations or other delusional symptoms. Furthermore, as noted in a review of the literature by McKinnon (1996), the hypersexuality often observed in the manic phases of bipolar disorder, as well as in the early onset of symptoms of schizophrenia, can increase consumers' participation in unsafe sex, suggesting that the phase of an individual's psychiatric illness may affect participation in higher-risk behaviours.

In addition to the HIV risks characteristic of psychiatric disability itself or SMP, many mental health consumers encounter other, social factors which increase their vulnerability to HIV infection. These include having a relatively small pool of eligible sexual partners, and lack of education about HIV from service providers who are reluctant to address HIV-related issues with consumers, conduct risk assessments, or encourage and support HIV testing (Brady and Carmen, 1990; Kalichman et al, 1994; Cook et al, 1994). Other social factors, such as poverty, limited access to physical health care, stigma and discrimination, and housing instability, also contribute to the vulnerability of mental health consumers to HIV infection (Cook et al, 1994).

Examinations of consumers' knowledge of HIV risks, modes of transmission, and other facts about the disease, as well as how to prevent it, indicate that there are looming misconceptions about HIV/AIDS among mental health consumers. In one study, 51% incorrectly believed that HIV could be spread through casual contact, while 37% thought it would be unsafe to be in the same room with a person who has AIDS (McKinnon et al, 1996). In general, these studies also have demonstrated the importance of addressing HIV/AIDS within mental health services programmes. Although Cook et al (1994) demonstrated that the majority of consumers reported some basic information regarding HIV, such as knowing what it is (68%), knowing how a person gets it (71%), and knowing how to prevent it (69%), overwhelmingly, the source of the information for consumers was from group or individual counselling within a psychosocial rehabilitation agency (25%). Only 7% reported getting information from written sources, 5% reported receiving it from other types of service providers, and only 4% of the consumers in this sample reported that they had received HIV/AIDS information from physicians (non-psychiatrists) or other health-care providers. These data indicate that it is essential that mental health providers who work directly with this group include HIV/AIDS in the array of the services available to consumers.

For integration of HIV-related activities into existing services models, it is important to focus on HIV education and prevention; this means conducting risk assessments with mental health consumers, counselling and HIV testing, and meeting the treatment needs of HIV+ consumers. It also is essential that service providers in all types of service settings examine their own stereotypes and attitudes surrounding mental health consumers' sexuality, substance use, and the influence of the stigma surrounding HIV/AIDS and the effects that it has on provider attitudes toward consumers who are infected. Many integrated services models are particularly successful with SMP clients because they address both conditions simultaneously, but also consider the synergistic relationship between chronic mental illness and substance abuse (Drake et al, 1998). These same integrated treatment settings would be ideal programmes in which to incorporate HIV/AIDS-related services, since not only can HIV-prevention and risk-reduction programmes be included in the array of services available for consumers, but also these programmes can be designed with a long-term approach, to strengthen the consistency of the treatment messages that consumers receive about substance use and recovery, harm reduction, and other HIV risks related to SMP status (Drake et al, 1998; Minkoff, 1989).

HIV/AIDS education and prevention

There are several strategies by which HIV-related activities can be integrated into institutional and community-based mental health services.

Within institutional facilities, it is important to conduct HIV risk assessments with inpatients, and to provide them with the option to be tested or the necessary referral and contact information for testing (or treatment) services within the community. If consumers request HIV testing while they are inpatients, it is essential to obtain informed consent, to conduct the pre- and post-test counselling with interested consumers, and to inform them of their test results *before* they are discharged. In community mental health settings, several studies have recommended the integration of HIV services as regular features of rehabilitation service plans, intensive case management, community support services, and housing and residential services, and have identified several effective methods for conducting education programmes with mental health consumers, regardless of the treatment setting (Cook et al, 1995; Cournos and Bakalar, 1996).

Successful education, prevention, and risk-reduction programmes for mental health consumers have included a number of similar elements. Overall, providers are encouraged to specify one central training objective or theme to be addressed in each session, provide concrete information and examples which are relevant to consumers' own behaviours and activities, schedule short sessions for each topic and repeat the sessions as required, limit the number of written materials and assignments, and provide a summary for each session so that consumers can develop a sense of "closure" as well as a "take-away" message from the session. In developing strategies for prevention, programmes should provide consumers with the most up-to-date information on the facts and myths about HIV transmission; address safer sex behaviours, IVDU, and other substance abuse; consider harm reduction strategies such as needle cleaning and needle exchange; and resolve concerns related to blood transfusions, medication-related injections, blood donations, and the use of other blood products. In the majority of cases, activities that focus on skills acquisition and development, role-plays, or simulations are considered among the best methods. In settings where face-to-face or group meetings are less feasible, providers can integrate HIV prevention and education into street and community outreach efforts, peer education and consumer-led support groups, and include families in education and prevention activities.

HIV/AIDS risk-assessment strategies

It is increasingly important to conduct risk assessments as a regular part of institutional and community mental health services with all consumers, not only those with comorbid substance use diagnoses. Staff must determine whether consumers can provide informed consent to complete the risk assessment, and should remind consumers that this information is private and confidential, and will not affect their access to services or benefits.

Providers not only must discuss activities and behaviours related to HIV transmission, but should be able to evaluate the extent of individual consumers' risks, as well as assist consumers in personalizing their HIV risks within a behavioural context. For example, many male consumers engage in sex with other men, yet, since they do not identify themselves as gay (or homosexual), they may not perceive any personal risk. Thus, it is essential to reframe the fact that risks are associated with specific behaviours, not with labels or stereotypes regarding sexual orientation. It also is important to remind consumers that there are numerous benefits in completing risk assessments, and that they can be an invaluable tool in the early detection and improved medical treatment of HIV. McKinnon (1996) identified several essential components to include in a basic HIV risk assessment for mental health consumers:

1. frequency of vaginal, anal, and oral intercourse
2. the number, gender, and known HIV risks of sexual partners
3. whether the consumer has exchanged sex for money, drugs, shelter, cigarettes, or other material gain
4. past history of and current symptoms related to other sexually transmitted diseases
5. consistent and appropriate use of condoms and other contraceptive methods
6. recreational/street drug use, specifically injection or sniffed substances
7. sharing of injection drug paraphernalia such as needles and syringes
8. use of alcohol
9. frequency of sexual intercourse while under the influence of alcohol and/or drugs.

Finally, there are numerous institutional and personal staff barriers to conducting risk assessments, as well as providing services to mental health consumers (Cook et al, 1994; Cournos and Bakalar, 1996; McKinnon, 1996). In addition to the aforementioned topical areas necessary for a comprehensive HIV risk assessment, McKinnon (1996) also suggests several strategies which providers should employ when completing assessments with this population. One is to limit the use of technical jargon without explaining these terms to the consumer, and to explore consumers' vocabulary and the types of sexual and drug terms consumers use in completing risk assessments. It is important, whenever possible, to use the consumers' language, as well as to clarify their descriptions of behaviours and practices. It is also important to complete risk assessments in safe and private settings, and to remind consumers constantly that their responses are confidential, and that the information will not be disclosed to anyone who is not directly involved in providing services to the consumer. It also is important for providers to acknowledge consumers' cultural background. Issues such as culture, religion and spirituality, and language can affect their openness to discussing sex and drug use behaviours.

Counselling and HIV testing for consumers

In order to ensure that consumers are receiving the highest quality of care possible, it is important for all services providers who work with mental health consumers to familiarize themselves with the guidelines for HIV counselling and testing for inpatient psychiatric units, as well as outpatient mental health facilities (provided by the American Psychiatric Association in the USA) before attempting to counsel consumers regarding a decision to have an HIV test (American Psychiatric Association, 1996; 1992, respectively). In providing services and support related to HIV test counselling, there are several issues upon which providers can rely in helping consumers to make an informed decision to have an HIV test. It is critically important for providers to assist consumers in understanding the meaning of the test, the information the tests provide, and how that information will be used. Providers should address specific issues in a pre-test counselling session, as well as be prepared to revisit these and to discuss additional topics in a post-test counselling session.

The pre-test counselling session should focus on a number of issues. First, in accordance with human subject guidelines and federal policy regulations, it is essential to obtain specific, written consent for an HIV blood screening from the consumer. Once consent has been secured, providers should address the meaning of the blood test(s), including the validity of the ELISA (enzyme-linked immunosorbent assay) and the Western blot, and the differences between confidential and anonymous testing. Futhermore, as regulations and laws vary throughout the USA, it is important to review with consumers whether their home state requires name or incidence reporting, and how this will affect them personally. It also is important for providers to assess each consumer's strengths and weaknesses, and to handle questions that consumers have about testing, confidentiality, and other relevant issues (Razzano et al, 1997).

In the post-test counselling session, there also are several topics on which to focus regardless of consumers' test results. These include the following: how consumers will notified of their test results; strategies to reduce immediate stress and anxiety related to receiving their test results; reviewing continued prevention, risk-assessment, and harm-reduction strategies to reduce spread of infection; handling new questions and concerns; and identifying whether any referral or follow-up services are necessary. For consumers whose test results are positive, providers will need to develop plans which address and overcome initial fears regarding HIV infection, identify ways to make lifestyle changes which promote good health, determine whether any of the consumers' relationships will need to be redefined, recognize needs related to adjustments in social relationships and ongoing physical changes, and make decisions about appropriate resources and medical treatments. In the USA, it also will be necessary to discuss with consumers any specific state laws regarding situations in which individuals with HIV have not notified their sexual partners of their HIV status. Many states have adopted statues supporting the idea that people living with HIV/AIDS have a "duty to warn" sexual partners in advance of intimate contact, including situations in which sex is exchanged for money or material gain. In some states in the USA (e.g., Nevada), failure to do so constitutes a felony and is subject to fines and/or incarceration (Nevada Revised Statutes, Chapter 201, Section 205 [NRS 201.205]; NRS 201.358).

Issues for service providers

In addition to traditional in- and outpatient services available to mental health consumers regarding mental illness and HIV/AIDS, there are several areas which have been identified as especially important for providers and other clinicians to consider. In general, staff must address their own attitudes and attributions related to HIV/AIDS. It is essential, however, that providers also examine their personal attitudes, biases, and prejudices about sexuality; specific sexual activities; consumers' choices regarding sexual partners; alcohol and drug use; using sex to obtain drugs, money, or other material gain; and other risky behaviours in general. This will require that providers determine their own "comfort zone" related to these issues, as well as, in some cases, resistance to openly discussing issues regarding sexuality, alcohol, and drug use with consumers (Razzano et al, 1997). Staff also must ascertain whether they are willing to provide consumers with the materials and information necessary to practise safer sex and harm-reduction strategies, such as latex condoms or needle cleaning/exchange resources. Furthermore, as it is well established that HIV/AIDS does not discriminate among people, service providers also must be sensitive to issues of cultural diversity among mental health consumers when providing test counselling, conducting risk assessments, and implementing education and prevention programmes.

WORKING WITH HIV/AIDS-AFFECTED CONSUMERS

The chronic nature of mental illness requires that service providers continue to emphasize health promotion, as well as strategies for consumers to monitor their illness progression. In working with HIV+ consumers, providers must first determine their level of disease progression. This is an essential component of service delivery, since consumers may present with HIV infection at various levels. Among asymptomatic consumers, ongoing case management, medication and treatment needs, appropriate treatment options, substance use and harm reduction, and residential and financial resources should be emphasized. For symptomatic consumers, the rate of disease progression, characterized by indicators such as CD4 cell count and viral load, diagnosis of opportunistic infections (such as oral candidiasis and Pneumocystis carinii pneumonia), and the impact of other, constitutional symptoms (e.g., sustained weight loss or persistent diarrhoea), must be determined.

Medical treatment for HIV+ consumers

Among HIV+ individuals, regardless of their mental health status, the presence of the virus will make experiences with any medication side effects more severe. Since the most common form of treatment for mental health consumers is use of specific medications to reduce and control the symptoms of their mental illnesses, providers must keep in mind that all consumers living with HIV are more sensitive to pharmacological treatment, as well as the side effects of those treatments. For example, if a psychotropic medication causes photosensitivity, the risk of sunburn is raised for HIV+ consumers taking the medication. Similarly, the effects of other recreational substances are exacerbated among consumers who are HIV+. For example, the sedating effects of alcohol will be more severe, such that consumers who use alcohol while they are taking medications such as Xanax®, Ativan®, or lithium risk lethal levels of CNS sedation.

Despite risks related to medications, as well as their potential side effects, there are numerous benefits in strengthening services related to medication compliance with HIV+ mental health consumers. In particular, the psychological stress of having HIV/AIDS may increase the risk of relapse of psychotic symptoms. Therefore, strategies to ensure compliance with psychotropic regimens may lessen the severity of these psychosocial responses to a positive HIV test or retard illness progression to full-blown AIDS. Furthermore, the onset of any of the neuropsychiatric syndromes associated with HIV and advancing AIDS will be more easily recognized and treated among consumers whose symptoms are known to be more under control. Finally, the adherence to complex antiretroviral regimens will be better. This is especially important for any consumers receiving highly active antiretroviral therapy (HAART), which includes protease inhibitors, since missing one dose or even taking these medications 1 h later than the scheduled time can result in the manufacture of treatment-resistant strains of HIV.

It also is essential to consider the risks associated with long-term use of psychotropic medications among HIV+ consumers. Aside from their increased sensitivity to medication side effects, consumers are often more likely to present signs of sedation, orthostatic hypotension, and extrapyramidal effects (e.g., akathisia, pseudoparkinsonism, etc.); demonstrate impaired cognitive functioning, particularly among those prescribed tricyclic antidepressants or lithium; be vulnerable to increased risk of adverse drug–drug interactions between many psychotropic medications and medications for HIV/AIDS that have been virtually unstudied in clinical trials; and develop immunosuppressive conditions (e.g., agranulocytosis) from the use of certain antipsychotics, including some of the atypical classes (e.g., olanzapine), an effect which can further compromise the health of HIV+ consumers who take them. Providers working with consumers with SMP must address the added risk of interactions between multiple types of medication (i.e., psychotropics and HIV regimens) and street drugs and alcohol. While published data regarding the interaction effects of two prescribed medications, such as psychotropics and antiretrovirals, are minimal, there are even fewer studies examining interactions effects for people taking multiple (i.e., more than two) drug regimens. Furthermore, although information regarding the interaction effects between medications commonly prescribed for mental health problems and recreational drugs and alcohol are available (Ford et al, 1992), very little is understood regarding the interaction of recreational drugs and HIV regimens, as well as of recreational drugs, HIV regimens, and psychotropic medications (Project Inform, 2000).

In general, there are several approaches to medication management that providers can discuss with consumers, as well as review with psychiatrists, pharmacologists, and other members of the treatment team. It is essential to be clear about target symptoms prior to treatment to ensure that the medication(s) is working properly. If it is necessary to begin consumers on new medications, dosages should be started at one-third to one-half the conventional starting levels, and then increased in smaller increments and at more frequent intervals. It also is extremely important to use serum drug levels to guide dosing whenever possible. While many HIV+ consumers who are in the early, asymptomatic stages of HIV may be able to tolerate typical dosages, others, with more advanced illness progression, may require lower doses.

The case of James

James is a 34-year-old man with an Axis I diagnosis of schizophrenia. He has had 18 psychiatric hospitalizations since the age of 23; most of these hospitalizations occurred when James stopped taking his psychotropic medications. Currently, he lives in one of the apartments in a community integrated living arrangement (CILA), along with seven other mental health consumers. James shares an apartment with one other male resident. In general, James' brother calls once a month, but otherwise he has no family contact. He attends a partial hospitalization programme on a regular basis. James' medications include Risperdal, Klonopin, Haldol, and Cogentin.

James has been arrested twice for disorderly conduct after drinking at a neighbourhood bar, and once he was found unconscious in the street outside the bar. When staff at the day programme and CILA counselled James on the dangers of drinking alcohol while taking medications, James became agitated and told them to "mind their own business". Recently, staff at the CILA have noticed the odour of marijuana on James's clothing when he returns from the day programme. James confided to one staff member that his medications are poison and that marijuana is the only thing that really makes him feel better. He said that smoking pot helps him sleep better, and "the voices don't bother me as much when I'm high. Things are better with girls too. I feel more comfortable with them after we've smoked a joint together." James also said that he frequently has sexual encounters with two female residents who live in the same building. However, he believes that he is "not a real man" if he uses condoms.

There are several services issues on which case managers working with James should focus. In many cases, these issues can be addressed within the context of completing an HIV risk assessment that focuses on the nature and frequency of sexual and substance use activities in which James engages, what he knows about them, and some of the patterns which support his participation in them. The steps to be taken may include, but are not limited to the following:

1. *Address James' unsafe sexual behaviours.* There may be several issues to discuss with James, and it is likely that these will need to be consistently revisited in order to reduce the likelihood that he will continue to engage in high-risk behaviours.
   - Educate James about all types of sexually transmitted diseases, including their modes of transmission, symptoms (and the fact that people may be unaware that they have a sexually transmitted disease (STD) and pass it on unknowingly), and available treatments.
   - Explore James's belief that he is not "manly" if he uses a condom during sex. A cognitive/behavioural approach may be effective in helping James to think differently about protecting himself during sex and the other ways that a man can express himself to maintain a positive self-image. One might explore the way that James might feel if he contracts an STD.
   - Determine whether James is sexually active with anyone else besides the two women who live in the building.

- Make condoms available to James.
- Encourage testing for HIV and STD in order to establish a baseline and to develop an ongoing, proactive risk-reduction plan with James.

2. *Address alcohol and other drug use.* It is especially important to address substance use with James, particularly within the context of HIV risk behaviours. It is important for James to try to make a connection between alcohol and other drug use and risky behaviours, such as having unsafe sex, in order to ensure that he can focus on HIV risks from substance use, which is not a direct mode of transmission.
  - Assess the extent of James's alcohol and other drug use, and the degree of his impairment in functioning resulting from this use, and make appropriate recommendations for intervention/treatment (SMP outpatient treatment, integrated SMP groups, detox ification, inpatient treatment, etc.).
  - Provide psychoeducation about the ways in which alcohol and other drugs can exacerbate symptoms of mental illness. This might be more effective if there is a peer educator who can do this type of work, or perhaps it could be done as part of a small group activity at the CILA.
  - Remind James that excessive use of alcohol or other drugs can adversely affect sexual performance rather than enhance it.
  - Identify any other drugs that James is using, especially IVDU, and find out whether he is using needles or having unprotected sex with partners who use (or have used) IVDUs or shared needles.
  - Explore issues related to where James gets money to buy alcohol, marijuana, or other drugs. Is he engaging in illegal activities to support his habit? It will be important to determine whether he engages in high-risk behaviours, such as trading sex for money or drugs.
  - Help James to identify all the reasons (in addition to wanting to reduce social inhibitions) that he uses alcohol or other drugs.
  - Cognitive/behavioural counselling may help James to think about other ways to feel more comfortable in social situations when he is sober. A *"strengths perspective"* may empower James to focus more on his positive attributes. Also draw attention to how alcohol and other drugs can make a person look more foolish in social situations because, while under the influence, one often lacks discretion and control.

3. *Identify the problems (past and present) that James is having with psychotropic medications and adhering to his medication treatment plan.*
  - Discuss with James the side effects that he has experienced.
  - Explore the issues or other reasons *James* gives for not wanting to take his medications.
  - Address the reasons that James gives for referring to his medications as "being poison". Determine whether this thinking is the result of physical issues related to medication side effects or the result of delusional thinking or other symptoms manifestations.

- Determine whether James's psychiatrist has been consulted regarding these medication compliance issues. Explore the possibility that there are other medications with fewer unpleasant side effects which might be appropriate for James in reducing or eliminating his symptoms.
- Provide psychoeducation and regularly check with James regarding medication and symptom management. Provide ongoing information about how alcohol or other drug use may interfere with the psychotropic medications, rendering them less effective, and support positive behaviours such as abstinence and harm reduction.

4. *Identify and explore other possible interventions for James which support and build upon these, and other, HIV risk-reduction strategies.*

- With James's consent, work on engagement with his brother to determine whether he can be more available for support. Encourage his brother to become more involved in James's treatment (family psychoeducation, family therapy, etc.).
- Help James determine and pursue other interests (employment, hobbies) so that he can engage in new social activities, besides drinking, smoking marijuana, and casual sex. Assist James to establish some short-term, attainable goals to strive for and a reasonable plan to reach those goals, as well as long-term issues that are important to him.
- Consider other treatment interventions besides the day programme. If James is using alcohol and marijuana, and not taking his psychotropic medications, perhaps other programmes/services may be able to help him address these issues more effectively.

SUMMARY AND CONCLUSIONS

The risks of HIV/AIDS among mental health consumers who also have substance abuse diagnoses are well documented. In order to address the growing education, risk-assessment, prevention, testing, and treatment needs of consumers living with HIV, service providers must continue to develop and integrate new programmes into existing service models. Overwhelmingly, previous research on clients with SMP indicates that the most successful of these endeavours are programmes which support the use of multidisciplinary treatment teams, integrated service delivery, and ongoing, long-term programming. In addition, however, consumers can and should take an active role in their protection from HIV. It is essential that consumers, providers, and other stakeholders form partnerships in addressing the need for relevant HIV education and prevention services. This form of collaboration can more fully support the *HIV-sensitive* services necessary to protect consumers from the ongoing effects of this devastating epidemic.

ACKNOWLEDGEMENTS

The author gratefully acknowledges the intellectual contributions of Marie M. Hamilton, LCSW; Chris Murray, MSW; and Colleen J. Murray to this chapter.

REFERENCES

American Psychiatric Association (1992) Policy Statement: Policy guidelines for outpatient psychiatric services. APA AIDS Resource Center, American Psychiatric Association, Washington, DC.

American Psychiatric Association (1996) Policy Statement: Policy guidelines for inpatient psychiatric units. APA AIDS Resource Center, American Psychiatric Association, Washington, DC.

Brady, S.M. and Carmen, E. (1990) AIDS risk in the chronically mentally ill: clinical strategies for prevention. *New Directions for Mental Health Services*, **48**: 83–95.

Carey, M.P., Carey, K.B. and Kalichman, S.C. (1997) Risk for human immunodeficiency virus (HIV) infection among persons with severe mental illness. *Clinical Psychology Review*, **17**: 271–291.

Centers for Disease Control and Prevention (2000) HIV prevalence estimates and AIDS case projections: results. *Morbidity and Mortality Weekly Report*, **12**: 7–11.

Centers for Disease Control and Prevention (1999) *AIDS Cases Reported to the Centers for Disease Control Through December 1998*. HIV/AIDS Surveillance Report: Exposure Categories [Web site: www.cdc.gov].

Cook, J., Razzano, L., Jayaraj, A., Myers, M., Nathanson, F., Stott, M. and Stein, M. (1994) HIV-risk assessment for psychiatric rehabilitation clientele: implications for community-based services. *Psychosocial Rehabilitation Journal*, **17**: 105–115.

Cournos, F., McKinnon, K., Meyer-Bahlburg, H., Guido, J.R. and Meyer, I. (1993) HIV risk activity among persons with severe mental illness: preliminary findings. *Hospital and Community Psychiatry*, **44**: 1104–1106.

Cournos, F. and Bakalar, N. (Eds.), (1996) *AIDS and People with Severe Mental Illness: A Handbook for Professionals*. New Haven, CT, Yale University Press.

Cournos, F. and McKinnon, K. (1997) HIV seroprevalence among people with severe mental illness in the United States: a critical review. *Clinical Psychology Review*, **17**: 259–269.

Drake, R.E., Mercer-McFadden, C., Mueser, K.T., McHugo, G.J. and Bond, G.R. (1998) Review of integrated mental health and substance abuse treatment for patients with dual diagnosis. *Schizophrenia Bulletin*, **24**: 589–608.

Ferrando, S. and Bataki, S. (2000) Substance abuse and HIV infection. In F. Cournos and M. Forstein (Eds.), *New Directions for Mental Health Services: What Mental Health Practitioners Need to Know About HIV and AIDS*, **87**(Fall), 69–76.

Ford, J.A., Rolfe, B., Moore, D. and Lucot, J. (1992) Disability related medications: side effects and interactions. SARDI Project, Wright State University.

Horwath, E., Cournos, F., McKinnon, K., Guido, J.R. and Herman, R. (1996) Illicit-drug injection among psychiatric patients without a primary substance use disorder. *Psychiatric Services*, **47**: 181–185.

Kalichman, S.C., Kelly, J.A., Johnson, J.R. and Bulto, M. (1994) Factors associated with risk for HIV infection among chronic mentally ill adults. *American Journal of Psychiatry*, **151**: 122–127.

McDermott, B.E., Sautter, F.J., Winstead, D.K. and Quirk, T. (1994) Diagnosis, health, beliefs, and risk of HIV infection in psychiatric patients. *Hospital and Community Psychiatry*, **45**: 580–585.

McKinnon, K. (1996) Sexual and drug-use risk behavior. In F. Cournos and N. Bakalar (Eds.), *AIDS and People with Severe Mental Illness: A Handbook for Professionals*. New Haven, CT, Yale, University Press.

McKinnon, K., Cournos, F., Sugden, R., Guido, J.R. and Herman, R. (1996) The relative contributions of psychiatric symptoms and AIDS knowledge to HIV risk behaviors among people with severe mental illness. *Journal of Clinical Psychiatry*, **57**: 506–513.

McKinnon, K. and Rosner, J. (2000) Severe Mental Illness and HIV-AIDS. In F. Cournos and M. Forstein (Eds.), *New Directions for Mental Health Services: What Mental Health Practitioners Need to Know About HIV and AIDS*, **87**(Fall): 69–76.

Minkoff, K. (1989) An integrated treatment model for dual diagnosis of psychosis and addiction. *Hospital and Community Psychiatry*, **40**: 1031–1036.

Project Inform (2000) Drug interactions (WWW.projectinform.org). San Francisco, CA.

Razzano, L.A., Mason, C.M., Callahan, J., Donnally, J., Richardson, N. and Murphy, M. (1997) *HIV/AIDS and People with Serious Mental Illness: Strategies for Providers Working with Mental Health Consumers*. Chicago, IL, Center for Mental Health Services HIV Illinois Mental Health Provider Education Program (CHIME), University of Illinois at Chicago.

Rosenberg, S.D., Goodman, L.A., Osher, F.C., Swartz, M.S., Essock, S.M., Butterfield, M.I., Constantine, N.T., Wolford, G.L. and Salyers, M.P., (2001). Prevalence of HIV, hepatitis B and hepatitis C in people with severe mental illness. *American Journal of Public Health*, **91**: 31–37.

Part V

THE EVOLVING EVIDENCE BASE

Chapter 20

COCHRANE REVIEW OF TREATMENT OUTCOME STUDIES AND ITS IMPLICATIONS FOR FUTURE DEVELOPMENTS

Ann Ley and David Jeffery

The context of this chapter is evidence-based medicine, which has been defined as "the conscientious and judicious use of the current best evidence from clinical care research to guide health care decisions" (Jadad, 1998: 98). Constructing an evidence base is a long and demanding task requiring, among other things, an enormous amount of energy and commitment, particularly in an area which is as challenging as substance misuse with psychosis (SMP). Our focus is on treatments, for which research evidence is gradually accumulating through the use of a variety of methods, most of which will have been illustrated in the preceding chapters. On the basis of many excellent sources (e.g., Jadad et al 1996; Oxman, 1994), we start the chapter with some suggestions to guide research consumers in their own judgements of research quality and the validity of the conclusions that can be drawn. We then outline the main features of the various research methods and report on our systematic review of randomized, controlled trials examining outcome studies of treatments for those with SMP. This work has already been published electronically in the Cochrane database of systematic reviews (Ley et al, 1999) and will be updated when the results of new trials are forthcoming. The chapter ends with some suggestions for both researchers and practitioners.

Substance Misuse in Psychosis: Approaches to Treatment and Service Delivery.
Edited by Hermine L. Graham, Alex Copello, Max J. Birchwood and Kim T. Mueser.
© 2003 John Wiley & Sons, Ltd.

EVALUATION OF EVALUATIVE RESEARCH

While it is important for both clinicians and researchers to be enthusiastic and optimistic about treatments in this challenging area (Drake et al, 1993), when coming to a judgement as to the value of these treatments, they must take a dispassionate view of the outcome research. The following checklist could be applied to reports of all types of quantitative research design:

1. What type of study was it? (systematic review, RCT, quasi-experimental, descriptive).
2. Were both the objectives of the study and the outcome measures clearly defined?
3. Was there a description of participants who dropped out?
4. Were rating scales of demonstrated reliability and validity? (e.g., their development had been reported in a peer-reviewed journal).
5. Was there a clear description of the inclusion and exclusion criteria?
6. Was the sample size justified (e.g., power calculations)?
7. Was there a clear description of the interventions?
8. Were the data reported adequately (e.g., means and standard deviations)?
9. Were the methods of statistical analysis appropriate to the data?
10. Did the conclusions follow from the evidence?
11. Were recommendations linked to the strength of the evidence?

The last two points are particularly important as they are dependent on the previous items and frequently appear in abstracts. We now briefly describe outcome research methods and demonstrate the application of the above checklist through our own systematic review.

Systematic reviews

The systematic review rests at the top of the traditional hierarchy of evidence, followed by individual randomized, controlled trials, and cohort studies, such as quasi-experimental and descriptive studies including demonstration projects (Greenhalgh, 1997). In the absence of strong evidence, expert opinion should be sought (Department of Health, 1996).

Systematic reviews differ from their traditional, narrative counterparts in a number of ways. The latter are usually written by people considered to be experts in the field and are particularly attractive to readers as a time-saving device. The disadvantage is that the reviewer can present and interpret the information in a subjective and idiosyncratic way. Systematic reviews use explicit and reproducible methods to locate and select studies, thus reducing the potential for bias and optimizing the potential for reliability of conclusions (Adams and Soares, 1997; Greenhalgh, 1997; Mulrow, 1994). Duplicate data when trials are reported in more than one paper can be eliminated through the careful examination of all the papers and, if necessary, contacting the authors. Publication bias (the well-documented tendency to publish only trials demonstrating a significant result) can be reduced by a thorough attempt to find unpublished studies—the so-called "grey" literature. Systematic reviews are published electronically by the Cochrane Collaboration, an international organization whose purpose is to supply high-quality evidence to inform people providing and receiving health care. An advantage of Cochrane reviews is that the information is corrected or updated when new or additional, possibly unpublished, trials come to light. Meta-analysis is an important feature of some paper and most Cochrane reviews; that is, data from appropriate studies are pooled and then statistically analysed all together. For continuous data (e.g., questionnaire scale data), weighted means can be combined in order to provide a reliable estimate of the effect of a treatment. For dichotomous/binary data (e.g., whether drinking or abstinent), the odds ratio is calculated. This is "the ratio of the odds of an event in the experimental (intervention) group to the odds of an event in the control group" (Mulrow and Oxman, 1997). In a research area where there are a lot of studies, some of which individually did not show a statistically significant result—perhaps because of a small sample size—meta-analysis can be very useful. Obviously, the studies have to have much in common in terms of the treatments and measures used.

Single randomized, controlled trials (RCTs)

The key feature of RCTs is that individuals are randomly assigned to either a treatment or control group at the start of the study. This process maximizes the probability that both known and unknown features of the participants will be similarly distributed in all groups, minimizing the likelihood of systematic differences between groups at the start of the study which could provide alternative explanations for the trial results (selection bias). In common with all methods of outcome research, RCTs vary in quality.

Quasi-experimental studies

The overall design of quasi-experimental studies can closely resemble that of RCTs, where two groups are compared at baseline and then at various times during or post-treatment. However, in quasi-experimental studies, participants are *not* randomly assigned to groups, thus increasing the probability of selection bias.

Descriptive studies/demonstration projects

Descriptive studies and demonstration projects consist of a *single* group of clients from whom measures can be taken before and at various times during or after treatment. This type of study can be useful in exploring treatment possibilities in an area. However, the lack of any control or comparison group means that no claims can be made for the superiority of the treatment over any other treatment, or no treatment. For example, they do not exclude other plausible reasons for change such as the passage of time. However, the results of such studies can be regarded as indications of useful avenues to pursue, which should be the focus of further, more rigorously conducted research.

Developing an evidence base

Each of the above research methods has its place in building an evidence base for a new treatment. A parallel can be drawn with the development of pharmaceutical products, whereby potentially beneficial treatments are subjected to a series of trials of increasing rigour (Jadad, 1998). It is only after acceptability and efficacy have been demonstrated among small groups of patients that a treatment is subjected to a fully fledged RCT. Assessing the ability of a SMP intervention to secure engagement, for example, as discussed in detail in the treatment section of this book, can be equated to a preliminary trial of acceptability to clients, which could be evaluated by means of descriptive studies. Once acceptability has been demonstrated, treatment efficacy could be evaluated in small, homogeneous groups. Finally, the reference standard of an RCT can be used to demonstrate effectiveness. Obviously, this is not as simple as we have made it sound, particularly with a client group who are difficult to engage and retain in treatment. However, the development of SMP treatments has been accompanied by active research, and, by 1998, there was a body of studies, primarily based on either descriptive or quasi-experimental methods, together with a number of narrative reviews (e.g., Drake et al, 1996, 1998). Most of the research came from the USA, but the topic was becoming of increasing interest to practitioners in the UK and other countries (see Lowe, 1999).

COCHRANE REVIEW

Clinicians had become aware of the necessity of devising a treatment response to the challenges posed by SMP and required guidance, not only on the effectiveness of specific interventions (Drake et al, 1998), and individual programme components (Winyard, 1995), but also on appropriate models of service delivery (Weaver et al, 1999). In the USA, the drive had been towards integrated programmes, with substance misuse and psychiatric treatment being provided concurrently by the same personnel in an attempt to avoid the problems of inadequate care which may arise if provided by two treatment systems (Ries, 1993). It was thought by some that these programmes, requiring additional resources and possibly radical redesign of service delivery systems may not be necessary in countries such as the UK, where care systems are more integrated (Johnson, 1997). It was also unclear whether such expenditure would be justified by research evidence. It was against this background that, under the aegis of the Cochrane Schizophrenia Group, we conducted our systematic Cochrane review of randomized, controlled trials to evaluate the effect of substance misuse treatment programmes within psychiatric care for people with problems of both substance misuse and serious mental illness.

METHOD

Identification of trials

We aimed to identify all relevant randomized, controlled trials which compared any programme of substance misuse treatment within standard psychiatric care to standard psychiatric care alone. Standard psychiatric care is defined as the normal level of psychiatric care in the area where the trial was conducted. Trial participants were any individuals presenting to adult psychiatric services with severe mental illness (however diagnosed) and current problems of substance misuse (however diagnosed).

We conducted extensive electronic searches of the following databases: Biological Abstracts, 1985 to February 1998; CINAHL, 1982 to February 1998; The Cochrane Library, Issue 3, 1998; The Cochrane Schizophrenia Group's Register, August 1998; EMBASE, January 1980 to February 1998; MEDLINE, January 1966 to February 1998; PsycLIT, January 1974 to February 1998; and SocioFile, January 1974 to February 1998. The search strategies used can be viewed via the Cochrane Library (Ley et al, 1999), or are available from the authors on request. Trials were also sought by cited reference searching, examination of reference lists, hand-searching and personal contact via a concurrent national survey of UK professionals working with this particular population (Jeffery et al, 2000). We asked all contacts whether they knew of any published or unpublished trials.

We also contacted authors of all potentially relevant studies identified from the electronic searches, asking them about any other published or unpublished trials.

No studies were identified by citation searching or from personal contact. We found 4806 citations using the electronic search strategy. This high number of "hits", the vast majority of which were irrelevant, demonstrates the problem of using the word "drug" in the context of medical databases. From inspection of the title, abstract and keywords, 240 appeared relevant to the project. Citations and, where possible, abstracts were independently inspected by the research team, who then obtained the papers, inspected their content and assessed their quality. On the basis of criteria described in *The Cochrane Collaboration Handbook* (Mulrow and Oxman, 1997), trials were included only if participants were thought to have been randomized.

Limitations

It is probable that there were a number of studies which we failed to find with our search. An experienced searcher may find only 50% of relevant material within MEDLINE (Adams and Soares, 1997). There were also difficulties in locating unpublished studies through standard bibliographic sources. We were unable to obtain two unpublished studies which we had located, in spite of repeated attempts to contact the authors.

OUTCOME MEASURES AND DATA EXTRACTION

The main outcome measures were numbers lost to treatment (a measure of treatment engagement), symptoms of severe mental illness, substance use, hospitalization, life satisfaction and homelessness. Post hoc, the outcome of "lost to evaluation" was also included. Lost to evaluation is the proportion of people leaving the study altogether. Lost to treatment, however, is the number who do not wish to carry on in the treatment. A proportion of this group will usually be willing to provide data for the study. Data from the selected trials were extracted independently by two of the authors. Disputes were resolved by discussion. Except for the analysis of loss to follow-up as a dependent variable per se, data from studies where attrition was greater than 50% were not used because of the strong likelihood of bias. For binary data, the initial analysis was the estimation of the Peto odds ratios at the 95% confidence interval. For outcomes based on rating scales, the minimum standards were that:

1. the psychometric properties of the scale should have been described in a peer-reviewed journal
2. the scale should either have been a self-report or have been completed by an independent rater or relative (not the therapist)
3. it should provide a global assessment of an area of functioning.

To avoid the pitfall of applying parametric tests to skewed continuous data, we applied the following standards:

1. Standard deviations and means were reported in the paper or obtainable from the authors.
2. the standard deviation, when multiplied by 2, was less than the mean, as otherwise the mean was unlikely to be an appropriate measure of the centre of the distribution (Altman and Bland, 1996).

Skewed data were not included in any meta-analysis, but reported separately.

Results

At the time, six randomized, controlled trials, all from the USA, met our inclusion criteria (Bond et al, 1991—two trials; Burnam et al, 1995;. Drake et al, 1998; Hellerstein et al, 1995; Lehman et al, 1993). Descriptions of each trial, together with individual results, are shown in Table 20.1.

The main result of the review was that there were few trials of adequate quality. As can be seen from Table 20.1, the most serious methodological problems were small samples, attrition, skewed data and the use of adapted, non-peer-reviewed scales. All of the trials investigated different interventions with different populations, and no trial showed a substantial treatment effect. Thus, there was no clear evidence supporting an advantage of any type of substance-misuse intervention for those with serious mental illness over the value of standard care. No one intervention was clearly superior to another.

A particular problem which we encountered was in deciding precisely *what* was being evaluated. At the beginning of this chapter, we referred to the needs of clinicians to identify specific treatments or individual programme components (Drake et al, 1998; Winyard, 1995), and appropriate models of service delivery (Weaver et al, 1999). It is the combination of these two elements which forms a programme. In the trials we reviewed, one evaluated a treatment (Bond, 1991) by comparing reference groups with standard care; and two evaluated programmes—group treatment in intensive case management (Lehman et al, 1993) and Assertive Community Treatment

Table 20.1 Summary of randomized controlled trials evaluating any programme of substance misuse for those with severe mental illness

Study	Participants	Interventions	Outcomes	Results (95% confidence interval)
Bond et al (1991) Anderson site Allocation: "randomly assigned", no further details Assessment: 6, 12, 18 months	Inclusion criteria: a) age 18–45; b) chronic mental illness (Indiana Dept. Mental Health Criteria); c) substance abuse or dependence (DSM-III-R), or documented evidence of substance abuse/use, extensive hospital/crisis service use over previous year $n = 42$ Of 21 who entered study: Diagnosis: 57% schizophrenia Age: mean 30 years Sex: 33% female Setting: Community Mental Health Center, Indiana, USA	1. Reference groups for substance misuse: engagement, stabilize residential situation. Peer support group, role models, plus standard psychiatric care. $n = 21$ 2. Standard psychiatric care. $n = 21$	Lost to evaluation Unable to use (attrition >50%) — Hospitalization Problems due to substance use Quality of life	No group differences at 6 months (OR 1.75, 0.53–5.77), 12 months (OR 1.75, 0.53–5.77), or 18 months (OR 2.14, 0.64–7.15) See combined result in text
Bond et al (1991) Evansville site Allocation: "randomly assigned", no further details Assessment: 6, 12, 18 months	Inclusion criteria as above $n = 42$ Of 30 who entered study: Diagnosis: 43% schizophrenia Age: mean 30 years Sex: 23% female Setting: Community Mental Health Center, Indiana, USA	1. Assertive Community Treatment (ACT) for substance misuse: emphasis on replacement activities (e.g., employment) Assistance in medication and money management, individual planning and client choice, plus standard psychiatric care $n = 21$ 2. Standard psychiatric care. $n = 21$	Lost to evaluation Hospitalization (hospital days at 6 months) Unable to use Hospitalization	No group differences at 6 months (OR 1.00, 0.27–3.75), 12 months (OR 1.00, 0.28–3.55), or 18 months (OR 0.66, 0.19–2.34) See combined result in text Skewed data.

Burnam et al (1995) Allocation: "randomly assigned" stratified by gender and primary mental disorder—no further details Assessment: 3, 6 and 9 months (participants paid $10 each interview)	$n = 276$ (all homeless) Diagnosis: 7% schizophrenia, 55% major affective, 38% both, 79% alcohol disorder in past year, 72% substance misuse in past year Age: mean 37 years Sex: 16% female Setting: residential, urban, mostly high-cost housing, large concentration of homeless people, Los Angeles, USA	1. Social model: residential programme, educational groups, 12-step programmes including AA or NA, discussion groups, individual counselling, case-management, psychiatric consultation, ongoing medication management, general community activities. $n = 67$ 2. Non-residential programme: above model 1–9 pm, 5 days/week, more case management for basic needs $n = 144$ 3. Control group: no special	(hospital admissions—no data for this site) Hospitalization (hospital days at > 6 months—no SD) Problems due to substance use (adapted version of DAPS—not peer-reviewed scale) Quality of life (adapted version of LSC—not peer-reviewed scale)	Authors' unpublished analysis indicated no group differences
			Lost to evaluation	Difference in favour of residential programme at 9 months (OR 0.46, 0.25–0.84) See combined result in text
			Lost to treatment	At 3 months, 87% lost overall, but difference in favour of the residential programme (OR 0.26, 0.11–0.61)
			Substance use: average change (self-reports of no. of days of alcohol consumption and illicit drug use in past 30 days)	Data skewed. Authors' analysis indicated no group differences at 9 months

continues overleaf

Table 20.1 (*continued*)

Study	Participants	Interventions	Outcomes	Results (95% confidence interval)
		intervention but free to access other services (shelters, mental health clinics, AA groups). $n = 65$	Homelessness (self-reports of percentage of nights in last 60 spent on streets or in independent housing) Unable to use Mental state (adapted measure taken from SCL-90 and PERI). Levels of alcohol in last 30 days—adapted measure	Data skewed. Authors' analysis indicated no group differences at 9 months
Lehman et al (1993) Allocation: randomized "using an urn randomization technique to balance the treatment groups in terms of primary mental disorder and gender"; no further details.	Inclusion criteria: age 18–40, informed consent, schizophrenia or schizoaffective disorder or bipolar or major depressive disorder and lifetime substance use or dependence disorder (DSM-III-R), referred by clinician for treatment of dual diagnosis $n = 29$ (substance use in past 30 days) Diagnosis: 67% schizophrenia	1. Intensive case management plus standard care: Stein and Test model, 1:15 staff-patient ratio, specialized group programme 5 h/week—sessions on substance abuse/mental illness education, experiential "rap" session, on-site self-help group, off-site self-help group (AA/NA), social activity. $n = 14$	Lost to evaluation Days in hospital Mental state (ASI-psychiatric) Substance use (ASI-alcohol, ASI-drug) Quality of life (QOLI)	At 12 months: None Data skewed. Authors' analysis indicated no group differences Data skewed. Authors' analysis indicated no group differences Data skewed. Authors' analysis indicated no group differences Difference in favour of standard care group (WMD −1.34, −2.47 to −0.21)

Assessment: 6, 12 months	Age: mean 30.5 years Sex: 26% female Setting: Community mental health centre and a psychosocial rehabilitation centre, Maryland, USA	2. Standard care: CMHC-based plus psychosocial rehabilitation services, routine outpatient services, supported housing if needed, 1:25 staff-patient ratio, no organized substance abuse treatment $n = 15$	Lost to evaluation Lost to treatment	At 8 months: None 64% lost overall. No group differences (OR 0.38, 0.12–1.23) Data skewed.
Hellerstein et al (1995) Allocation: "randomly assigned"—no further details Assessment: 4, 8 months.	Inclusion criteria: age 18–50, schizophrenia-continuum disorder (Research Diagnostic Criteria) plus psychoactive substance abuse/dependence (DSM-III-R), desire for substance abuse treatment $n = 47$ Diagnosis: 30% schizophrenia Age: mean 31.9 years Sex: 23% female Setting: outpatient department of urban substance abuse unit, New York, USA	1. Integrated treatment: group outpatient psychotherapy and psychoeducation plus drug treatment—all at same site, twice a week $n = 24$ 2. Non-integrated standard treatment: comparable levels of substance abuse and psychiatric service from separate sites without formal case coordination $n = 23$	Mental state (ASI-psychiatric) Substance use (ASI-drug). Unable to use. Days in hospital (data skewed and parametric test applied)	Authors' analysis indicated no group differences Data skewed. Authors' analysis indicated no group differences
Drake et al (1998) Allocation: "randomly assigned within site"—no further details Assessment: 6, 12, 18, 24, 30 and 36 months	Inclusion criteria: schizophrenia, schizoaffective or bipolar disorder (DSM-III-R), active substance use disorder (DSM-III-R) in past 6 months, age 18–60, no additional medical conditions or mental	1. ACT: community-based, assertive engagement, high intensity, caseload ~12, 24-h responsibility, multidisciplinary team, close work with support system and continuity of staffing plus direct substance abuse treatment by team members,	Lost to evaluation Loss to treatment Hospitalization Community days—no. of days	At 3 years: Difference in favour of ACT (OR 0.17, 0.06–0.53) No group differences (OR 1.66, 0.77–3.58) Data skewed. Authors' analysis indicated no group differences No group differences in last 6 months of study (WMD 3.7, *continues overleaf*

Table 20.1 (continued)

Study	Participants	Interventions	Outcomes	Results (95% confidence interval)
Outcome assessment: case managers ratings assessed by three independent raters, blind to group allocation	retardation, informed consent given Diagnosis: 53% schizophrenia, 73% alcohol abuse 42% drug abuse $n = 223$. Age: mean 34 years Sex: 26% female Setting: two predominantly rural and two urban areas in New Hampshire, USA	use of stage-wise, dual-disorder model, dual-disorder treatment groups and exclusive team focus on patients with dual disorders $n = 109$ 2. Standard Case Management: community-based, multidisciplinary team approach, worked with client's support system and vigorously addressed co-occurring substance use, caseload ~25. $n = 114$	living in stable community residences	-11.58 to -18.98) or at any other time
			Mental state (BPRS total scores)	No group differences in last 6 months of study (WMD -0.22, -3.32 to -2.88) or at any other time
			Substance use (SATS)	No group differences in last 6 months of study (WMD 0.11, -0.41 to -0.63) or at any other time
			Substance misuse (days)	Skewed data. Authors' analysis indicated no group differences
			Substance use (AUS)	No group differences in last 6 months of study (WMD -0.12, -0.49 to -0.25) or at any other time
			Substance use (DUS)	No group differences in last 6 months of study (WMD -0.28, -0.78 to -0.22) or at any other time
			Substance use (remission/alcohol)	No group differences in last 6 months of study (OR 0.75, 0.39–1.44) or at any other time
			Substance use (remission/drugs)	No group differences in last 6 months of study (OR 1.35, 0.57–3.22) or at any other time
			Quality of life (QOLI)	No group differences in last 6 months of study (WMD 0.1, -0.28 to -0.45) or any other time

with substance misuse treatment based on replacement activities (Bond, 1991)—both of which were compared with standard care. Three compared different models of delivery by offering similar substance misuse treatment in both conditions (Burnam et al, 1995; Drake et al, 1998; Hellerstein et al, 1995).

Summary

Our review draws on a large research effort and presents an accurate picture of the results of RCTs at that time. Explanations by the authors of the trials for the lack of effect include a failure to engage clients in the programme (Lehman et al, 1993; Burnam et al, 1995); contamination of the control group (Bond et al, 1991); the similarity of the two programmes and problems in the fidelity of implementation (Drake et al, 1998); and "sufficient" rather than "comprehensive" programmes providing a limited range of services (Hellerstein et al, 1995).

At the present time, our review can offer little guidance on the relative merits of different interventions for current practitioners. Indeed, one cannot yet be sure that *any* specialized treatment is better than standard mental health treatment. However, it is important to be clear that the current lack of evidence of effectiveness is *not* evidence of lack of effectiveness. It may be that these treatments *do* work, but until we have more well-designed RCTs, and strong evidence from other evaluations, the jury must remain out.

WHAT ABOUT NON-RCT EVIDENCE?

Given the lack of suitable RCTs, it is reasonable to seek guidance from other types of studies (Department of Health, 1996). It is interesting to note that the Cochrane Drug and Alcohol Group (Cochrane Library, 2001) are using less stringent criteria for including studies and are working on a system for combining data from types of design other than RCTs into a meta-analysis. Another approach is suggested by the American Psychological Association's Task Force on Promotion and Dissemination of Psychological Procedures (Task Force, 1995). They describe criteria for empirically validated "well-established" and "probably efficacious" treatments, an abbreviated version of which is shown in Table 20.2. With this method, quality criteria are applied, but the studies are simply counted. There is no attempt to combine the data into a meta-analysis.

We attempted an expansion of criteria ourselves in the form of a review of the non-RCT outcome studies found in the course of our literature search (Ley et al, unpublished paper). However, at the present time, even with

Table 20.2   Abbreviated American Psychological Association Task Force criteria for empirically validated treatments

Well-established treatments	Probably efficacious treatments
1. At least two good group design studies (different investigators), demonstrating treatment is: a) superior to pill or psychological placebo, or to another treatment b) equivalent to an already-established treatment in studies with adequate statistical power (about 30 per group) OR 2. A large series of single case design studies demonstrating efficacy—comparing the intervention to another treatment as in 1a For both 1 and 2: 3. Studies conducted with treatment manuals 4. Client samples clearly specified	1. Two studies showing the treatment is more effective than a waiting-list control group OR 2. Two studies otherwise meeting the well-established treatment criteria 1, 3 and 4, but conducted by the same investigator, or one good study demonstrating effectiveness by these same criteria OR 3. At least two good studies demonstrating effectiveness but flawed by heterogeneity of the client samples OR 4. A small series of single case design studies otherwise meeting the well-established treatment criteria 1, 3 and 4.

all the studies, including demonstration projects, we would not have been able to meet the American Psychological Association Task Force criteria for one empirically validated treatment.

A WAY FORWARD FOR OUTCOME RESEARCH

As many chapters in this book show, the development of a treatment likely to be successful in an RCT is a lengthy business. Our review can be seen as a contribution to the long process of developing an evidence base in this area. It illustrates the difficulties faced by researchers into treatments for substance misuse and severe mental illness—a combination of two areas which are themselves problematic (McHugo et al, 1998; Perl et al, 2000).

It is obvious that many more well-designed RCTs are needed. They should take into account all the methodological issues raised here, be large enough to offer sufficient statistical power and be designed so that data can easily be combined into a meta-analysis. The main evaluative effort should be invested in assessing the effectiveness of the many *specific* treatments and programme elements that have been recently developed, and which are described in this volume. Treatments such as motivational groups (Drake et al, 1995), drug education and coping skills (Bennett et al, 2001), and cognitive-behavioural therapy for substance misuse (Kavanagh et al, 1998) should be compared with attention placebos and standard care. Aimed at particular outcomes, they will yield results in a shorter time frame than the programmes into which they are put, and therefore should pose fewer organizational and methodological problems. The question of the superiority of integrated services should be set aside in the short term. Until they are delivering treatments of demonstrated efficacy, it is not likely that RCT comparisons of such service delivery models will reward the enormous organizational effort and cost involved. Similarly, large-scale intervention programmes should also await the empirical demonstration of the effectiveness of their elements, since the design requirements of component analysis within large programmes are very onerous. It may not be possible to evaluate some specific treatments in isolation. In this case, they should be evaluated in as small a number of combinations as possible.

A way forward for clinicians and other users of outcome research

The tide of opinion among leaders in the field (Bellack and Gearon, 1998; Drake et al, 2001), including UK practitioners (Jeffery et al, 2000), is that, despite the current lack of clear evidence, drug/alcohol treatment should be offered in addition to standard mental health care. Moreover, the current view is that there are encouraging indications that the developments to date are valuable. As there is currently no clear direction from the outcome research, those seeking to offer interventions to those with SMP should turn to this expert opinion. They may implement whole programmes as they have been developed, or select particular elements from a programme to meet the needs of the populations they serve. However, we do not yet know which elements are effective; that is, which parts of the New Hampshire comprehensive integrated treatment programme are the active ingredients for securing engagement with the service. It is therefore particularly important for practitioners and service managers to collect process and outcome data, and to evaluate critically their local implementation of these treatments (Sackett et al, 2000).

We will update our Cochrane review at regular intervals. Meanwhile, we encourage practitioners to evaluate critically for themselves any new outcome studies, using our checklist as a starting place.

ACKNOWLEDGEMENTS

We thank Clive Adams (Cochrane Schizophrenia Group) for advice and support for the Cochrane review, Ian Bennun (Head of Psychology Service,

South Devon Healthcare Trust) for support, and those authors who kindly supplied us with unpublished information regarding their trials. The review was supported by the South Devon Healthcare Trust, UK; the South and West Regional Health Authority Research and Development Directorate, UK; and Central Sydney Area Mental Health Services, Australia.

REFERENCES

Adams, C. and Soares, K. (1997) The Cochrane Collaboration and the process of systematic reviewing. *Advances in Psychiatric Treatment*, **3**: 240–246.

Bellack, A.S. and Gearon, J.S. (1998) Substance abuse treatment for people with schizophrenia. *Addictive Behaviours*, **23**: 749–766.

Bennett, M.E., Bellack, A.S. and Gearon, J.S. (2001) Treating substance abuse in schizophrenia. An initial report. *Journal of Substance Abuse Treatment*, **20**: 163–175.

Bond, G.R., McDonel, E.C., Miller, L.D. and Pensec, M. (1991) Assertive community treatment and reference groups: an evaluation of their effectiveness for young adults with serious mental illness and substance abuse problems. *Psychosocial Rehabilitation Journal*, **15**: 31–43.

Burnam, M.A., Morton, S.C., McGlynn, E.A., Peterson, L.P., Stecher, B.M., Hayes, C. and Vaccaro, J.V. (1995) An experimental evaluation of residential and non-residential treatment for dually diagnosed homeless adults. *Journal of Addictive Diseases*, **14**: 111–134.

Cochrane Library, Issue 4, 2001. Oxford: Update Software. Updated quarterly.

Department of Health (1996) *Promoting Clinical Effectiveness: A Framework for Action in and Through the NHS*. NHS Executive Report.

Drake, R.E., Bartels, S.J., Teague, G.B., Noordsy, D.L. and Clark, R.E. (1993) Treatment of substance abuse in severely mentally ill patients. *Journal of Nervous and Mental Disease*, **181**: 606–611.

Drake, R.E., Essock, S.M., Shaner, A., Carey, K.B., Minkoff, K., Kola, L., Lynde, D., Osher, F.C., Clark, R.E. and Rickards, L. (2001) Implementing dual diagnosis services for clients with severe mental illness. *Psychiatric Services*, **52**: 469–476.

Drake, R.E., McHugo, G.J., Clark, R.E., Teague, G.B., Xie, H., Miles, K. and Ackerson, T.H. (1998) Assertive community treatment for patients with co-occurring severe mental illness and substance use disorder: a clinical trial. *American Journal of Orthopsychiatry*, **68**: 201–215.

Drake, R.E., Mercer McFadden, C., Mueser, K.T., McHugo, G.J. and Bond, G.R. (1998) A review of integrated mental health and substance abuse treatment for patients with dual disorders. *Schizophrenia Bulletin*, **24**: 589–608.

Drake, R.E., Mueser, K.T., Clark, R.E. and Wallach, M.A. (1996) The course, treatment, and outcome of substance disorder in persons with severe mental illness. *American Journal of Orthopsychiatry*, **66**: 42–51.

Drake, R.E., Noordsy, D.L. and Ackerson, T. (1995) Integrating mental health and substance abuse treatments for persons with chronic mental disorders: a model. In A.F. Lehman and L.B. Dixon (Eds.), *Double Jeopardy: Chronic Mental Illness and Substance Use Disorders*, pp. 251–264. Chur, Switzerland, Harwood Academic Publishers.

Greenhalgh, T. (1997) *How To Read a Paper: The Basics of Evidence Based Medicine*. London, BMJ Publishing Group.

Hellerstein, D.J., Rosenthal, R.N. and Miner, C.R. (1995) A prospective study of integrated outpatient treatment for substance-abusing schizophrenic patients. *American Journal on Addictions*, **4**: 33–42.

Jadad, A. (1998) *Randomised Controlled Trials*. London, BMJ Books.

Jadad, A.R., Moore, R.A., Carroll, D., Jenkinson, C., Reynolds, D.J.M., Gavaghan, D.J. and McQuay, H.J. (1996) Assessing the quality of reports of randomized clinical trials: is blinding necessary? *Controlled Clinical Trials*, **17**: 1–12.

Jeffery, D.P., Ley, A., Bennun, I. and McLaren, S. (2000) Delphi survey of opinion on interventions for severe mental illness and substance misuse problems. *Journal of Mental Health*, **9**: 371–384.

Johnson, S. (1997) Dual diagnosis of severe mental illness and substance misuse: a case for specialist services? *British Journal of Psychiatry*, **171**: 205–208.

Kavanagh, D.J., Young, R., Boyce, L., Clair, A., Sitharthan, T., Clark, D. and Thompson, K. (1998) Substance treatment options in psychosis (STOP): a new intervention for dual diagnosis. *Journal of Mental Health*, **7**: 135–143.

Lehman, A.F., Herron, J.D., Schwartz, R.P. and Myers, C.P. (1993) Rehabilitation for adults with severe mental illness and substance use disorders: a clinical trial. *Journal of Nervous and Mental Disease*, **181**: 86–90.

Ley, A., Jeffery, D.P., McLaren, S. and Siegfried, N. (1999) Treatment programmes for people with both severe mental illness and substance misuse. The Cochrane Library [2]. Oxford, Update Software.

Lowe, A. (1999) Drug abuse and psychiatric comorbidity. *Current Opinion in Psychiatry*, **12**: 291–295.

McHugo, G.J., Hargreaves, W.A., Drake, R.E., Clark, R.E., Xie, H., Bond, G.R. and Burns, B.J. (1998) Methodological issues in assertive community treatment studies. *American Journal of Orthopsychiatry*, **68**: 246–260.

Mulrow, C.D. (1994) Rationale for systematic reviews. *British Medical Journal*, **309**: 597–599.

Mulrow, C.D. and Oxman, A.D. (1997) *The Cochrane Collaboration Handbook* (Version 4.0).

Oxman, A.D. (1994). Checklists for review articles. *British Medical Journal*, **309**, 648–651.

Perl, H.I., Dennis, M.L. and Huebner, R.B. (2000) State-of-the-art methodologies in alcohol-related health services research. *Addiction*, **95** *Suppl 3:* S275–S280.

Ries, R. (1993) Clinical treatment matching models for dually diagnosed patients. *Psychiatric Clinics of North America*, **16***:* 167–175.

Sackett, D.L., Straus, S.E., Richardson, W.S., Rosenberg, W. and Haynes, R.B. (2000) *Evidence-Based Medicine* (2nd edn). Edinburgh, Churchill Livingstone.

Task Force on Promotion and Dissemination of Psychological Procedures, Division of Clinical Psychology, American Psychological Association (1995) Training in and dissemination of empirically validated psychological treatments: report and recommendations. *Clinical Psychologist*, **48**: 3–23.

Weaver, T., Renton, A., Stimson, G. and Tyrer, P. (1999) Severe mental illness and substance misuse. *British Medical Journal*, **318**: 137–138.

Winyard, G. (1995) Improving clinical effectiveness: a co-ordinated approach. In M. Deighan and S. Hitch (Eds.), *Clinical Effectiveness from Guidelines to Cost-Effective Practice*, pp. 1–10. Brentwood, Earlybrave Publications.

EPILOGUE: FUTURE DIRECTIONS

CONCLUDING REMARKS

*Hermine L. Graham, Alex Copello, Max J. Birchwood
and Kim T. Mueser*

It has been a delight to edit this book. We have been inspired by the richness of the material provided by our distinguished contributors, who have, between them, been largely responsible for trailblazing an area increasingly recognized as central to the management of people with serious mental health problems. In Chapter 20, Ley and Jeffery remind us that there is still a lot of work to be done: we hope that this book will stimulate debate and lead to further developments.

We would like to conclude with a few reflections on the current state of the field and some personal thoughts on possible future directions. In order to advance our scientific understanding, we will need to continue to develop approaches based on clear conceptual frameworks and evaluate the impact of these approaches rigorously. In Chapter 20, Ley and Jeffery make proposals for further evaluation while suggesting that the question of the "superiority of integrated services" should be set aside in the short term until we can prove the efficacy of particular treatments. This certainly sets out one possible research agenda.

However, in setting aside the integrated aspects of the treatment, do we now run the risk of losing the essence of what makes a difference to this client group? As we have argued elsewhere (Copello et al, 2001), we feel that there are two important features of the design of a trial that need to be considered in future evaluation of interventions with this client group.

First, we need to consider carefully the extent to which results based on highly selective samples and clinical conditions that are very different from

Substance Misuse in Psychosis: Approaches to Treatment and Service Delivery.
Edited by Hermine L. Graham, Alex Copello, Max J. Birchwood and Kim T. Mueser.
© 2003 John Wiley & Sons, Ltd.

routine practice can be later generalized. It is important to consider the issue of the representativeness of the clinical conditions within which a particular intervention works. This issue is more fully discussed in a review of meta-analyses that includes 486 psychotherapy studies. Using carefully defined criteria for "clinical representativeness", Shadish et al (1997) found that none of the 486 studies reviewed met the most stringent level of criteria for clinical representativeness. The authors highlight the need for more evaluation of interventions as they are used in clinical practice (i.e., effectiveness studies). Effectiveness trials, in contrast to efficacy trials, are concerned with external validity, that is, the extent to which results can be generalized to "real world" conditions. Whereas in an efficacy trial every attempt is made to maximize internal validity, in an effectiveness trial, conditions are kept as close as possible to those present in clinical situations. This is done while at the same time attempts are made to preserve internal validity. Within such trials, for example, existing clinicians deliver treatments following carefully designed training and supervision, and exclusion criteria are kept to a minimum in order to test the treatments with those clients who normally present to services. Even though setting up such a trial is complex, the design features facilitate its integration into routine clinical practice.

The second issue relates to the fact that in the management of people with substance misuse in psychosis, most interventions are also directed at the mental health team within which other services are delivered. This is partly done in an effort to change the "whole team" approach. The aim is to increase the extent to which substance misuse issues are addressed in all aspects of care as well as the specific components of any particular intervention. The result of this process is that there are changes within the team that seriously compromise the extent to which an individual client treated by that team can be seen as the unit of randomization in a randomized controlled trial, given the contamination effects that may arise from exposure to the service as a whole. It becomes more appropriate therefore to treat *the team* as the unit of randomization, and therefore to use a cluster randomization design. Cluster randomized trials are increasingly being used in the health service in the UK to deal with this type of situation.

A cluster-randomized trial has the potential to address some important questions for this area: the challenge is to develop the resources and level of collaboration that such an enterprise may require.

REFERENCES

Copello, A., Graham, H. and Birchwood, M. (2001) Evaluating substance misuse interventions in psychosis: the limitations of the RCT with "patient" at the unit of analysis. *Journal of Mental Health*, **10**: 585–587.

Shadish, W.R., Matt, G.E., Navarro, A.M., Siegle, G., Crits-Christoph, P., Hazelrigg, M.D., Jorm, A.F., Lyons, L.C., Nietzel, M.T., Prout, H.T., Robinson, L., Lee Smith, M., Svartberg, M. and Weiss, B. (1997) Evidence that therapy works in clinically representative conditions. *Journal of Consulting and Clinical Psychology*, **65**: 355–365.

INDEX

Page numbers in *italics* refer to figures and tables
Page numbers in **bold** refer to entire chapters

Index compiled by Judith Reading

The Wiley Series in

CLINICAL PSYCHOLOGY